Liver Transplantation

Editor

ROBERTO J. FIRPI

CLINICS IN LIVER DISEASE

www.liver.theclinics.com

Consulting Editor
NORMAN GITLIN

May 2017 • Volume 21 • Number 2

ELSEVIER

1600 John F. Kennedy Boulevard ● Suite 1800 ● Philadelphia, Pennsylvania, 19103-2899

http://www.theclinics.com

CLINICS IN LIVER DISEASE Volume 21, Number 2
May 2017 ISSN 1089-3261, ISBN-13: 978-0-323-52844-3

Editor: Kerry Holland
Developmental Editor: Meredith Madeira

Clinics in Liver Disease (ISSN 1089-3261) is published quarterly by Elsevier Inc., 360 Park Avenue South, New York, NY 10010-1710. Months of issue are February, May, August, and November. Business and Editorial Offices: 1600 John F. Kennedy Blvd., Ste. 1800, Philadelphia, PA 19103-2899. Customer Service Office: 3251 Riverport Lane, Maryland Heights, MO 63043. Periodicals postage paid at New York, NY and additional mailing offices. Subscription prices are $281.00 per year (U.S. individuals), $100.00 per year (U.S. student/resident), $476.00 per year (U.S. institutions), $403.00 per year (international individuals), $200.00 per year (international student/resident), $590.00 per year (international instituitions), $347.00 per year (Canadian individuals), $200.00 per year (Canadian student/resident), and $590.00 per year (Canadian institutions). Foreign air speed delivery is included in all *Clinics* subscription prices. All prices are subject to change without notice. **POSTMASTER:** Send address changes to *Clinics in Liver Disease*, Elsevier Health Sciences Division, Subscription Customer Service, 3251 Riverport Lane, Maryland Heights, MO 63043. **Customer Service: Telephone: 1-800-654-2452 (U.S. and Canada); 314-447-8871 (outside U.S. and Canada). Fax: 314-447-8029. E-mail: journalscustomer service-usa@elsevier.com (for print support); journalsonlinesupport-usa@elsevier.com (for online support).**

Reprints. For copies of 100 or more of articles in this publication, please contact the Commercial Reprints Department, Elsevier Inc., 360 Park Avenue South, New York, NY 10010-1710. Tel.: 212-633-3874; Fax: 212-633-3820; E-mail: reprints@elsevier.com.

Clinics in Liver Disease is covered in *MEDLINE/PubMed (Index Medicus)*, Science Citation Index Expanded, Journal Citation Reports/Science Edition, and Current Contents/Clinical Medicine.

Contributors

CONSULTING EDITOR

NORMAN GITLIN, MD, FRCP (LONDON), FRCPE (EDINBURGH), FAASLD, FACP, FACG
Formerly, Professor of Medicine, Chief of Hepatology, Emory University, Currently, Consultant, Atlanta Gastroenterology Associates, Atlanta, Georgia

EDITOR

ROBERTO J. FIRPI, MD, MS, AGAF, FAASLD, FACG
Associate Professor of Medicine, Section of Hepatobiliary Diseases and Transplantation, University of Florida, Gainesville, Florida

AUTHORS

MANAL ABDELMALEK, MD, MPH
Associate Professor of Medicine, Division of Gastroenterology, Duke University, Durham, North Carolina

ELIZA W. BEAL, MD
Postdoctoral Research Fellow, Division of Transplantation, Department of Surgery, The Ohio State University Wexner Medical Center, Columbus, Ohio

MARINA BERENGUER, MD
Servicio de Medicina Digestivo (Torre F-5), La Fe University Hospital, Ciberehd, University of Valencia, Valencia, Spain

JENNIFER BERUMEN, MD
Assistant Professor of Abdominal Transplantation and Hepatobiliary Surgery, University of California, San Diego, La Jolla, California

SYLVESTER M. BLACK, MD, PhD
Assistant Professor of Surgery, Division of Transplantation, Department of Surgery, The Ohio State University Wexner Medical Center, Columbus, Ohio

RONIEL CABRERA, MD, MS
Associate Professor of Medicine, Medical Director, Liver Transplant Program, Section of Hepatobiliary Diseases (Liver Unit), Division of Gastroenterology, Hepatology and Nutrition, Department of Medicine, University of Florida, Gainesville, Florida

MICHAEL R. CHARLTON, MD, FRCP
Professor of Medicine, Chief of Hepatology, Medical Director of Liver Transplantation, Intermountain Transplant Center, Intermountain Medical Center, Murray, Utah

VIRGINIA C. CLARK, MD, MS
Assistant Professor of Medicine, Division of Gastroenterology, Hepatology, and Nutrition, University of Florida, Gainesville, Florida

RENUMATHY DHANASEKARAN, MD
Instructor, Division of Gastroenterology and Hepatology, Stanford University, Palo Alto, California

ERIK DUTSON, MD
Department of Surgery, University of California at Los Angeles, Los Angeles, California

FABRIZIO FABRIZI, MD
Division of Nephrology, Maggiore Hospital, IRCCS Foundation, Milano, Italy

JUAN F. GALLEGOS-OROZCO, MD
Assistant Professor of Medicine, Medical Director of Liver Transplantation, Division of Gastroenterology, Hepatology and Nutrition, University of Utah School of Medicine, Salt Lake City, Utah

ALAN HEMMING, MD
Professor and Chief of Abdominal Transplant and Hepatobiliary Surgery, University of California, San Diego, La Jolla, California

MATTHEW KAPPUS, MD
Assistant Professor of Medicine, Division of Gastroenterology, Duke University, Durham, North Carolina

ALEXANDER KUO, MD
Associate Professor of Clinical Medicine, Division of Gastroenterology and Hepatology, University of California, San Diego, San Diego, California

CYNTHIA LEVY, MD
Division of Hepatology, Miller School of Medicine, University of Miami, Miami, Florida

ESTER COELHO LITTLE, MD
Banner Transplant Institute, Banner University Medical Center Phoenix, Phoenix, Arizona

VICTOR ILICH MACHICAO, MD
Associate Professor of Medicine, Medical Director Liver Transplantation, Division of Gastroenterology, Hepatology and Nutrition, McGovern Medical School, University of Texas Health Science Center at Houston, Houston, Texas

ERIC F. MARTIN, MD
Assistant Professor of Medicine, Division of Hepatology, Miller School of Medicine, University of Miami, Miami, Florida

PIERGIORGIO MESSA, MD
Division of Nephrology, Maggiore Hospital, IRCCS Foundation, Milano, Italy

ANTHONY MICHAELS, MD
Assistant Professor of Medicine, Division of Gastroenterology, Hepatology and Nutrition, The Ohio State University Wexner Medical Center, Columbus, Ohio

PATRICK G. NORTHUP, MD, MHS
Associate Professor of Medicine, Division of Gastroenterology and Hepatology, Department of Medicine, Center for the Study of Coagulation Disorders in Liver Disease, University of Virginia, Charlottesville, Virginia

NATHALIE A. PENA POLANCO, MD
Division of Internal Medicine, Miller School of Medicine, University of Miami, Miami, Florida

SAMMY SAAB, MD, MPH, AGAF, FAASLD
Departments of Surgery and Medicine, University of California at Los Angeles, Los Angeles, California

JONATHAN G. STINE, MD, MSc, FACP
Associate Professor of Medicine, Division of Gastroenterology and Hepatology, Department of Medicine, Center for the Study of Coagulation Disorders in Liver Disease, University of Virginia, Charlottesville, Virginia

DUMINDA SURAWEERA, MD
Department of Medicine, Olive-View Medical Center, Sylmar, California

ALBERTO UNZUETA, MD
Gastroenterology-Transplant Hepatology Fellow, Division of Gastroenterology, Hepatology and Nutrition, Department of Medicine, University of Florida, Gainesville, Florida

IRINE VODKIN, MD
Assistant Professor of Clinical Medicine, Division of Gastroenterology and Hepatology, University of California, San Diego, San Diego, California

Contents

Liver Transplantation and Bariatric Surgery: Best Approach   215

Duminda Suraweera, Erik Dutson, and Sammy Saab

> Obesity has become increasingly prevalent, and the number of obese patients in need of liver transplant is expected to continue to increase. In addition, liver disease due to nonalcoholic fatty liver disease is expected to become the leading cause of liver transplantation in the near future. However, obesity remains a relative contraindication in liver transplant. New strategies in managing this patient population are clearly needed. To this end, the authors review the current literature on the efficacy of bariatric surgery in the setting of liver transplantation in obese patients.

Treatment Options in Patients Awaiting Liver Transplantation with Hepatocellular Carcinoma and Cholangiocarcinoma   231

Alberto Unzueta and Roniel Cabrera

> Liver transplantation (LT) provides a good chance of cure for selected patients with hepatocellular carcinoma (HCC) and perihilar cholangiocarcinoma (pCCA). Patients with HCC on a waiting list for LT are at risk for tumor progression and dropout. Treatment of HCC with locoregional therapies may lessen dropout due to tumor progression. Strict selection and adherence to the LT criteria for patients with pCCA before and after neoadjuvant chemotherapy are critical for optimal outcome with LT. This article reviews the existing data for the various treatment strategies used for patients with HCC and pCCA awaiting LT.

Coagulopathy Before and After Liver Transplantation: From the Hepatic to the Systemic Circulatory Systems   253

Jonathan G. Stine and Patrick G. Northup

> The hemostatic environment in patients with cirrhosis is a delicate balance between prohemostatic and antihemostatic factors. There is a lack of effective laboratory measures of the hemostatic system in patients with cirrhosis. Many are predisposed to pulmonary embolus, deep vein thrombosis, and portal vein thrombosis in the pretransplantation setting. This pretransplantation hypercoagulable milieu seems to extend for at least several months post-transplantation. Patients with nonalcoholic fatty liver disease, inherited thrombophilia, portal hypertension in the absence of cirrhosis, and hepatocellular carcinoma often require individualized approach to anticoagulation. Early reports suggest a potential role for low-molecular-weight heparins and direct-acting anticoagulants.

pathophysiology, and treatment of de novo and recurrence of NASH after liver transplantation.

Management of Immunosuppression in Liver Transplantation

Renumathy Dhanasekaran

Liver transplantation outcomes have significantly improved over the past few decades owing largely to the introduction of effective immunosuppression medications. Further comprehension of the unique immune microenvironment of the liver has led to the development of newer molecular targeted therapeutics. Understanding the mechanism of action and adverse effect profiles of these medications is crucial for appropriate management of posttransplant patients. In this review, the author describes the immunologic response elicited by liver transplantation, chronicles the various immunosuppressant drug classes, discusses the evidence behind their use, and evaluates the management of special subpopulations of posttransplantation patients.

Liver Transplantation in Alpha-1 Antitrypsin Deficiency

Virginia C. Clark

Alpha-1 antitrypsin (AAT) deficiency is a common inherited metabolic disorder caused by a point mutation in the SERPIN1A gene. A small portion of homozygous PI*ZZ individuals develop severe liver disease that requires liver transplantation. Posttransplant survival is excellent. The largest burden of advanced liver disease lies within the adult population rather than children. Evaluation of lung function in adults before transplant is essential because of the underlying risk for chronic obstructive pulmonary disease. Post–liver transplantation lung function should also be monitored for decline. Although uncommon, cases of simultaneous lung and liver transplant for AAT deficiency have been reported.

Predictors of Cardiovascular Events After Liver Transplantation

Juan F. Gallegos-Orozco and Michael R. Charlton

Indications for liver transplant have been extended, and older and sicker patients are undergoing transplantation. Infectious, malignant, and cardiovascular diseases account for the most posttransplant deaths. Cirrhotic patients can develop heart disease through systemic diseases affecting the heart and the liver, cirrhosis-specific heart disease, or common cardiovascular. No single factor can predict posttransplant cardiovascular complications. Patients with history of cardiovascular disease, and specific abnormalities on echocardiography, electrocardiography, or serum markers of heart disease seem to be at increased risk of complications. Pretransplant cardiovascular evaluation is essential to detecting these risk factors so their effects can be mitigated through appropriate intervention.

Autoimmune Hepatitis in the Liver Transplant Graft

Eliza W. Beal, Sylvester M. Black, and Anthony Michaels

Recurrent autoimmune hepatitis (AIH) and de novo AIH are 2 important causes of late graft failure after liver transplantation (LT). Recurrent AIH

CLINICS IN LIVER DISEASE

THE CLINICS ARE AVAILABLE ONLINE!
Access your subscription at:
www.theclinics.com

CLINICS IN LIVER DISEASE

Erratum

In the November 2016 issue (Volume 20, number 4), in the article on pages 607-628, "Epidemiology and Impact of Vaccination on Disease," by Noele P. Nelson, Philippa J. Easterbrook, and Brian J. McMahon, the following disclosure statement should have been included for Dr. Easterbrook: "The author alone is responsible for the views expressed in this publication and they do not necessarily represent the views, decisions or policies of the World Health Organization."

A corrected version of this article can be found online at http://www.liver.theclinics.com/.

Clin Liver Dis 21 (2017) xiii
http://dx.doi.org/10.1016/j.cld.2017.02.002
1089-3261/17

Preface

Liver Transplantation in the Twenty-First Century

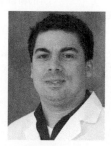

Roberto J. Firpi, MD, MS, AGAF, FAASLD, FACG
Editor

Thanks to Dr Tom Starzl, the pioneer surgeon in liver transplantation in the early 1960s, liver transplant has become one of the most effective therapies to treat patients with chronic liver diseases all over the world. Back in the earliest days of liver transplantation, the survival rates were dismal. But the discovery of cyclosporine and tacrolimus led to significant improvement in rejection rates. Better immunosuppression and better patient outcomes led to a proliferation of liver transplant centers across the United States so that this life-saving surgery is widely available. Since the initial days of transplant, many important changes have occurred that affect clinical practice in liver transplantation. Most notably was the adoption of the Model for End-Stage Liver Disease and the Pediatric Model for End-Stage Liver Disease to allocate organs and the subsequent modifications to the allocation system over time. All are in efforts to improve wait-list mortality and survival after transplantation. The impact of chronic hepatitis C cirrhosis on organ demand cannot be overstated, which now may be mitigated somewhat by highly effective therapies that report cure rates close to 100%. Now, we are even expanding the criteria for liver transplant by considering malignant conditions such as cholangiocarcinoma and hepatocellular carcinoma. With that come the challenges and limits of organ availability, which transplant programs have met by extending donor criteria and new allocation policies for deceased donor livers.

Since 1988, close to 150,000 liver transplants have been performed in the United States based on Organ Procurement and Transplantation Network data as of November 11, 2016. The number of transplants performed for the indications of nonalcoholic fatty liver disease and cryptogenic liver disease will soon surpass the current major indication of viral hepatitis c in the United States. Given the complexity of the patients awaiting liver transplant, this discipline has become a delicate one. One that needs very dedicated physicians to care for very sick patients. In this issue, an

Clin Liver Dis 21 (2017) xv–xvi
http://dx.doi.org/10.1016/j.cld.2017.02.001
1089-3261/17/© 2017 Published by Elsevier Inc.

internationally renowned group of authors (hepatologists and transplant surgeons) provide an update in important topics in liver transplantation in the twenty-first century.

Roberto J. Firpi, MD, MS, AGAF, FAASLD, FACG
Section of Hepatobiliary Diseases and Transplantation
University of Florida
1600 SW Archer Road, MSB Room M440
Gainesville, FL 32610, USA

E-mail address:
Roberto.Firpi@medicine.ufl.edu

Liver Transplantation and Bariatric Surgery
Best Approach

Duminda Suraweera, MD[a], Erik Dutson, MD[b],
Sammy Saab, MD, MPH[b,c],*

KEYWORDS

- Obesity • Liver transplantation • Bariatric surgery • Cirrhosis • NASH

KEY POINTS

- Bariatric surgery has been shown to be an effective means to not only lower body mass index but also reduce obesity-related comorbidities.
- Although the use of bariatric surgery in the setting of liver transplant (LT) is not yet extensively studied, preliminary data are promising.
- Bariatric surgery before or during liver transplantation seems ideal in most patients because surgical procedures after LT can be technically difficult because of adhesions and have increased risk of several complications due to post-LT medications.

INTRODUCTION

The prevalence of obesity has increased dramatically in the United States, with an overwhelming impact on health and health care. Obesity is defined as a body mass index (BMI) equal to or greater than 30 kg/m^2.[1] In 2016, it is estimated that the prevalence of obesity in the United States was 34.7 as compared with 15% in 1987.[2,3] The obesity epidemic has gradually expanded from an adult-onset disorder to affecting many children. From 2011 to 2012, it is estimated that 32% of children were overweight or obese at 2 years of age in the United States.[4] This high prevalence will likely lay the foundation for future increases in rates of obesity-related comorbidities, such as diabetes, heart disease, and liver disease, including end-stage liver disease (ESLD).

Liver transplant (LT) has long been the gold standard for the treatment of ESLD, acute liver failure, and primary hepatic malignancy.[5] Transplantation not only extends survival

Disclosure: The authors have nothing to disclose.
[a] Department of Medicine, Olive-View Medical Center, 14445 Olive View Drive, 2B-182, Sylmar, CA 91342, USA; [b] Department of Surgery, University of California at Los Angeles, 200 Medical Plaza, Suite 214, Los Angeles, CA 90095, USA; [c] Department of Medicine, University of California at Los Angeles, 200 Medical Plaza, Suite 214, Los Angeles, CA 90095, USA
* Corresponding author. Pfleger Liver Institute, UCLA Medical Center, 200 Medical Plaza, Suite 214, Los Angeles, CA 90095.
E-mail address: SSaab@mednet.ucla.edu

Clin Liver Dis 21 (2017) 215–230
http://dx.doi.org/10.1016/j.cld.2016.12.001
1089-3261/17/© 2016 Elsevier Inc. All rights reserved.

liver.theclinics.com

but also improves quality of life and psychological well-being of patients.[6] However, despite its success, LT remains a surgically demanding procedure. Organ availability is limited, with most transplanted livers acquired from a deceased donor. Organ allocation in the United States is managed by The United Network for Organ Sharing. Because of limitations in organs and complexity of LT, careful patient selection is essential. Contraindications are generally center specific, but common contraindications include cardiopulmonary disease that cannot be corrected, acquired immunodeficiency syndrome, malignancy outside of the liver or metastatic hepatocellular carcinoma, and lack of social care or history of nonadherence with medical care.[5] A BMI greater than 40 kg/m^2 is considered to be a relative contraindication in many transplant centers.[5]

A growing number of obese patients are being evaluated for LT.[7–9] It is estimated that the prevalence of obesity is 20% to 30% in LT recipients in the United States.[10,11] At waiting list and transplantation, prevalence of morbid obesity was 3.8% and 3.4%, respectively, in 2007.[12] Obesity has been shown to be an independent risk factor in the progression of liver disease in patients with cirrhosis of all causes.[13,14] In addition, nonalcoholic fatty liver disease (NAFLD) has become the third leading cause of liver disease in the United States.[15] Although rates of alcoholic and viral liver disease are on the decline, rates of NAFLD are on the increase and may become the leading cause of liver transplantation in the next decade.[16,17] Nonalcoholic steatohepatitis (NASH) is already the second leading cause of liver disease among adult waiting-list registrants in the United States.[18] Furthermore, these estimates of NASH prevalence may be underestimated given that most cryptogenic cirrhosis is thought to be unrecognized NASH.[19,20] It has become clear that techniques to improve outcomes in liver transplantation in obese patients are urgently needed. Bariatric surgery may be of benefit in this setting. The authors review the current literature on the use of bariatric surgery in the setting of LT.

IMPACT OF OBESITY IN LIVER TRANSPLANT

The increased prevalence of obesity has presented many challenges in LT. Obese LT patients have been found to have higher rates of primary graft dysfunction and significantly higher mortality when compared with nonobese counterparts, primarily due to worse cardiovascular outcomes.[11,21] Obese patients undergoing LT have been shown to have increased perioperative complications than nonobese patients. Higher rates of infection, transfusion requirements, increased operative times, and longer intensive care unit stays were all associated with obesity.[22,23] Patients with BMI greater than 40 kg/m^2 have significantly higher rates of mortality after LT.[24] Perioperative mortality was increased at 1, 2, and 5 years after LT primarily due to cardiovascular complications.[11] Thus, obesity has historically been considered a contraindication for liver transplantation.[25] Severely obese patients have a 10% higher likelihood of being turned down for organ offers, whereas morbidly obese patients are 16% more likely to be turned down.[26] However, other studies have shown mixed results or no significant difference in perioperative morbidity and mortality in obese patients.[27,28]

Patients with NAFLD present a unique challenge to LT because most usually have a metabolic syndrome with associated conditions, such as diabetes mellitus, hypertension, and hyperlipidemia. One study evaluating the causes of liver diseases among patients awaiting LT found that patients with NASH were more likely to be older and have diabetes, a higher median BMI, and a lower glomerular filtration rate when compared with patients with liver disease from other causes.[18] Coronary artery disease is also a major factor complicating the management of these patients. Patel and colleagues[29] compared patients with alcoholic and nonalcoholic ESLD and found that alcoholic patients had a coronary artery disease incidence of 2% as compared with 13% in the nonalcoholic group (P<.005). Patients with NAFLD also have significantly higher perioperative cardiovascular mortality when compared with alcoholic patients.[30] Another study evaluated the impact of type 2 diabetes and obesity on long-term outcomes in LT and found that the presence of type 2 diabetes pretransplant and posttransplant as well as presence of type 2 diabetes in the donors was associated with increased mortality.[31] However, although patients with NASH tend to have higher comorbidities, overall grouped mortality after LT is comparable to that of other causes for ESLD.[17,32,33] Subgroup analysis of NASH patients with increased mortality found that patients with age 60 years or greater and BMI equal to or greater than 30 kg/m^2 with diabetes and hypertension had an immediate mortality in post-LT of 25% with the 30-day mortality of 31% and 1-year mortality of 50%.[34] This finding was significantly higher than other causes and the overall NASH mortality, which was 21.4%.[34]

Recurrence of NAFLD is common posttransplant with estimates ranging from 30% to 100%, depending on patient's individual risk factors.[35,36] However, the risk of developing advanced fibrosis or cirrhosis is low, around 4%, with no significant difference in short- or long-term survival when compared with other cohorts.[37] Dureja and colleagues[38] evaluated NAFLD recurrence in 88 recipients after LT for NAFLD and found that BMI pre-LT and post-LT correlated with recurrence rate. Other factors, such as post-LT triglyceride levels and average steroid dose at 6 months, were also correlated with recurrence. However, there was no significant difference in overall mortality. Contos and colleagues[39] found that the risk of allograft steatosis approached 100% at 5 years in patients with LT for NASH compared with 25% in non-NASH controls.

Not only has NAFLD been shown to reoccur post-LT but also patients may develop NAFLD even if their initial liver failure was due to a different cause.[40-46] Seo and colleagues[47] conducted a retrospective analysis of 68 patients with LT and found de novo NAFLD development in 18% of patients at 28 ± 18 months, and 9% developed of NASH. Multivariable logistic regression analysis revealed that an increase in BMI greater than 10% after LT was associated with increased risk of developing de novo NAFLD, whereas the use of angiotensin–converting-enzyme inhibitors was associated with reduced risk. Other factors that have been shown to increase the risk of de novo NAFLD development after LT include tacrolimus-based immunosuppression regimen, diabetes mellitus, hyperlipidemia, hypertension, and alcoholic liver disease as primary indication for initial LT and pretransplant liver graft steatosis.[46] Prevalence of some of these risk factors tends to be significantly greater in patients after LT than in the general population (Table 1). There has been an increasing prevalence of NAFLD

Table 1
Comparison of risk factors of nonalcoholic fatty liver disease in patients after liver transplantation compared with the general US population

Disease	Prevalence Post–LT, %	Prevalence in US Population, %
Diabetes mellitus	21–32	3–12
Hypertension	41–81	15–34
Hyperlipidemia	20–66	15–30
Obesity	39–43	16–38

Data from Burke A, Lucey MR. Non-alcoholic fatty liver disease, non-alcoholic steatohepatitis and orthotopic liver transplantation. Am J Transplant 2004;4(5):686–93; and Ford ES, Giles WH, Dietz WH. Prevalence of the metabolic syndrome among US adults: findings from the third National Health and Nutrition Examination Survey. JAMA 2002;287(3):356–9.

in both deceased and living liver donor populations. Because of the limitations of organ resources, there has been a push to use marginal donors or "extended criteria donors"[48]; this has resulted in the increasing use steatotic allografts. Allografts with 30% to 60% fat have been associated with graft dysfunction, decreased graft survival, and increased mortality.[49] The distribution of fat has also been shown to be an important factor, with macrovascular steatosis resulting in greater dysfunction than microvascular distribution.[50,51] Obesity will likely continue to play a significant role in affecting outcomes in the LT setting.

NONSURGICAL INTERVENTIONS FOR OBESITY

Lifestyle interventions such as exercise and dietary modifications have not been fully evaluated in obese patients with cirrhosis. Some studies suggest oral branched chain amino acids can decrease incidence of hepatocellular carcinoma and increase serum albumin levels in overweight and obese patient.[14,52] Although the mechanism is not fully understood, it may lead to improved insulin sensitivity in muscle and reduced oxidative stress.[53] Increasing physical activity has been shown to be more difficult in patients with cirrhosis.[54,55] Moderate levels of physical exercise has also been shown to increase portal pressure in patients with cirrhosis, potentially increasing the risk of bleeding in patients with varices.[56] However, aerobic exercise in cirrhotic patients has been shown to improve insulin resistance, decrease body fat, improve liver enzymes, and increase quality of life.[57,58] One study suggests walking 5000 or more steps per day and maintaining a total energy intake of 30 kcal/ideal body weight are appropriate goals for compensated cirrhotic patients.[55]

TYPES OF BARIATRIC SURGERY

Bariatric surgery is currently the only therapy for severe obesity that has been shown to result in significant weight loss and is more effective than nonsurgical interventions.[59] Furthermore, substantial improvements of not only physical but also mental health have been associated with bariatric surgery spanning up to 25 years after surgery.[60] Patients qualify for surgical intervention if BMI equal to or greater than 40 kg/m^2 or equal to or greater than 34 kg/m^2 with at least one obesity-related comorbidity.[61] Furthermore, patients should be screened carefully with an interdisciplinary approach involving medical, surgical, psychiatric, and nutritional professionals (**Table 2**).[62] There are several bariatric procedures currently being practiced, each with its advantages and disadvantages (**Table 3**). Traditionally, it was thought that bariatric surgery decreases body weight either through a restrictive or malabsorptive process; however, it is now thought that neurohormonal exposure plays a prominent role in the weight loss and resolution of obesity-associated comorbidities that is achieved.

The gastric band is an adjustable band placed high in the stomach to produce a 30 mL pouch and is currently the only purely restrictive procedure available (**Fig. 1**A).[63,64] An inflatable cuff with a subcutaneous port allows for easy adjustability of the band. Mean excess weight loss of 45% to 65% was seen at 7 to 10 years after the procedure.[65–67] Common complications include band erosion, band infection, band slippage, esophagitis, esophageal dilation, and port problems. Complication rates have ranged from 50% to 80% at 5 to 12 years after the procedure.[65,66,68] Reoperation rates range from 20% to 50% at 5 to 10 years.[65–67,69] Inadequate weight loss has been seen in 30% to 45% in 5-year follow-up.[68,70,71] Although being safe and less invasive, the adjustable gastric band has high reoperation rates and results in significant less weight loss than the Roux-en-Y gastric bypass, resulting in a significant decline in its use.

Table 2
Preoperative assessment before bariatric surgery

Consultant	Role
Bariatric surgeon	Primary person to coordinate the interdisciplinary team and evaluate candidacy for surgery
Primary care physician	Evaluation and treatment of comorbidities both before and after bariatric surgery; consider advanced diagnostic testing and expert consultation when indicated
Psychiatrist	Assess psychological well-being and ability/willingness to participate in postoperative treatments/rehabilitation
Nutritionist	Assess patient's nutrition status and provide education

Test	Indication
Complete blood cell count Basic metabolic panel Live function test Coagulation panel Thyroid-stimulating hormone Hemoglobin A1c Fasting lipid panel Iron panel Vitamin B12, folate, thiamine levels	All patients
Hypercoagulable workup	Personal or family history of thromboembolism or hypercoagulable disorder
Chest radiograph	Age $\geq$50 y, known/suspected cardiopulmonary disease
Electrocardiogram	Men $\geq$40 y, women $\geq$50 y, known cardiac history, hypertension, diabetes, or hyperlipidemia
Echocardiogram	Known heart murmur or valvular disease
Polysomnography	Suspected sleep apnea
Esophagogastroduodenoscopy	Known gastroesophageal reflux disease/peptic ulcer disease or symptoms
Colonoscopy	Regular malignancy screening
Prostate-specific antigen	Men $\geq$40 y
Urine pregnancy test	Woman of childbearing age
Pap smear/mammogram	Regular female malignancy screening

Data from Kuruba R, Koche LS, Murr MM. Preoperative assessment and perioperative care of patients undergoing bariatric surgery. Med Clin North Am 2007;91(3):339–51, ix.

In contrast, a sleeve gastrectomy is the permanent removal of most of the body and fundus of the stomach, typically 60% to 75% (**Fig. 1B**).[59,64] It has become the most common bariatric procedure in the United States. Although sleeve gastrectomy reduces the gastric volume, its primary mechanism may be via alteration of neurohormonal pathways. This theory is supported by studies showing comparable reduction in body weight and improvements in glycemic tolerance between sleeve gastrectomy and Roux-en-Y gastric bypass even though Roux-en-Y is a more rigorous procedure.[72] Although the exact neurohormonal mechanism is still under investigation, several possible agents have been identified. Studies have shown a reduction in the levels of ghrelin secreted by the stomach after sleeve gastrectomy, thereby decreasing the sensation of hunger.[72] Furthermore, levels of peptide-YY and GLP-1, neuropeptides known to induce satiety, have been found to increase in

Table 3
Advantages and disadvantages of different types of bariatric surgeries

Procedure	Advantages	Disadvantages
Gastric band	Minimally invasive, reversible	Relatively less weight loss with high rates of complications
Sleeve gastrectomy	Gastric function maintained, significant weight loss, and resolution of obesity comorbidities, no issues with malabsorption	Possible bleeding or leakage from staple line
Roux-en-Y	Significant weight loss and resolution of obesity comorbidities	Higher complication rates, malabsorption of certain vitamins/minerals
Biliopancreatic diversion with duodenal switch	Significant weight loss and resolution of obesity comorbidities	Highest rates of complications, severe malabsorption

patients after sleeve gastrectomy.[72] Recently, yet another molecular target, farsenoid-X receptor (FXR), has been shown to play a key role. Bile acids are known to regulate metabolism by binding to FXR, and sleeve gastrectomy is thought to increase circulating bile acids, thereby promoting FXR activation and leading to improved glucose tolerance and weight loss.[73,74] Sleeve gastrectomy leaves the pylorus intact to allow for normal gastric function. Mean excess weight loss of 40% to 70% is typically achieved 12 months after the procedure.[72,75,76] Complications are minimized by keeping the pylorus intact. Patients may still have vomiting because of overeating, and there is a risk of leaking from the surgically altered stomach. With time, the stomach may become atonic, thereby reducing the intake restriction, at which time a gastric bypass may be pursued.

Roux-en-Y gastric bypass is considered the gold standard of bariatric surgery in the United States and achieves significant weight loss via restrictive, malabsorptive, and neurohormonal means (**Fig. 1C**).[64] Although traditionally its effectiveness was thought to be volume restriction combined with malabsorption, new data suggest that it may be more closely related to neurohormonal effects related to altered exposure of various anatomic gastrointestinal mucosa.[77–82] Roux-en-Y involves creation of a small gastric pouch, typically 30 mL in size, by segmentation of the stomach with staples or division.[83] The proximal jejunum is then divided about 30 cm below the ligament of Treitz with the proximal end joining the small bowel about 100 cm below the point of division and the distal end brought up to form a gastroenterostomy. Mean excess weight loss was 60% to 68% at 4 to 7 years after the procedure.[66,70,71] Inadequate weight loss was seen in 4% to 5% at 5 to 10 years.[70,71] Complications occur in about 25% to 40% of patients at 10 years and include leaking at anastomotic sites, acute gastric dilation, delayed gastric emptying, and dumping syndrome.[66,70] Nutritional deficiencies can also occur, typically deficiencies in calcium, vitamin B1, vitamin B12, and iron.

Biliopancreatic diversion with duodenal switch is a primarily malabsorptive procedure that involves significant intestinal modification (**Fig. 1D**).[64] The procedure does involve some removal of the stomach but less than that seen in Roux-en Y bypass, thus allowing for patients to have larger meals. An enteric limb, approximately 250 cm in length, is then anastomosed to the postpyloric duodenum. The duodenobiliopancreatic limb is subsequently anastomosed to the Roux limb about 100 cm

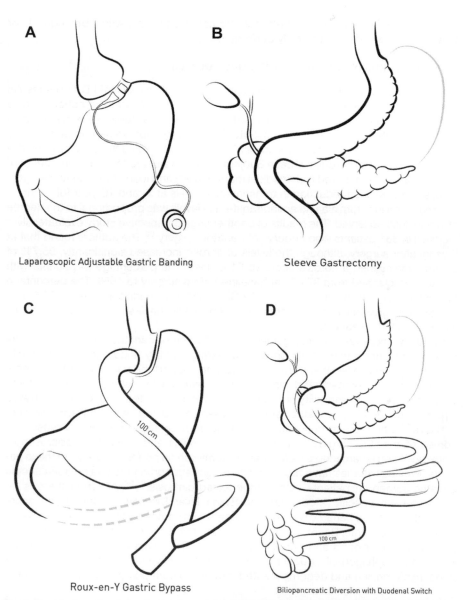

Fig. 1. Surgical methods for bariatric surgery. (*A*) Laparoscopic adjustable gastric banding. (*B*) Sleeve gastrectomy. (*C*) Roux-en-Y gastric bypass. (*D*) Biliopancreatic diversion with duodenal switch. (*From* Vu L, Switzer NJ, De Gara C, et al. Surgical interventions for obesity and metabolic disease. Best Pract Res Clin Endocrinol Metab 2013;27(2):241–4; with permission.)

proximal to the ileocecal valve. Documented operative mortality is about 1% and can be as high as 2.5% when surgery is performed laparoscopically.[84] Typically, these patients have high complication rates, including bowel obstruction, dumping syndrome, bile reflux, diarrhea, and nutritional deficiencies in fat-soluble vitamins, protein, calcium, zinc, and iron. Because of the high rates of complications, biliopancreatic diversion with duodenal switch is reserved for patients typically with a BMI equal to or greater than 55 and is infrequently performed.

BARIATRIC SURGERY IN PATIENTS WITH LIVER DISEASE

Most patients undergoing bariatric surgery have some degree of NAFLD.[85] The results of a *Cochrane Review* in 2010 found 21 prospective or retrospective cohort studies evaluating bariatric surgery in treating NASH, but none of the studies were randomized controlled trials.[86] The results of most studies showed improvement in steatosis or inflammation scores; however, 4 studies also described some deterioration in the degree of fibrosis. The Swedish Obese Subjects study evaluated the long-term effect of bariatric surgery compared with medical management and found that bariatric surgery results in a sustained reduction in transaminase levels at 2- and 10-year follow-up.[87] The reduction in serum alanine aminotransferase levels was proportional to the degree of weight loss observed. The results of another large prospective study evaluated liver biopsies in 381 patients who underwent bariatric surgery.[88] The authors found that at 5 years after surgery, although the levels of fibrosis increased significantly, 95.7% of patients maintained a fibrosis score of F1 or less. The percentage of patients with steatosis decreased from 37.4% at baseline before surgery to 16%. The percentage of patients with probable or definite NASH decreased significantly from 27.4% to 14.2%. The greatest improvements occurred within the first year, but the results were sustained 5 years later.

Currently, there are no clear guidelines on the use of bariatric surgery in patients with cirrhosis nor a consensus on what bariatric modality is best for a patient with cirrhosis.[89,90] However, there are limited data to support the use of bariatric surgery in patients with compensated cirrhosis. One retrospective study found that there was an increase in mortality in patients with compensated and decompensated cirrhosis undergoing bariatric surgery when compared with patients without cirrhosis.[91] Shimizu and colleagues[92] conducted a database review to assess outcomes of bariatric surgery in patients with cirrhosis and found that laparoscopic Roux-en-Y and laparoscopic sleeve gastrectomy can be performed safely in these patients. Previous studies have found similar results supporting the use of laparoscopic bariatric surgery in patients with compensated cirrhosis.[93,94] Although there is no consensus on specific Model for End-Stage Liver Disease or Child-Pugh score threshold, pursuing bariatric surgery in patients with compensated cirrhosis is reasonable in select patients. Bariatric surgery should not be pursued in patients with decompensated liver cirrhosis and portal hypertension. The authors recommend obtaining screening esophagogastroduodenoscopy and abdominal ultrasound to evaluate for portal hypertension and decompensated cirrhosis before pursuing bariatric surgery.

BARIATRIC SURGERY AND LIVER TRANSPLANT

Preliminary results of bariatric surgery performed before, during, or after LT have been promising and an area of active research (**Table 4**). Before LT, bariatric surgery had been typically performed at least 1 year before LT, which allowed time to reach BMI goals and improvement in obesity-related comorbidities. In contrast, if bariatric surgery is scheduled after LT, the authors recommend waiting at least 1 year after LT to minimize the risk of acute cellular rejection from interruptions in immunosuppressant regimen. Furthermore, BMI tends to fluctuate immediately after LT with one study finding on average patients gaining 5.1 kg over the first year after LT and 9.5 kg at 3 years.[95] The authors review the benefits and drawbacks on perioperative timing of bariatric surgery in the setting of LT in later discussion.

Table 4		
Advantages and disadvantages of timing of bariatric surgery in the setting of liver transplantation		
Timing	Advantages	Disadvantages
Before LT	Decreased weight and resolution of comorbidities before LT with benefits remaining after transplant	Increased cost with 2 separate hospitalizations, increased patient discomfort, delay of LT
During LT	Minimizes cost and patient discomfort, resolution of obesity-related comorbidities after LT	Complex procedure
After LT	Decreases obesity related comorbidities after LT	Increased risk of wound dehiscence and infection in the setting of post–LT immunosuppression, increased adhesions

BARIATRIC SURGERY BEFORE LIVER TRANSPLANTATION

Bariatric surgery before transplantation aims to optimize patient's obesity-associated medical conditions before LT. However, attempting bariatric surgery before liver transplantation does delay transplant because patients will often have to wait until BMI responds adequately, and complications from bariatric surgery may further delay transplantation. Furthermore, by separating the 2 procedures, there are increased financial costs and increased hospitalizations. Lin and colleagues[96] conducted a retrospective analysis of 20 patients with ESLD and 6 patients with end-stage renal disease who underwent laparoscopic sleeve gastrectomy as a weight loss method before liver or kidney transplantation. Mean percentage of excess weight loss at 1, 3, and 12 months was 17%, 26%, and 50%, respectively. Six patients experienced postoperative complications, which included infections, staple line leak, bleeding, and kidney injury. There was no perioperative mortality. All patients reached BMI goals for liver transplantation within 1 year, with a mean time between gastrectomy to transplant of 16.6 months. Takata and colleagues[97] evaluated the safety and efficacy of laparoscopic Roux-en-Y gastric bypass in 7 patients with end-stage renal disease and laparoscopic sleeve gastrectomy in 6 patients with cirrhosis and 2 patients with end-stage lung disease. The mean percentage of excess weight loss at 9 months was 61% in end-stage renal patients, 33% in patients with cirrhosis, and 61.5% in patients with ESLD. Obesity-associated comorbidities improved or resolved in all patients. Fourteen of 15 (93%) patients reached goal BMI for transplantation. Several other case reports have been published with successful sleeve gastrectomy before liver transplantation.[98]

BARIATRIC SURGERY DURING TRANSPLANTATION

Benefits of combining bariatric surgery with liver transplantation include immediately undergoing transplant and avoiding delays with surgery before LT described above, decreased hospital stay, reduced cost, and decreased stress and pain. Heimbach and colleagues[99] compared the use of noninvasive pretransplant weight loss with sleeve gastrectomy during liver transplantation. A total of 37 patients achieved weight loss and underwent LT alone, and 7 patients underwent transplantation combined with sleeve gastrectomy. In those who were enrolled in the noninvasive weight loss program alone, weight gain to BMI greater than 35 was seen in 60% (21 of 34), post-LT diabetes in 35% (12 of 34), and steatosis in 21% (7 of 34), with 3 deaths plus 3 graft losses. In patients who underwent sleeve gastrectomy, there was substantial weight loss with mean BMI of 29. No patients developed post-LT diabetes or steatosis. There were no deaths or graft losses. One patient developed a leak from the gastric staple line, and one had excess weight loss.

BARIATRIC SURGERY AFTER TRANSPLANTATION

Goal of performing bariatric surgery after LT would be to improve survival by reducing obesity-related comorbidities as well as to reduce incidence of NASH. A serious draw-back in performing bariatric surgery in a LT recipient is the increased risk of wound complications and dehiscence due to the use of steroids and other immunosuppressant medications, such as mammalian target of rapamycin (mTOR). In fact, chronic and active use of steroid or immunosuppressant medications has been shown to be a strong predictor of 30-day postoperative morbidity and mortality following primary bariatric surgery.[100] Major adhesions can also make bariatric surgery technically difficult in post-LT patients.[101] Lin and colleagues[102] performed sleeve gastrectomy on 9 obese LT recipients with the goal of improving diabetes and steatohepatitis. Mean time between LT and bariatric surgery was 5.9 (±2.4) years. At 6 months, excess weight loss averaged 55.5%. Three patients had complications of mesh dehiscence after a synchronous incisional hernia repair, bile leak from the liver surface requiring laparoscopic drainage, and postoperative dysphagia that required reoperation. There were no episodes of graft rejection. Hepatic and renal functions were unchanged. Calcineurin inhibitor levels remained stable with no need for dose adjustments.

SUMMARY

Bariatric surgery has been shown to be an effective means to not only lower BMI but also reduce obesity-related comorbidities. Although the use of bariatric surgery in the setting of LT is not yet extensively studied, preliminary data are promising. Bariatric surgery before or during liver transplantation seems ideal in most patients because surgical procedures after LT can be technically difficult due to adhesions and have increased risk of several complications due to post-LT medications.

REFERENCES

1. Kopelman PG. Obesity as a medical problem. Nature 2000;404(6778):635–43.
2. Ogden CL, Carroll MD, Kit BK, et al. Prevalence of obesity in the United States, 2009-2010. NCHS Data Brief 2012;(82):1–8.
3. Ward ZJ, Long MW, Resch SC, et al. Redrawing the US obesity landscape: bias-corrected estimates of state-specific adult obesity prevalence. PLoS One 2016;11(3):e0150735.
4. Moss BG, Yeaton WH. Young children's weight trajectories and associated risk factors: results from the Early Childhood Longitudinal Study-Birth Cohort. Am J Health Promot 2011;25(3):190–8.
5. Martin P, DiMartini A, Feng S, et al. Evaluation for liver transplantation in adults: 2013 practice guideline by the American Association for the Study of Liver Diseases and the American Society of Transplantation. Hepatology 2014;59(3):1144–65.
6. Duffy JP, Kao K, Ko CY, et al. Long-term patient outcome and quality of life after liver transplantation: analysis of 20-year survivors. Ann Surg 2010;252(4):652–61.

7. Singal AK, Guturu P, Hmoud B, et al. Evolving frequency and outcomes of liver transplantation based on etiology of liver disease. Transplantation 2013;95(5): 755–60.
8. Agopian VG, Kaldas FM, Hong JC, et al. Liver transplantation for nonalcoholic steatohepatitis: the new epidemic. Ann Surg 2012;256(4):624–33.
9. Stepanova M, Wai H, Saab S, et al. The portrait of an adult liver transplant recipient in the United States from 1987 to 2013. JAMA Intern Med 2014;174(8): 1407–9.
10. Zaydfudim V, Feurer ID, Moore DE, et al. The negative effect of pretransplant overweight and obesity on the rate of improvement in physical quality of life after liver transplantation. Surgery 2009;146(2):174–80.
11. Nair S, Verma S, Thuluvath PJ. Obesity and its effect on survival in patients undergoing orthotopic liver transplantation in the United States. Hepatology 2002; 35(1):105–9.
12. Pelletier SJ, Schaubel DE, Wei G, et al. Effect of body mass index on the survival benefit of liver transplantation. Liver Transpl 2007;13(12):1678–83.
13. Berzigotti A, Garcia-Tsao G, Bosch J, et al. Obesity is an independent risk factor for clinical decompensation in patients with cirrhosis. Hepatology 2011;54(2): 555–61.
14. Muto Y, Sato S, Watanabe A, et al. Overweight and obesity increase the risk for liver cancer in patients with liver cirrhosis and long-term oral supplementation with branched-chain amino acid granules inhibits liver carcinogenesis in heavier patients with liver cirrhosis. Hepatol Res 2006;35(3):204–14.
15. Schreuder TC, Verwer BJ, van Nieuwkerk CM, et al. Nonalcoholic fatty liver disease: an overview of current insights in pathogenesis, diagnosis and treatment. World J Gastroenterol 2008;14(16):2474–86.
16. Mandell MS, Zimmerman M, Campsen J, et al. Bariatric surgery in liver transplant patients: weighing the evidence. Obes Surg 2008;18(12):1515–6.
17. Charlton MR, Burns JM, Pedersen RA, et al. Frequency and outcomes of liver transplantation for nonalcoholic steatohepatitis in the United States. Gastroenterology 2011;141(4):1249–53.
18. Wong RJ, Aguilar M, Cheung R, et al. Nonalcoholic steatohepatitis is the second leading etiology of liver disease among adults awaiting liver transplantation in the United States. Gastroenterology 2015;148(3):547–55.
19. Caldwell SH, Oelsner DH, Iezzoni JC, et al. Cryptogenic cirrhosis: clinical characterization and risk factors for underlying disease. Hepatology 1999;29(3): 664–9.
20. Liou I, Kowdley KV. Natural history of nonalcoholic steatohepatitis. J Clin Gastroenterol 2006;40(Suppl 1):S11–6.
21. Hillingso JG, Wettergren A, Hyoudo M, et al. Obesity increases mortality in liver transplantation–the Danish experience. Transpl Int 2005;18(11):1231–5.
22. LaMattina JC, Foley DP, Fernandez LA, et al. Complications associated with liver transplantation in the obese recipient. Clin Transplant 2012;26(6):910–8.
23. Hakeem AR, Cockbain AJ, Raza SS, et al. Increased morbidity in overweight and obese liver transplant recipients: a single-center experience of 1325 patients from the United Kingdom. Liver Transpl 2013;19(5):551–62.
24. Dick AA, Spitzer AL, Seifert CF, et al. Liver transplantation at the extremes of the body mass index. Liver Transpl 2009;15(8):968–77.
25. Thuluvath PJ. Morbid obesity with one or more other serious comorbidities should be a contraindication for liver transplantation. Liver Transpl 2007; 13(12):1627–9.

26. Segev DL, Thompson RE, Locke JE, et al. Prolonged waiting times for liver transplantation in obese patients. Ann Surg 2008;248(5):863–70.

27. Perez-Protto SE, Quintini C, Reynolds LF, et al. Comparable graft and patient survival in lean and obese liver transplant recipients. Liver Transpl 2013;19(8): 907–15.

28. Saab S, Lalezari D, Pruthi P, et al. The impact of obesity on patient survival in liver transplant recipients: a meta-analysis. Liver Transpl 2015;35(1):164–70.

29. Patel S, Kiefer TL, Ahmed A, et al. Comparison of the frequency of coronary artery disease in alcohol-related versus non-alcohol-related endstage liver disease. Am J Cardiol 2011;108(11):1552–5.

30. Vanwagner LB, Bhave M, Te HS, et al. Patients transplanted for nonalcoholic steatohepatitis are at increased risk for postoperative cardiovascular events. Hepatology 2012;56(5):1741–50.

31. Younossi ZM, Stepanova M, Saab S, et al. The impact of type 2 diabetes and obesity on the long-term outcomes of more than 85 000 liver transplant recipients in the US. Aliment Pharmacol Ther 2014;40(6):686–94.

32. Afzali A, Berry K, Ioannou GN. Excellent posttransplant survival for patients with nonalcoholic steatohepatitis in the United States. Liver Transpl 2012;18(1): 29–37.

33. Wong RJ, Chou C, Bonham CA, et al. Improved survival outcomes in patients with non-alcoholic steatohepatitis and alcoholic liver disease following liver transplantation: an analysis of 2002-2012 United Network for Organ Sharing data. Clin Transplant 2014;28(6):713–21.

34. Malik SM, deVera ME, Fontes P, et al. Outcome after liver transplantation for NASH cirrhosis. Am J Transplant 2009;9(4):782–93.

35. Patel YA, Berg CL, Moylan CA. Nonalcoholic fatty liver disease: key considerations before and after liver transplantation. Dig Dis Sci 2016;61(5):1406–16.

36. Czaja AJ. Recurrence of nonalcoholic steatohepatitis after liver transplantation. Liver Transpl Surg 1997;3(2):185–6.

37. Yalamanchili K, Saadeh S, Klintmalm GB, et al. Nonalcoholic fatty liver disease after liver transplantation for cryptogenic cirrhosis or nonalcoholic fatty liver disease. Liver Transpl 2010;16(4):431–9.

38. Dureja P, Mellinger J, Agni R, et al. NAFLD recurrence in liver transplant recipients. Transplantation 2011;91(6):684–9.

39. Contos MJ, Cales W, Sterling RK, et al. Development of nonalcoholic fatty liver disease after orthotopic liver transplantation for cryptogenic cirrhosis. Liver Transpl 2001;7(4):363–73.

40. Patil DT, Yerian LM. Evolution of nonalcoholic fatty liver disease recurrence after liver transplantation. Liver Transpl 2012;18(10):1147–53.

41. Burke A, Lucey MR. Non-alcoholic fatty liver disease, non-alcoholic steatohepatitis and orthotopic liver transplantation. Am J Transplant 2004;4(5):686–93.

42. Saab S, Cho D, Lassman RC, et al. Recurrent non-alcoholic steatohepatitis in a living related liver transplant recipient. J Hepatol 2005;42(1):148–9.

43. Lim LG, Cheng CL, Wee A, et al. Prevalence and clinical associations of posttransplant fatty liver disease. Liver Transpl 2007;27(1):76–80.

44. Laish I, Braun M, Mor E, et al. Metabolic syndrome in liver transplant recipients: prevalence, risk factors, and association with cardiovascular events. Liver Transpl 2011;17(1):15–22.

45. McAlister VC, Haddad E, Renouf E, et al. Cyclosporin versus tacrolimus as primary immunosuppressant after liver transplantation: a meta-analysis. Am J Transplant 2006;6(7):1578–85.

46. Dumortier J, Giostra E, Belbouab S, et al. Non-alcoholic fatty liver disease in liver transplant recipients: another story of "seed and soil". Am J Gastroenterol 2010; 105(3):613–20.
47. Seo S, Maganti K, Khehra M, et al. De novo nonalcoholic fatty liver disease after liver transplantation. Liver Transpl 2007;13(6):844–7.
48. McCormack L, Dutkowski P, El-Badry AM, et al. Liver transplantation using fatty livers: always feasible? J Hepatol 2011;54(5):1055–62.
49. Perkins JD. Saying "Yes" to obese living liver donors: short-term intensive treatment for donors with hepatic steatosis in living-donor liver transplantation. Liver Transpl 2006;12(6):1012–3.
50. Selzner N, Selzner M, Jochum W, et al. Mouse livers with macrosteatosis are more susceptible to normothermic ischemic injury than those with microsteatosis. J Hepatol 2006;44(4):694–701.
51. Spitzer AL, Lao OB, Dick AA, et al. The biopsied donor liver: incorporating macrosteatosis into high-risk donor assessment. Liver Transpl 2010;16(7):874–84.
52. Yatsuhashi H, Ohnishi Y, Nakayama S, et al. Anti-hypoalbuminemic effect of branched-chain amino acid granules in patients with liver cirrhosis is independent of dietary energy and protein intake. Hepatol Res 2011;41(11):1027–35.
53. Ohno T, Tanaka Y, Sugauchi F, et al. Suppressive effect of oral administration of branched-chain amino acid granules on oxidative stress and inflammation in HCV-positive patients with liver cirrhosis. Hepatol Res 2008;38(7):683–8.
54. Hayashi F, Momoki C, Yuikawa M, et al. Nutritional status in relation to lifestyle in patients with compensated viral cirrhosis. World J Gastroenterol 2012;18(40): 5759–70.
55. Hayashi F, Matsumoto Y, Momoki C, et al. Physical inactivity and insufficient dietary intake are associated with the frequency of sarcopenia in patients with compensated viral liver cirrhosis. Hepatol Res 2013;43(12):1264–75.
56. Garcia-Pagan JC, Santos C, Barbera JA, et al. Physical exercise increases portal pressure in patients with cirrhosis and portal hypertension. Gastroenterology 1996;111(5):1300–6.
57. Hickman IJ, Jonsson JR, Prins JB, et al. Modest weight loss and physical activity in overweight patients with chronic liver disease results in sustained improvements in alanine aminotransferase, fasting insulin, and quality of life. Gut 2004;53(3):413–9.
58. Konishi I, Hiasa Y, Tokumoto Y, et al. Aerobic exercise improves insulin resistance and decreases body fat and serum levels of leptin in patients with hepatitis C virus. Hepatol Res 2011;41(10):928–35.
59. Colquitt JL, Picot J, Loveman E, et al. Surgery for obesity. Cochrane Database Syst Rev 2009;(2):CD003641.
60. Driscoll S, Gregory DM, Fardy JM, et al. Long-term health-related quality of life in bariatric surgery patients: a systematic review and meta-analysis. Obesity (Silver Spring) 2016;24(1):60–70.
61. Obesity: Preventing and managing the global epidemic. Report of a WHO consultation. World Health Organ Tech Rep Ser 2000;894(i–xii):1–253.
62. Kuruba R, Koche LS, Murr MM. Preoperative assessment and perioperative care of patients undergoing bariatric surgery. Med Clin North Am 2007;91(3): 339–51, ix.
63. Toolabi K, Golzarand M, Farid R. Laparoscopic adjustable gastric banding: efficacy and consequences over a 13-year period. Am J Surg 2016;212(1):62–8.
64. Vu L, Switzer NJ, De Gara C, et al. Surgical interventions for obesity and metabolic disease. Best Pract Res Clin Endocrinol Metab 2013;27(2):239–46.

65. Mittermair RP, Obermuller S, Perathoner A, et al. Results and complications after Swedish adjustable gastric banding—10 years experience. Obes Surg 2009; 19(12):1636–41.

66. Spivak H, Abdelmelek MF, Beltran OR, et al. Long-term outcomes of laparoscopic adjustable gastric banding and laparoscopic Roux-en-Y gastric bypass in the United States. Surg Endosc 2012;26(7):1909–19.

67. Lanthaler M, Aigner F, Kinzl J, et al. Long-term results and complications following adjustable gastric banding. Obes Surg 2010;20(8):1078–85.

68. Boza C, Gamboa C, Perez G, et al. Laparoscopic adjustable gastric banding (LAGB): surgical results and 5-year follow-up. Surg Endosc 2011;25(1):292–7.

69. Tran TT, Pauli E, Lyn-Sue JR, et al. Revisional weight loss surgery after failed laparoscopic gastric banding: an institutional experience. Surg Endosc 2013; 27(11):4087–93.

70. Nguyen NT, Slone JA, Nguyen XM, et al. A prospective randomized trial of laparoscopic gastric bypass versus laparoscopic adjustable gastric banding for the treatment of morbid obesity: outcomes, quality of life, and costs. Ann Surg 2009; 250(4):631–41.

71. Angrisani L, Lorenzo M, Borrelli V. Laparoscopic adjustable gastric banding versus Roux-en-Y gastric bypass: 5-year results of a prospective randomized trial. Surg Obes Relat Dis 2007;3(2):127–32 [discussion: 132–3].

72. Karamanakos SN, Vagenas K, Kalfarentzos F, et al. Weight loss, appetite suppression, and changes in fasting and postprandial ghrelin and peptide-YY levels after Roux-en-Y gastric bypass and sleeve gastrectomy: a prospective, double blind study. Ann Surg 2008;247(3):401–7.

73. Ryan KK, Tremaroli V, Clemmensen C, et al. FXR is a molecular target for the effects of vertical sleeve gastrectomy. Nature 2014;509(7499):183–8.

74. Kuipers F, Groen AK. FXR: the key to benefits in bariatric surgery? Nat Med 2014;20(4):337–8.

75. Lee SY, Lim CH, Pasupathy S, et al. Laparoscopic sleeve gastrectomy: a novel procedure for weight loss. Singapore Med J 2011;52(11):794–800.

76. Paluszkiewicz R, Kalinokwski P, Wroblewski T, et al. Prospective randomized clinical trial of laparoscopic sleeve gastrectomy versus open Roux-en-Y gastric bypass for the management of patients with morbid obesity. Wideochir Inne Tech Maloinwazyjne 2012;7(4):225–32.

77. Laferrere B, Heshka S, Wang K, et al. Incretin levels and effect are markedly enhanced 1 month after Roux-en-Y gastric bypass surgery in obese patients with type 2 diabetes. Diabetes Care 2007;30(7):1709–16.

78. Laferrere B, Teixeira J, McGinty J, et al. Effect of weight loss by gastric bypass surgery versus hypocaloric diet on glucose and incretin levels in patients with type 2 diabetes. J Clin Endocrinol Metab 2008;93(7):2479–85.

79. Morinigo R, Moize V, Musri M, et al. Glucagon-like peptide-1, peptide YY, hunger, and satiety after gastric bypass surgery in morbidly obese subjects. J Clin Endocrinol Metab 2006;91(5):1735–40.

80. Korner J, Inabnet W, Conwell IM, et al. Differential effects of gastric bypass and banding on circulating gut hormone and leptin levels. Obesity (Silver Spring) 2006;14(9):1553–61.

81. Rodieux F, Giusti V, D'Alessio DA, et al. Effects of gastric bypass and gastric banding on glucose kinetics and gut hormone release. Obesity (Silver Spring) 2008;16(2):298–305.

82. le Roux CW, Aylwin SJ, Batterham RL, et al. Gut hormone profiles following bariatric surgery favor an anorectic state, facilitate weight loss, and improve metabolic parameters. Ann Surg 2006;243(1):108–14.

83. Pories WJ. Bariatric surgery: risks and rewards. J Clin Endocrinol Metab 2008; 93(11 Suppl 1):S89–96.

84. Moshiri M, Osman S, Robinson TJ, et al. Evolution of bariatric surgery: a historical perspective. AJR Am J Roentgenol 2013;201(1):W40–8.

85. Dixon JB, Bhathal PS, O'Brien PE. Nonalcoholic fatty liver disease: predictors of nonalcoholic steatohepatitis and liver fibrosis in the severely obese. Gastroenterology 2001;121(1):91–100.

86. Chavez-Tapia NC, Tellez-Avila FI, Barrientos-Gutierrez T, et al. Bariatric surgery for non-alcoholic steatohepatitis in obese patients. Cochrane Database Syst Rev 2010;(1):CD007340.

87. Burza MA, Romeo S, Kotronen A, et al. Long-term effect of bariatric surgery on liver enzymes in the Swedish Obese Subjects (SOS) study. PLoS One 2013;8(3): e60495.

88. Mathurin P, Hollebecque A, Arnalsteen L, et al. Prospective study of the long-term effects of bariatric surgery on liver injury in patients without advanced disease. Gastroenterology 2009;137(2):532–40.

89. Wu R, Ortiz J, Dallal R. Is bariatric surgery safe in cirrhotics? Hepat Mon 2013; 13(2):e8536.

90. Dixon JB. Surgical management of obesity in patients with morbid obesity and nonalcoholic fatty liver disease. Clin Liver Dis 2014;18(1):129–46.

91. Mosko JD, Nguyen GC. Increased perioperative mortality following bariatric surgery among patients with cirrhosis. Clin Gastroenterol Hepatol 2011;9(10): 897–901.

92. Shimizu H, Phuong V, Maia M, et al. Bariatric surgery in patients with liver cirrhosis. Surg Obes Relat Dis 2013;9(1):1–6.

93. Dallal RM, Mattar SG, Lord JL, et al. Results of laparoscopic gastric bypass in patients with cirrhosis. Obes Surg 2004;14(1):47–53.

94. Cobb WS, Heniford BT, Burns JM, et al. Cirrhosis is not a contraindication to laparoscopic surgery. Surg Endosc 2005;19(3):418–23.

95. Richards J, Gunson B, Johnson J, et al. Weight gain and obesity after liver transplantation. Liver Transpl 2005;18(4):461–6.

96. Lin MY, Tavakol MM, Sarin A, et al. Laparoscopic sleeve gastrectomy is safe and efficacious for pretransplant candidates. Surg Obes Relat Dis 2013;9(5): 653–8.

97. Takata MC, Campos GM, Ciovica R, et al. Laparoscopic bariatric surgery improves candidacy in morbidly obese patients awaiting transplantation. Surg Obes Relat Dis 2008;4(2):159–64 [discussion: 164–5].

98. Taneja S, Gupta S, Wadhawan M, et al. Single-lobe living donor liver transplant in a morbidly obese cirrhotic patient preceded by laparoscopic sleeve gastrectomy. Case Rep Transplant 2013;2013:279651.

99. Heimbach JK, Watt KD, Poterucha JJ, et al. Combined liver transplantation and gastric sleeve resection for patients with medically complicated obesity and end-stage liver disease. Am J Transplant 2013;13(2):363–8.

100. Andalib A, Aminian A, Khorgami Z, et al. Early postoperative outcomes of primary bariatric surgery in patients on chronic steroid or immunosuppressive therapy. Obes Surg 2016;26(7):1479–86.

101. Tichansky DS, Madan AK. Laparoscopic Roux-en-Y gastric bypass is safe and feasible after orthotopic liver transplantation. Obes Surg 2005;15(10): 1481–6.
102. Lin MY, Tavakol MM, Sarin A, et al. Safety and feasibility of sleeve gastrectomy in morbidly obese patients following liver transplantation. Surg Endosc 2013;27(1): 81–5.

Treatment Options in Patients Awaiting Liver Transplantation with Hepatocellular Carcinoma and Cholangiocarcinoma

Alberto Unzueta, MD[a], Roniel Cabrera, MD, MS[a,b],*

KEYWORDS

- Locoregional therapies • Bridging • Down-staging • Neoadjuvant therapies
- Outcomes

KEY POINTS

- The management of patients with hepatocellular carcinoma (HCC) on a waiting list (WL) for liver transplant (LT) includes several types of locoregional therapies (LRTs) that need to be selected based on patient and tumor characteristics as well as center expertise.
- The radiological response to LRT, level of α-fetoprotein (AFP), response of AFP to LRT, and tumor size/multifocality are factors associated with dropout from a WL for LT.
- The radiologic and AFP responses to LRT are important predictors of tumor biology and can predict outcomes after LT.
- LRT could be beneficial to preventing dropout from a WL when the waiting time for LT is greater than 6 months.
- Thermal ablation strategies (radiofrequency ablation [RFA] and microwave ablation [MWA]) and transarterial chemoembolization [TACE] are commonly used strategies as a bridge or down-staging for LT.
- The use of neoadjuvant protocols for liver transplantation in perihilar cholangiocarcinoma (pCCA) is necessary for optimal outcomes.

The authors have nothing to disclose.
[a] Division of Gastroenterology, Hepatology and Nutrition, Department of Medicine, University of Florida, 1600 Southwest Archer Road, P.O. Box 100277, Gainesville, FL 32610, USA; [b] Liver Transplant Program, Section of Hepatobiliary Diseases (Liver Unit), Division of Gastroenterology, Hepatology and Nutrition, Department of Medicine, University of Florida, 1600 Southwest Archer Road, MSB Room M440, Gainesville, FL 32610, USA
* Corresponding author. Liver Transplant Program, Section of Hepatobiliary Diseases (Liver Unit), Division of Gastroenterology, Hepatology and Nutrition, Department of Medicine, University of Florida, 1600 Southwest Archer Road, MSB Room M440, Gainesville, FL 32610, USA.
E-mail address: roniel.cabrera@medicine.ufl.edu

Clin Liver Dis 21 (2017) 231–251
http://dx.doi.org/10.1016/j.cld.2016.12.002
1089-3261/17/© 2017 Elsevier Inc. All rights reserved.

liver.theclinics.com

INTRODUCTION

HCC is one of the most common malignancies worldwide and its prevalence is expected to increase over the next 2 decades mainly due to the rising incidence of cirrhosis from nonalcoholic fatty liver disease.[1] HCC develops in the background of cirrhosis in approximately 80% of cases. LT is considered the best treatment for cure in patients with HCC because it removes both the tumor and the underlying chronic liver disease. Approximately 5% of patients listed for LT in the United States have HCC.[2] Due to a limited number of organs, listing for HCC is restricted to patients with tumor burden within the Milan criteria defined as 1 tumor greater than 2 cm but less than or equal to 5 cm or 2 to 3 tumors less than or equal to 3 cm. For those patients with tumors beyond the Milan criteria various down-staging criteria and strategies have been studied. The LRT options for patients listed or considered for LT with HCC are based on the degree of hepatic dysfunction, tumor burden, tumor location, and the transplant center experience (**Fig. 1**).[2,3]

High-level evidence in the form of randomized controlled trials is lacking that examines the role of LRT as bridge or down-staging strategies to LT. Most of the published studies are heterogeneous with variable reported outcomes. A majority of the reports are single-center studies with a low number of patients. The studies that have not shown differences between treated and untreated patients usually have waiting times for LT that are less than 6 months.[4–6]

Although the use of LRT prior to LT is common in most transplant centers, the evidence for a clear post-transplant survival advantage with LRT is not a consistent finding.[4,7–9] The rationale for the use of LRT as a bridge or down-staging therapy is to decrease the dropout rate before transplantation from tumor progression and to

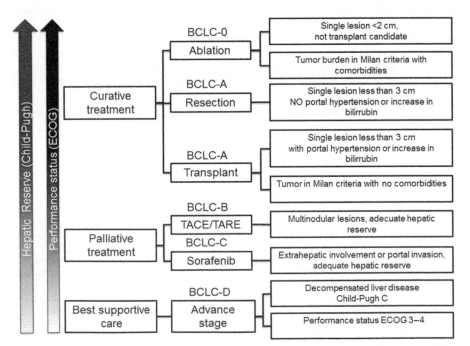

Fig. 1. Management of HCC. BCLC staging system for HCC; BCLC-0, very early stage; BCLC-A, early stage; BCLC-B, intermediate stage; BCLC-C, advance stage; BCLC-D, terminal stage; ECOG, Eastern Cooperative Oncology Group performance status.

decrease recurrence after transplantation. The degree of response to LRT is considered an important factor and surrogate marker of a more favorable tumor biology[10–12] whereas an inadequate tumor response to therapy predicts a stronger probability for dropout.[13–15] The time on a WL is also associated with dropout from the WL for HCC patients due to intrahepatic or extrahepatic tumor progression at a rate of 7% to 11% at 6 months and 38% at 12 months.[16,17] Radiographic tumor progression over 3 months to 6 months with or without LRT is associated with tumor recurrence and a decreased survival after LT.[10–12] Serum AFP level and the AFP response to LRT also predict tumor recurrence and a worse post-LT survival.[18] Patients with a lack of response and elevated AFP (>20 ng/mL) showed higher dropout rates (21.6% at 1 year and 26.5% at 2 years) compared with patients with a complete response and AFP level less than 20 ng/mL (2% dropout at 1 year and 2 years). HCC patients with a high AFP levels can achieve acceptable LT outcomes if their AFP levels are reduced with LRT during the waiting period.[19,20]

PATIENT EVALUATION OVERVIEW

The United Network for Organ Sharing (UNOS) regulates the allocation of organs in the United States (**Boxes 1** and **2**, **Table 1**). The UNOS policy allows patients with Milan T2 (2 tumors 2–5 cm or 2–3 tumors ≤3 cm) to receive priority listing for LT. In the UNOS new allocation policy in effect since October 2015, patients within Milan criteria are listed for 6 months at their calculated MELD and patients are given 28 points if the tumor remains within Milan criteria for 6 months, with MELD increases of 3 points every 3 months thereafter equivalent to 10% mortality risk (maximum 34 points).[2]

LOCOREGIONAL THERAPIES

The Barcelona Clinic Liver Cancer (BCLC) staging system is commonly used as the standard algorithm to stage patients with HCC and select the best evidence-based LRT for those on a WL (see **Fig. 1**, **Table 1**).[8] Ablation is recommended for patients with early-stage disease (BCLC 0-A) when they are not candidates for surgical resection (eg, patients with clinically significant portal hypertension). TACE is the recommended treatment of patients with intermediate-stage disease (BCLC B—unresectable, multifocal hepatic lesions, no evidence of portal vein thrombosis, asymptomatic patients).[8] Other treatments still considered too experimental are high-intensity focused ultrasound (HIFU) and external radiation with stereotactic body radiation therapy

---

Box 1
Selection criteria for liver transplantation

UNOS

- Stage T1 (1 tumor <2 cm) and stage T2 (1 tumor 2–5 cm or 2–3 tumors ≤3 cm)

Milan criteria

- Most common eligibility criteria for LT among patients with HCC

- Single lesion ≤5 cm or 2 to 3 lesions each ≤3 cm

Expanded criteria

- UCSF: a single HCC ≤6.5 cm or ≤3 tumors, with the largest ≤4.5 cm and a total tumor burden ≤8 cm[21]

- Up to 7: HCC with 7 as the sum of the size of the largest tumor (in cm) and the number of tumors[22]

Box 2
Definitions used in the management of patients with hepatocellular carcinoma on a waiting list

Neoadjuvant treatments (bridging/down-staging)

- Treatments that are used before LT to improve the outcomes after LT, for example, LRTs (TACE and RFA)

Bridging (stages T1 and T2)

- Patients who are already on WL based on Milan criteria
- Potential advantages: decreases WL dropout by preventing progression of the tumor outside Milan criteria, decreases recurrence, and improves survival after LT

Down-staging (stage T3 or higher)[12,23]

- Patient is outside Milan criteria
- Makes patients eligible for LT after successful down-staging with similar survival than patients within Milan criteria
- Successful down-staging: LRT has resulted in tumor shrinkage and/or devitalization (tumors no longer exhibit arterial phase enhancement on imaging)
- Goal to select patients with more favorable tumor biology, because down-staged patients have a higher risk of dropout from WL[24]

Dropout

- Patient is withdrawn from WL
- Death, increase in size of tumor outside Milan/USCF criteria, worsening of severity of disease

Ablate and wait strategy[25]

- Observation time after LRT with subsequent restaging (Milan or UCSF criteria), usually 3 months to 6 months
- Time as a surrogate of tumor biology: detect aggressive tumors with high risk of recurrence

Tumor-node-metastasis staging system: T0, no tumor; T1, 1 nodule less than 2 cm in diameter; T2, 1 nodule 2 cm to 5 cm in diameter or 3 nodules less than 3 cm in diameter; T3, 1 nodule greater than 5 cm in diameter or up to 3 nodules with 1 nodule greater than 3 cm; T4a, 4 or more nodules of any size; T4b, 4 or more nodules of any size plus intrahepatic portal vein or hepatic vein involvement. University of California, San Francisco (UCSF), criteria: solitary tumor <6.5 cm in diameter or 3 or fewer nodules with each <4.5 cm in diameter and a total tumor diameter <8 cm.
Data from Cescon M, Cucchetti A, Ravaioli M, et al. Hepatocellular carcinoma locoregional therapies for patients in the waiting list. Impact on transplantability and recurrence rate. J Hepatol 2013;58(3):609–18; and Majno P, Lencioni R, Mornex F, et al. Is the treatment of hepatocellular carcinoma on the waiting list necessary? Liver Transpl 2011;17(2):S98–108.

(SBRT).[26,27] The guidelines based on an international consensus conference do not recommend any specific LRT over the others for patients listed for LT or for patients on a down-staging protocol[9] (**Table 2**). A consensus statement recommends that LRTs be considered, however, in patients expected to wait more than 6 months to decrease dropout from a WL because of tumor progression.

ABLATION TREATMENTS

Percutaneous ethanol injection (PEI) was the first LRT used to treat small HCCs (**Tables 3** and **4**). PEI has now been largely replaced by thermal ablation (RFA and MWA) as the preferred ablation technique because it requires fewer session, allows

Table 1		
Therapies used in the management of hepatocellular carcioma		
1. Locoregional therapy		
Transarterial catheter	Chemoembolization	TACE, DEB-TACE
	Radioembolization	TARE, Y^{90}
Ablation	PEI	
	RFA	
	MWA	Percutaneous/laparoscopic
	HIFU	Extracorporeal therapy
2. Surgical resection		
3. Systemic therapy	Sorafenib	
4. Radiotherapy	SBRT	Extracorporeal therapy

for better local tumor control, and has superior overall survival. RFA has been shown to result in optimal tumor control for tumors less than 3 cm and can performed via the percutaneous or laparoscopic routes, depending on location. The size of the HCC is one of the key predictors of response to RFA. HCC lesions less than 2.5 cm show 90% complete necrosis and this response decreases to 50% for lesions exceeding 5 cm. RFA has an increased rate of complete response in terms of tumor necrosis (46%–74%)[28,29] compared with TACE (22%–29%).[5,6,30,31] In addition, RFA has been shown to decrease dropout from the WL compared with other ablation therapies.[32] Ablation and surgical resection have higher rates of complete response and tumor control compared with TACE.[14]

Other novel ablation techniques HIFU, an extracorporeal ablation therapy with high-frequency sound waves that has been used mainly in some Asian centers. HIFU has shown comparable tumor necrosis on explant with TACE when used as a bridge therapy to LT.[27,33]

TRANSCATHETER ARTERIAL TREATMENTS
Transarterial Chemoembolization

TACE is the most common LRT used as bridge therapy for patients awaiting LT alone or in combination with surgical resection or ablation [5,10,11,13–15,30,32,34–42] (**Tables 5** and **6**). TACE with doxorubicin or cisplatin can be done on a scheduled basis, repeated every 3 to 4 months or on an on-demand basis with frequent monitoring of liver function

Table 2	
International consensus conference report recommendations for liver transplantation for management of hepatocellular carcinoma patients on a waiting list	
1. UNOS T1 ($\leq$2 cm)	Bridging therapy—no recommendation made
2. UNOS T2 (Milan criteria) + waiting time longer than 6 months	LRT may be beneficial
3. Preferred LRT	No recommendation made
4. Patients beyond Milan criteria	Consider down-staging
5. Progressive disease, LRT not considered	Remove from WL

Data from European Association for The Study Of The Liver; European Organisation For Research And Treatment Of Cancer. EASL-EORTC Clinical Practice Guidelines: management of hepatocellular carcinoma. J Hepatol 2012;56(6):908–43; and Clavien P-A, Lesurtel M, Bossuyt PMM, et al. Recommendations for liver transplantation for hepatocellular carcinoma: an international consensus conference report. Lancet Oncol 2012;13(1):E11–22.

Table 3 Ablation treatments used as bridging therapies in patients on a waiting list		
RFA	• Second most widely used and reported LRT for patients awaiting LT • Insertion of 1 or more narrow probes (under ultrasound or CT guidance) into a target liver lesion, usually with the patient anesthetized • Probes are connected to an alternating current that generates heat at their tip causing thermal injury to tissue • Relatively long time (16–18 min) to achieve adequate thermal injury to fully ablate a 3–4 cm lesion • Heat sink effect: potential loss of heat energy (and treatment effect) if large blood vessels are near the treatment zone	
MWA	• Greater heating with shorter treatment time as well as a larger zone of ablation	
Contraindications	• Lesions high in the dome of the liver or near the gall bladder, due the risk of pulmonary injury or gall bladder necrosis	
Complications	• Abdominal pain and anorexia with or without fever • Severe (rare): serious bleeding (<2%), abscess formation, portal vein thrombosis, thoracic injury, and severe liver decompensation • Tumoral seeding by ablation probes (2%) • Overall mortality (<1%)	77
Bridging and down-staging	• RFA is effective as a bridge to LT with very low dropout rates (0%–6%) • Very small (≤3 cm) HCCs, RFA can achieve complete response equivalent in efficacy to resection • Down-staging of larger diameter tumors (>3–4 cm) limited role	78,79 80,81

to avoid treatment-related liver toxicity. Furthermore, the use of selective TACE during treatment can decrease the ischemic insult to surrounding nontumor liver tissue and more effectively target the tumor.[8,43] TACE with drug-eluting beads (DEB-TACE) has shown similar efficacy to TACE with a better safety profile (decrease liver toxicity and systemic adverse events), particularly in patients with more advanced disease.[44,45]

Transarterial Radioembolization

Transarterial radioembolization (TARE) with yttrium-90 (Y^{90}) glass beads induces tumor necrosis with high dose of Y^{90} radiation when micron-sized beads become trapped in the capillary beds of the tumor and preserve the patency of the hepatic artery. TARE is considered an option in patients with compromised blood supply of the portal vein (portal vein thrombosis, hepatofugal flow, or transjugular intrahepatic portosystemic shunt) who need down-staging to LT or resection.[46–50] Although TARE has shown a good safety profile with comparable outcomes to TACE, studies are lacking that directly compare both treatment strategies.[51,52] Retrospective studies have shown no differences in overall survival in BCLC B patients between TARE and TACE. The benefits of TARE compared with TACE include decrease in the number of required treatments, decrease in postembolic symptoms (due to increase patency of hepatic artery), and increase in time to tumor progression as well as increase in complete tumor necrosis on explant.[53,54] Patients treated with TARE do not require hospitalization and can receive treatment 7 days to 10 days after the pretreatment staging angiogram if there is no evidence of shunts to the lungs or gastrointestinal tract.[55] A prospective study of TARE versus TACE demonstrated an increase in quality of life in patients who received TARE, even if they had a more advanced disease compared with TACE.[56]

Table 4
Studies that use radiofrequency ablation/percutaneous ethanol injection as bridging therapy in hepatocellular carcinoma patients before liver transplantation

Author, Year	Treatment	Study Design	Patients	Liver Transplantation	Tumor Stage, %	Dropout Waiting List Number, (%)	Hepatocellular Carcinoma Recurrence, %	Intention to Treat Survival, %
Fontana et al,[82] 2002	RFA	Prosp	33	15	MC (30)	N/A	13	N/A
Mazzaferro et al,[78] 2004	RFA	Prosp	50	50	MC (40)	0	70	83 at 3 y
Lu et al,[79] 2005	RFA	Retro	52	41	MC (42)	3 (6)	0	74 at 3 y
Castroagudín et al,[83] 2005	PEI	Retro	34	23	T1-T2 (30)	5 (15)	4	NA
Pompili et al,[29] 2006	RFA, PEI	Retro	40	40	MC (37)	N/A	8	N/A
Brillet et al,[84] 2006	RFA	Prosp	21	16	MC	5 (24)	6	N/A
Rodríguez-Sanjúan et al,[85] 2008	RFA	Retro	28	28	MC (25)	N/A	7	N/A
Branco et al,[86] 2009	PEI	Retro	62	59	MC	3 (5)	5	64.4 at 3 y
DuBay et al,[87] 2011	RFA, no tx	Retro	77	51	MC	19 (25) vs 16 (21) NS	2	N/A

Abbreviations: MC, Milan criteria; N/A, not available; PEI, percutaneous ethanol injection; Prosp, prospective; Retro, retrospective; RFA, radiofrequency ablation; tx, treatment.

Table 5 Transcatheter arterial treatments used as bridging therapies in patients on the waiting list	
TACE	• Catheterization of the artery branches supplying the tumor blood flow • Infusion of chemotherapy/embolic agents into the branches • Chemotherapy agents: mixture of doxorubicin, cisplatin, and mitomycin-C, often premixed with ethiodized oil (Lipiodol) • Embolic agents: polyvinyl alcohol particles or Gelfoam • Intended duration of arterial occlusion is not permanent • Varying degrees of tumor necrosis
Outcomes	• Complete necrosis has not necessarily been predictive of post-LT survival [88] • No evidence of a clear post-transplant survival benefit • Short duration from TACE to LT (<3 months) in patients with biologically unfavorable tumors: increased HCC recurrence and reduced survival • Waitlist dropout rates of 3%–13% [11,30,40,89] • Improves survival in nontransplant candidates vs supportive care
DEB-TACE	• Uses microspheres beds (100–700 μm) impregnated with a chemotherapeutic agent (eg, doxorubicin) [44] • Efficacy, safety, and survival similar to TACE [44,90] • Can be used as bridging therapy before LT [91]
Advantages of DEB-TACE vs traditional TACE	• More concentrated delivery of chemotherapy in the targeted area • Longer duration • Less induced arterial ischemia • Potential use in patients with partially or completely thrombosed portal vein branches • Could benefit patients with worse liver function at baseline
PRECISION-V (Prospective Randomized Study of Doxorubicin-Eluting-Bead Embolization in the Treatment of Hepatocellular Carcinoma) study	• Lower incidence of alopecia, degree of post-treatment aminotransferase elevation, and frequency of decreased left ventricular function with DEB-TACE vs conventional TACE [44]
TARE	• Y^{90} microspheres delivered intra-arterially • Staging visceral angiography with technetium-99 to detect clinically relevant shunting to the gastrointestinal tract or lung [52] • If shunts to the gastrointestinal tract cannot be embolized, or if the lung-shunt fraction is elevated, Y^{90} is contraindicated • Bilobar disease: wait 1 month before treating the opposite side • Overall tolerance and safety seem comparable to TACE

(continued on next page)

Table 5 (continued)	
• Postembolization syndrome similar than TACE with less severity	92
• Radiation-induced liver disease, 4%–20%, jaundice/ascites 2–8 wk after treatment, risk increases with repeated treatments	55,93
• Radiation-induced biliary stricturing <10%	94
• Radiographic response and survival in nonoperative candidates seem comparable or possibly superior to TACE	95
• Utility as a bridge to LT, in selected series show that TARE is effective	52,96

Another use of TARE is in the setting of potential surgical resection to increase the size of the future liver remnant because it has been associated with hypertrophy of the contralateral lobe. The degree of hypertrophy directly correlates with the time since treatment and can be noticed as early as 1 month post-treatment.[57] This effect can benefit patients with BCLC criteria for resection that have not been previously considered for resection due to anatomic factors.

COMBINATION THERAPIES
Transarterial Chemoembolization Plus Radiofrequency Ablation

The synergistic effect of TACE followed by RFA has been evaluated as a bridge therapy in patients with HCC awaiting LT. A nonrandomized study reported complete necrosis in 77% of tumors on explant and a cumulative dropout rate of 17% at 2 years.[58]

Locoregional Therapies with Sorafenib

Vascular endothelial growth factor (VEGF) levels have been show to increase significantly after TACE treatment and the increase in levels is associated with a worse prognosis.[59] Several studies have tested the hypothesis that combination therapy with an anti-VEGF (multikinase inhibitor and sorafenib) treatment and LRT (TACE or Y^{90}) could be beneficial.[51,60–64] The SPACE trial (sorafenib or placebo plus TACE with doxorubicin-eluting beads for intermediate stage HCC) was a randomized controlled trial comparing DEB-TACE alone or in combination with sorafenib. The combination therapy in the SPACE trial did not improve time to tumor progression compared with DEB-TACE alone.[62] Another randomized study in patients with HCC on WL compared Y^{90} plus sorafenib versus Y^{90} alone. The patients who received sorafenib required dose reductions and the combination treatment was associated with more peritransplant biliary complications and acute rejections.[51] Based on current evidence, there is no clear benefit of combination therapy with sorafenib and the combinations seem associated with higher adverse events.

EMERGING THERAPIES
Stereotactic Body Radiation Therapy

SBRT is an extracorporeal radiation treatment that delivers a large dose of radiation to a highly targeted area using confocal beams. The sessions usually last 30 minutes to 60 minutes and the treatment is completed in 1 day to 5 days. SBRT can be used instead of ablation to treat lesions in the dome of the liver, near the gallbladder or nearby large blood vessels.[65] The use of SBRT as a bridge therapy to LT has been reported in a small series of patients with no evidence of HCC progression after treatment. Analysis of the

Table 6
Studies that use transarterial chemoembolizaiton as bridging therapy in hepatocellular carcinoma patients before liver transplantation

Author, Year	Treatment	Study Design	Patients	Liver Transplantation	Tumor Stage	Dropout Waiting List, Number, (%)	Hepatocellular Carcinoma Recurrence, %	Intention-to-Treat Survival, %
Graziadei et al,[35] 2003	TACE	Prosp	48	41	MC	0	2	94 at 5 y
Hayashi et al,[37] 2004	TACE	Retro	20	12	MC (100%)	6 (35)	0	62 at 3 y
Maddala et al,[39] 2004	TACE	Retro	54	45	MC (81%)	8 (15)	13	61 at 5 y
Decaens et al,[6] 2005	TACE vs none	Retro/case control	100 TACE 100 None	100	MC (71%)	N/A	13 vs 23	59 at 5 y
Perez-Saborido et al,[97] 2005	TACE vs none	Retro	18 28	18	MC (72%)	N/A	17 vs 36 NS	61 vs 38 at 5 y
Otto et al,[10] 2006	TACE	Prosp	34	23	MC	7 (20)	6	81 at 5 y
Millonig et al,[11] 2007	TACE	Prosp	68	66	MC	2 (3)	8	70 at 5 y
Alba et al,[89] 2008	TACE	Retro	63	56	MC	7 (11)	11	N/A
De Luna et al,[40] 2009	TACI	Retro	95	68	MC	17 (18)	N/A	85 at 3 y
Frangakis et al,[98] 2010	TACE vs none	Retro/case-control	43 22	43	MC (100%)	1 (3) 3 (15)	N/A	76 vs 57 at 2 y
Tsochatzis et al,[99] 2013	TACE, TAE	Retro	67	67	MC	N/A	6	N/A
Nicolini et al,[100] 2013	DEB-TACE vs TACE	Retro	22 16	N/A	MC	N/A	18	74 vs 59 at 3 y

Abbreviations: DEB-TACE, drug-eluting beads transarterial chemoembolization; MC, Milan criteria; N/A, not available; NS, P = not significant; Prosp, prospective; retro, retrospective; TACE, transarterial chemoembolization; TACI, transarterial chemoinfusion; Tx, treatment.

explant pathology, however, showed a low rate of complete tumor necrosis (27%).[26] Early experience shows good safety profile with mild, manageable side effects.[66]

SURGICAL TREATMENT OPTIONS

Surgical resection is a curative option for patients with adequate hepatic reserve and no evidence of clinically significant portal hypertension (**Table 7**). Resection can be used as a bridge therapy to LT to identify patients with a more favorable histology (absence of microvascular invasion) and who could benefit from LT even if outside the Milan criteria. The histologic characteristics can also select patients within Milan criteria with a poor prognosis who are at high risk for HCC recurrence after LT.[67] A major unmet need in patients with HCC after resection is the need for beneficial adjuvant treatments to decrease the well-known risk of recurrence after surgery. HCC recurrence after surgical resection is common, and unfortunately there are no proved therapies to lessen this risk after resection. The phase III multicenter, randomized controlled trial (STORM [adjuvant sorafenib for hepatocellular carcinoma after resection or ablation]) evaluated the benefit of sorafenib as adjuvant treatment after resection or ablation in more than 1000 patients and found no difference in recurrence-free survival between the sorafenib versus placebo groups.[68]

EVALUATION OF OUTCOME AND RECOMMENDATIONS FOR TREATMENT OF HEPATOCELLULAR CARCINOMA

Several factors influence outcomes and need careful consideration during the evaluation and treatment of patients with HCC on a WL for LT (**Boxes 3** and **4**, see **Fig. 1**; **Figs. 2** and **3**). Relevant outcomes include radiological response to treatment, dropout

Table 7 Surgical resection as bridging therapy in patients with hepatocellular carcinoma on a waiting list		

Advantages	1. Possible best control of tumor growth
	2. Select patients with poor prognosis in terms of tumor recurrence based on pathology
	  ○ Undifferentiated histotype
	  ○ Satellitosis
	  ○ Microvascular invasion
	  ○ Capsular effraction
		101

Disadvantages	• Higher costs • Periprocedural risks • Only considered in well-compensated patients without severe portal hypertension • Can make LT technically more difficult with a higher risk of post-operative complications	102
Salvage LT	• LT as a rescue treatment in cases of tumor recurrence or liver function failure after liver resection • Favorable results for salvage LT in patients within the Milan criteria or the UCSF criteria • Option of salvage LT cannot be offered to all patients initially treated by resection (HCC recurrence outside conventional LT criteria, comorbidities)	103 104,105
LDLT	• Surgical resection and a living donor liver graft has excellent long-term survival	106,107

Box 3
Outcome measures for locoregional therapies reported in neoadjuvant therapies

1. Radiological response to treatment
2. Dropout rate of a WL (0%–35%)
3. Tumor progression rate (0%–20%)
4. Tumor necrosis on explant
5. Waiting time for LT (4–12 months)
6. Proportion of patients transplanted (54%–100%)
7. Posttransplant survival (76% at 3 years, 94% at 5 years)
8. Intention-to-treat survival (57%–94%)
9. Posttransplant recurrence rate

Factors that have a negative impact on outcomes[13–15,28,29]:

- Size of tumor
- More advanced tumor stage
- HCC outside Milan criteria
- Down-staging (negative predictor of post-LT survival, HCC recurrence, and intention-to-treat survival)[11,35]
- No response to neoadjuvant treatments
- Elevated serum AFP
  - Patients with HCC on a WL for transplantation with a baseline serum AFP level of greater than 200 ng/mL have significantly worse outcomes.[70]
  - The most significant adverse determinant is a steady increase of AFP level greater than 15 ng/mL per month.[41]
  - Cutoff AFP levels of 300 ng/mL, 400 ng/mL, and 1000 ng/mL have been proposed for removal of patients from a WL for LT.[71,72]

Data from Cescon M, Cucchetti A, Ravaioli M, et al. Hepatocellular carcinoma locoregional therapies for patients in the waiting list. Impact on transplantability and recurrence rate. J Hepatol 2013;58(3):609–18.

Box 4
Radiological evaluation of locoregional treatment response: modified response evaluation criteria in solid tumors for hepatocellular carcinoma

Complete response

- No intra-arterial enhancement in all target lesions

Partial response

- Decrease of viable target lesions (arterial enhancement) at least of 30% (baseline sum of diameters of target lesions)

Stable disease

- Any lesion that is not considered as partial response or progressive disease

Progressive disease

- Increase of at least 20% in the sum of the diameters of viable target lesions (from baseline)

Data from Lencioni R, Llovet JM. Modified RECIST (mRECIST) Assessment for Hepatocellular Carcinoma. Semin Liver Dis 2010;30(1):52–60.

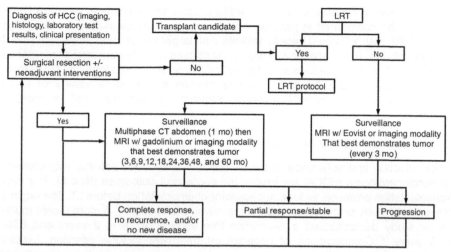

Fig. 2. University of Florida protocol for management of patients with HCC considered for LT.

rate on a WL, tumor progression rate, tumor necrosis on explant, waiting time for LT, post-LT survival, intention-to-treat survival, and post-LT recurrence rate.[69]

Although LRT is commonly used across LT centers for down-staging and as a bridge to LT, the selection of the type of LRT varies depending on center experience and expertise.[65] At the authors' institution, the preferred LRTs are MWA and TARE with Y[90] (see **Figs. 2** and **3**). In general, ablation therapies (RFA and MWA) are considered for lesions less than 3 cm. MWA (percutaneous or laparoscopic) is used for tumors near the dome of the liver, blood vessels, or gallbladder. SBRT can also be used in these settings. TACE is the most preferred modality

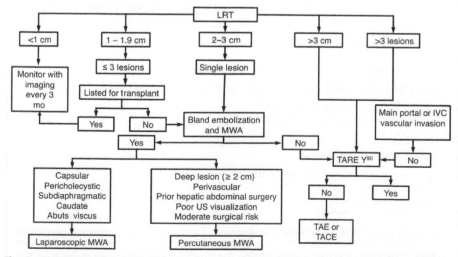

Fig. 3. University of Florida LRT protocol for management of HCC in patient candidates for LT. IVC, inferior vena cava; MWA, microwave ablation; TAE, transarterial embolization.

across centers in patients with preserved liver function. In addition, selective DEB-TACE can be considered in patients with some compromise in liver function. The use of TARE with Y^{90} could benefit patients with larger tumors and those with portal vein thrombosis. In the absence of high-level studies directly comparing the various forms of LRT as a bridge or down-staging for LT, no single strategy can be recommended. Until head-to-head prospective studies are done, a variety of LRTs continue to be used in HCC patients awaiting LT with the goal to improve outcomes.

PERIHILAR CHOLANGIOCARCINOMA

Strict selection and adherence to the LT protocol criteria for patients with perihilar cholangiocarcinoma (pCCA) are crucial for successful outcomes (**Box 5**). The new transplantation protocols include neoadjuvant chemoradiation before LT. The original Mayo Clinic study protocol had a 5-year survival rate of 82%.[73] A more recent multicenter study demonstrated a recurrence-free survival of 78 at 2 years and 65% at 5 years.[74] Complications of neoadjuvant treatment include infection, toxicity secondary to chemoradiotherapy and early or late vascular complications. Hepatic artery or portal vein stenosis and thrombosis has been reported in up to 40% of patients after LT.[75]

Box 5
Mayo Clinic neoadjuvant protocol for liver transplantation in perihilar cholangiocarcinoma

- Includes unresectable de novo pCCA or in the setting of primary sclerosing cholangitis
- Tumor size: radial tumor diameter ≤3 cm
- Tumor localized to biliary tree with no intrahepatic or extrahepatic metastasis
- Criteria for unresectability
  - Unresectable hiliar tumor—above the cystic duct
  - Cholangiocarcinoma in a primary sclerosing cholangitis patient
- Endoscopic ultrasound-guided fine-needle aspirate of suspected positive lymph nodes
- Patients with negative lymph nodes are enrolled in the neoadjuvant treatment
  1. External beam radiation (4000–4500 cGy)
  2. 5-Fluorouracil or gemcitabine brachytherapy
  3. Oral capecitabine (Xeloda) after external beam radiation and brachytherapy until the day of LT
  4. Staging laparotomy to rule out disease progression
- Listing for LT (MELD with exception points for pCCA) or living donor liver transplant

Prognostic factors of dropout before LT[76]
  - Carbohydrate antigen (CA) 19-9 >500 U/mL
  - Tumor >3 cm
  - MELD >20
  - Malignant brushing or biopsy

Prognostic factors of tumor recurrence after LT[76]
  - Elevated CA 19-9
  - Portal vein encasement
  - Residual tumor on explant

Data from Rizvi S, Gores GJ. Pathogenesis, diagnosis, and management of cholangiocarcinoma. Gastroenterology 2013;145(6):1215–29; and Hong JC, Jones CM, Duffy JP, et al. Comparative analysis of resection and liver transplantation for intrahepatic and hilar cholangiocarcinoma. Arch Surg 2011;146(6):683–9.

SUMMARY

The management of patients with HCC on a WL for LT includes several types of LRT that need to be selected based on patient and tumor characteristics as well as center expertise. The radiological response to LRT, level of AFP, response of AFP to LRT, and tumor size/multifocality are factors associated with dropout from a WL for LT. The radiologic and AFP responses to LRT are important predictors of tumor biology and can predict outcomes after LT. LRTs could be beneficial to prevent dropout from a WL when the waiting time for LT is greater than 6 months. Thermal ablation strategies (RFA and MWA) and TACE are commonly used strategies as a bridge or down-staging for LT. Transarterial radiotherapy with Y^{90} can be another LRT option for patients with HCC on a WL with compromised portal vein flow. Down-staging protocols like the UCSF can have comparable outcomes with patients with a tumor burden within the Milan criteria.

No single form of LRT can be recommended over another given the lack of prospective studies directly comparing them in patients with HCC waiting for an LT. The strict selection of patients who undergo neoadjuvant chemoradiotherapy for pCCA is necessary for optimal outcomes in patients selected for LT.

REFERENCES

1. El-Serag H, Davila JA, Petersen NJ, et al. The continuing increase in the incidence of hepatocellular carcinoma in the United States: an update. Ann Intern Med 2003;139(10):817–23.
2. Wedd JP, Nordstrom E, Nydam T, et al. Hepatocellular carcinoma in patients listed for liver transplantation: current and future allocation policy and management strategies for the individual patient. Liver Transpl 2015;21(12):1543–52.
3. Pompili M, Francica G, Ponziani FR, et al. Bridging and downstaging treatments for hepatocellular carcinoma in patients on the waiting list for liver transplantation. World J Gastroenterol 2013;19(43):7515–30.
4. Cabrera R, Dhanasekaran R, Caridi J, et al. Impact of transarterial therapy in hepatitis C-Related hepatocellular carcinoma on long-term outcomes after liver transplantation. Am J Clin Oncol 2012;35(4):345–50.
5. Porrett PM, Peterman H, Rosen M, et al. Lack of benefit of pre-transplant locoregional hepatic therapy for hepatocellular cancer in the current MELD era. Liver Transpl 2006;12(4):665–73.
6. Decaens T, Roudot-Thoraval F, Bresson-Hadni S, et al. Impact of pretransplantation transarterial chemoembolization on survival and recurrence after liver transplantation for hepatocellular carcinoma. Liver Transpl 2005;11(7):767–75.
7. Bruix J, Sherman M. Management of hepatocellular carcinoma: an update. Hepatology 2011;53(3):1020–2.
8. European Association For The Study Of The Liver, European Organisation For Research And Treatment Of Cancer. EASL-EORTC Clinical Practice Guidelines: management of hepatocellular carcinoma. J Hepatol 2012;56(6):908–43.
9. Clavien P-A, Lesurtel M, Bossuyt PMM, et al. Recommendations for liver transplantation for hepatocellular carcinoma: an international consensus conference report. Lancet Oncol 2012;13(1):E11–22.
10. Otto G, Herber S, Heise M, et al. Response to transarterial chemoembolization as a biological selection criterion for liver transplantation in hepatocellular carcinoma. Liver Transpl 2006;12(8):1260–7.

11. Millonig G, Graziadei IW, Freund MC, et al. Response to preoperative chemo-embolization correlates with outcome after liver transplantation in patients with hepatocellular carcinoma. Liver Transpl 2007;13(2):272–9.

12. Yao FY, Mehta N, Flemming J, et al. Downstaging of hepatocellular cancer before liver transplant: long-term outcome compared to tumors within Milan criteria. Hepatology 2015;61(6):1968–77.

13. Vitale A, D'Amico F, Frigo AC, et al. Response to therapy as a criterion for awarding priority to patients with hepatocellular carcinoma awaiting liver transplantation. Ann Surg Oncol 2010;17(9):2290–302.

14. Cucchetti A, Cescon M, Bigonzi E, et al. Priority of candidates with hepatocellular carcinoma awaiting liver transplantation can Be reduced after successful bridge therapy. Liver Transpl 2011;17(11):1344–54.

15. De Giorgio M, Vezzoli S, Cohen E, et al. Prediction of progression-free survival in patients presenting with hepatocellular carcinoma within the milan criteria. Liver Transpl 2010;16(4):503–12.

16. Llovet JM, Fuster J, Bruix J. Barcelona Clinic Liver Canc G. Intention-to-treat analysis of surgical treatment for early hepatocellular carcinoma: resection versus transplantation. Hepatology 1999;30(6):1434–40.

17. Yao FY, Bass NM, Nikolai B, et al. Liver transplantation for hepatocellular carcinoma: analysis of survival according to the intention-to-treat principle and dropout from the waiting list. Liver Transpl 2002;8(10):873–83.

18. Lai Q, Avolio AW, Graziadei I, et al. Alpha-fetoprotein and modified response evaluation criteria in solid tumors progression after locoregional therapy as predictors of hepatocellular cancer recurrence and death after transplantation. Liver Transpl 2013;19(10):1108–18.

19. Merani S, Majno P, Kneteman NM, et al. The impact of waiting list alpha-fetoprotein changes on the outcome of liver transplant for hepatocellular carcinoma. J Hepatol 2011;55(4):814–9.

20. Mailey B, Artinyan A, Khalili J, et al. Evaluation of absolute serum alpha-fetoprotein levels in liver transplant for hepatocellular cancer. Arch Surg 2011; 146(1):26–33.

21. Yao FY, Ferrell L, Bass NM, et al. Liver transplantation for hepatocellular carcinoma: Expansion of the tumor size limits does not adversely impact survival. Hepatology 2001;33(6):1394–403.

22. Mazzaferro V, Llovet JM, Miceli R, et al. Predicting survival after liver transplantation in patients with hepatocellular carcinoma beyond the Milan criteria: a retrospective, exploratory analysis. Lancet Oncol 2009;10(1):35–43.

23. Mehta N, Yao FY. Hepatocellular cancer as indication for liver transplantation. Curr Opin Organ Transplant 2016;21(2):91–8.

24. Mazzaferro V. Squaring the circle of selection and allocation in liver transplantation for HCC: an adaptive approach. Hepatology 2016;63(5):1707–17.

25. Roberts JP, Venook A, Kerlan R, et al. Hepatocellular carcinoma: ablate and wait versus Rapid transplantation. Liver Transpl 2010;16(8):925–9.

26. O'Connor JK, Trotter J, Davis GL, et al. Long-term outcomes of stereotactic body radiation therapy in the treatment of hepatocellular cancer as a bridge to transplantation. Liver Transpl 2012;18(8):949–54.

27. Chok KS, Cheung TT, Lo RC, et al. Pilot study of high-intensity focused ultrasound ablation as a bridging therapy for hepatocellular carcinoma patients wait-listed for liver transplantation. Liver Transpl 2014;20(8):912–21.

28. Lu DSK, Yu NC, Raman SS, et al. Radiofrequency ablation of hepatocellular carcinoma: treatment success as defined by histologic examination of the explanted liver. Radiology 2005;234(3):954–60.

29. Pompili M, Mirante VG, Rondinara G, et al. Percutaneous ablation procedures in cirrhotic patients with hepatocellular carcinoma submitted to liver transplantation: assessment of efficacy at explant analysis and of safety for tumor recurrence. Liver Transpl 2005;11(9):1117–26.

30. Majno PE, Adam R, Bismuth H, et al. Influence of preoperative transarterial lipiodol chemoembolization on resection and transplantation for hepatocellular carcinoma in patients with cirrhosis. Ann Surg 1997;226(6):688–701.

31. Jang JW, You CR, Kim CW, et al. Benefit of downsizing hepatocellular carcinoma in a liver transplant population. Aliment Pharmacol Ther 2010;31(3):415–23.

32. Huo TI, Huang YH, Su CW, et al. Validation of the HCC-MELD for dropout probability in patients with small hepatocellular carcinoma undergoing locoregional therapy. Clin Transplant 2008;22(4):469–75.

33. Ng KKC, Poon RTP, Chan SC, et al. High-intensity focused ultrasound for hepatocellular carcinoma a single-center experience. Ann Surg 2011;253(5):981–7.

34. Herrero JI, Sangro B, Quiroga J, et al. Influence of tumor characteristics on the outcome of liver transplantation among patients with liver cirrhosis and hepatocellular carcinoma. Liver Transpl 2001;7(7):631–6.

35. Graziadei IW, Sandmueller H, Waldenberger P, et al. Chemoembolization followed by liver transplantation for hepatocellular carcinoma impedes tumor progression while on the waiting list and leads to excellent outcome. Liver Transpl 2003;9(6):557–63.

36. Yao FY, Bass NM, Nikolai B, et al. A follow-up analysis of the pattern and predictors of dropout from the waiting list for liver transplantation in patients with hepatocellular carcinoma: implications for the current organ allocation policy. Liver Transpl 2003;9(7):684–92.

37. Hayashi PH, Ludkowski M, Forman LM, et al. Hepatic artery chemoembolization for hepatocellular carcinoma in patients listed for liver transplantation. Am J Transplant 2004;4(5):782–7.

38. Fisher RA, Maluf D, Cotterell AH, et al. Non-resective ablation therapy for hepatocellular carcinoma: effectiveness measured by intention-to-treat and dropout from liver transplant waiting list. Clin Transplant 2004;18(5):502–12.

39. Maddala YK, Stadheim L, Andrews JC, et al. Drop-out rates of patients with hepatocellular cancer listed for liver transplantation: outcome with chemoembolization. Liver Transpl 2004;10(3):449–55.

40. De Luna W, Sze DY, Ahmed A, et al. Transarterial chemoinfusion for hepatocellular carcinoma as downstaging therapy and a bridge toward liver transplantation. Am J Transplant 2009;9(5):1158–68.

41. Vibert E, Azoulay D, Hoti E, et al. Progression of alphafetoprotein before liver transplantation for hepatocellular carcinoma in cirrhotic patients: a critical factor. Am J Transplant 2010;10(1):129–37.

42. Ciccarelli O, Lai QR, Goffette P, et al. Liver transplantation for hepatocellular cancer: UCL experience in 137 adult cirrhotic patients. Alpha-foetoprotein level and locoregional treatment as refined selection criteria. Transpl Int 2012;25(8):867–75.

43. Golfieri R, Cappelli A, Cucchetti A, et al. Efficacy of selective transarterial chemoembolization in inducing tumor necrosis in small (< 5 cm) hepatocellular carcinomas. Hepatology 2011;53(5):1580–9.

44. Lammer J, Malagari K, Vogl T, et al. Prospective randomized study of doxorubicin-eluting-bead embolization in the treatment of hepatocellular carcinoma: results of the PRECISION V study. Cardiovasc Intervent Radiol 2010; 33(1):41–52.
45. Varela M, Real MI, Burrel M, et al. Chemoembolization of hepatocellular carcinoma with drug eluting beads: efficacy and doxorubicin pharmacokinetics. J Hepatol 2007;46(3):474–81.
46. Salem R, Lewandowski RJ, Mulcahy MF, et al. Radioembolization for hepatocellular carcinoma using Yttrium-90 microspheres: a comprehensive report of long-term outcomes. Gastroenterology 2010;138(1):52–64.
47. Hilgard P, Hamami M, El Fouly A, et al. Radioembolization with Yttrium-90 glass microspheres in hepatocellular carcinoma: european experience on safety and long-term survival. Hepatology 2010;52(5):1741–9.
48. Sangro B, Carpanese L, Cianni R, et al. Survival after Yttrium-90 Resin microsphere radioembolization of hepatocellular carcinoma across Barcelona clinic liver cancer stages: a European evaluation. Hepatology 2011;54(3):868–78.
49. Mazzaferro V, Sposito C, Bhoori S, et al. Yttrium-90 radioembolization for intermediate-advanced hepatocellular carcinoma: a phase 2 study. Hepatology 2013;57(5):1826–37.
50. Lewandowski RJ, Kulik LM, Riaz A, et al. A comparative analysis of transarterial downstaging for hepatocellular carcinoma: chemoembolization versus radioembolization. Am J Transplant 2009;9(8):1920–8.
51. Kulik L, Vouche M, Koppe S, et al. Prospective randomized pilot study of Y90+/-sorafenib as bridge to transplantation in hepatocellular carcinoma. J Hepatol 2014;61(2):309–17.
52. Tohme S, Sukato D, Chen HW, et al. Yttrium-90 radioembolization as a bridge to liver transplantation: a single-institution experience. J Vasc Interv Radiol 2013; 24(11):1632–8.
53. Riaz A, Kulik L, Lewandowski RJ, et al. Radiologic-pathologic correlation of hepatocellular carcinoma treated with internal radiation using Yttrium-90 microspheres. Hepatology 2009;49(4):1185–93.
54. Riaz A, Lewandowski RJ, Kulik L, et al. Radiologic-pathologic correlation of hepatocellular carcinoma treated with chemoembolization. Cardiovasc Intervent Radiol 2010;33(6):1143–52.
55. Sangro B, Salem R. Transarterial chemoembolization and radioembolization. Semin Liver Dis 2014;34(4):435–43.
56. Salem R, Gilbertsen M, Butt Z, et al. Increased quality of life among hepatocellular carcinoma patients treated with radioembolization, compared with chemoembolization. Clin Gastroenterol Hepatol 2013;11(10):1358–65.e1.
57. Vouche M, Lewandowski RJ, Atassi R, et al. Radiation lobectomy: time-dependent analysis of future liver remnant volume in unresectable liver cancer as a bridge to resection. J Hepatol 2013;59(5):1029–36.
58. Ashoori N, Bamberg F, Paprottka P, et al. Multimodality treatment for early-stage hepatocellular carcinoma: a bridging therapy for liver transplantation. Digestion 2012;86(4):338–48.
59. Sergio A, Cristofori C, Cardin R, et al. Transcatheter arterial chemoembolization (TACE) in hepatocellular carcinoma (HCC): the role of angiogenesis and invasiveness. Am J Gastroenterol 2008;103(4):914–21.
60. Kudo M, Imanaka K, Chida N, et al. Phase III study of sorafenib after transarterial chemoembolisation in Japanese and Korean patients with unresectable hepatocellular carcinoma. Eur J Cancer 2011;47(14):2117–27.

61. Sansonno D, Lauletta G, Russi S, et al. Transarterial chemoembolization plus sorafenib: a sequential therapeutic scheme for HCV-related intermediate-stage hepatocellular carcinoma: a randomized clinical trial. Oncologist 2012;17(3): 359–66.

62. Lencioni R, Llovet JM, Han G, et al. Sorafenib or placebo plus TACE with doxorubicin-eluting beads for intermediate stage HCC: the SPACE trial. J Hepatol 2016;64(5):1090–8.

63. Cabrera R, Pannu DS, Caridi J, et al. The combination of sorafenib with transarterial chemoembolisation for hepatocellular carcinoma. Aliment Pharmacol Ther 2011;34(2):205–13.

64. Vouche M, Kulik L, Atassi R, et al. Radiological-Pathological analysis of WHO, RECIST, EASL, mRECIST and DWI: imaging analysis from a prospective randomized trial of Y90 +/- sorafenib. Hepatology 2013;58(5):1655–66.

65. Byrne T, Rakela J. Loco-regional therapies for patients with hepatocelullar carcinoma awaiting liver transplantation: selecting an optimal therapy. World J Transplant 2016;6(2):306–12.

66. Bibault JE, Dewas S, Vautravers-Dewas C, et al. Stereotactic body radiation therapy for hepatocellular carcinoma: prognostic factors of local control, overall survival, and toxicity. PLoS One 2013;8(10):e77472.

67. Mazzaferro V, Lencioni R, Majno P. Early hepatocellular carcinoma on the procrustean bed of ablation, resection, and transplantation. Semin Liver Dis 2014;34(4):415–26.

68. Bruix J, Takayama T, Mazzaferro V, et al. Adjuvant sorafenib for hepatocellular carcinoma after resection or ablation (STORM): a phase 3, randomised, double-blind, placebo-controlled trial. Lancet Oncol 2015;16(13):1344–54.

69. Cescon M, Cucchetti A, Ravaioli M, et al. Hepatocellular carcinoma locoregional therapies for patients in the waiting list. Impact on transplantability and recurrence rate. J Hepatol 2013;58(3):609–18.

70. Bruix J, Reig M, Sherman M. Evidence-based Diagnosis, staging, and treatment of patients with hepatocellular carcinoma. Gastroenterology 2016;150(4): 835–53.

71. Pomfret EA, Washburn K, Wald C, et al. Report of a National conference on liver allocation in patients with hepatocellular carcinoma in the United States. Liver Transpl 2010;16(3):262–78.

72. Duvoux C, Roudot-Thoraval F, Decaens T, et al. Liver transplantation for hepatocellular carcinoma: a model including alpha-fetoprotein improves the performance of milan criteria. Gastroenterology 2012;143(4):986–94.

73. Rea DJ, Heimbach JK, Rosen CB, et al. Liver transplantation with neoadjuvant chemoradiation is more effective than resection for hilar cholangiocarcinoma. Ann Surg 2005;242(3):451–61.

74. Darwish Murad S, Kim WR, Harnois DM, et al. Efficacy of neoadjuvant chemoradiation, followed by liver transplantation, for perihilar cholangiocarcinoma at 12 US centers. Gastroenterology 2012;143(1):88–98.e3.

75. Mantel HTJ, Rosen CB, Heimbach JK, et al. Vascular complications after orthotopic liver transplantation after neoadjuvant therapy for hilar cholangiocarcinoma. Liver Transpl 2007;13(10):1372–81.

76. Murad SD, Kim WR, Therneau T, et al. Predictors of pretransplant dropout and posttransplant recurrence in patients with perihilar cholangiocarcinoma. Hepatology 2012;56(3):972–81.

77. Livraghi T, Meloni F, Solbiati L, et al, Collaborative Italian Group using AMICA system. Complications of microwave ablation for liver tumors: Results of a multi-center study. Cardiovasc Intervent Radiol 2012;35(4):868–74.
78. Mazzaferro V, Battiston C, Perrone S, et al. Radiofrequency ablation of small hepatocellular carcinoma in cirrhotic patients awaiting liver transplantation: a prospective study. Ann Surg 2004;240(5):900–9.
79. Lu DSK, Yu NC, Raman SS, et al. Percutaneous radiofrequency ablation of hepatocellular carcinoma as a bridge to liver transplantation. Hepatology 2005; 41(5):1130–7.
80. Livraghi T, Meloni F, Di Stasi M, et al. Sustained complete response and complications rates after radiofrequency ablation of very early hepatocellular carcinoma in cirrhosis: is resection still the treatment of choice? Hepatology 2008; 47(1):82–9.
81. Chen MS, Li JQ, Zheng Y, et al. A prospective randomized trial comparing percutaneous local ablative therapy and partial hepatectomy for small hepatocellular carcinoma. Ann Surg 2006;243(3):321–8.
82. Fontana RJ, Hamidullah H, Nghiem H, et al. Percutaneous radiofrequency thermal ablation of hepatocellular carcinoma: a safe and effective bridge to liver transplantation. Liver Transpl 2002;8(12):1165–74.
83. Castroagudin JF, Delgado M, Villanueva A, et al. Safety of percutaneous ethanol injection as neoadjuvant therapy for hepatocellular carcinoma in waiting list liver transplant candidates. Transplant Proc 2005;37(9):3871–3.
84. Brillet PY, Paradis V, Brancatelli G, et al. Percutaneous radiofrequency ablation for hepatocellular carcinoma before liver transplantation: a prospective study with histopathologic comparison. AJR Am J Roentgenol 2006;186(5 Suppl): S296–305.
85. Rodriguez-Sanjuan JC, Gonzalez F, Juanco C, et al. Radiological and pathological assessment of hepatocellular carcinoma response to radiofrequency. A study on removed liver after transplantation. World J Surg 2008;32(7):1489–94.
86. Branco F, Bru C, Vilana R, et al. Percutaneous ethanol injection before liver transplantation in the hepatocellular carcinoma. Ann Hepatol 2009;8(3):220–7.
87. DuBay DA, Sandroussi C, Kachura JR, et al. Radiofrequency ablation of hepatocellular carcinoma as a bridge to liver transplantation. HPB (Oxford) 2011; 13(1):24–32.
88. Stampfl U, Bermejo JL, Sommer CM, et al. Efficacy and nontarget effects of transarterial chemoembolization in bridging of hepatocellular carcinoma patients to liver transplantation: a histopathologic study. J Vasc Interv Radiol 2014;25(7):1018–26.
89. Alba E, Valls C, Dominguez J, et al. Transcatheter arterial chemoembolization in patients with hepatocellular carcinoma on the waiting list for orthotopic liver transplantation. AJR Am J Roentgenol 2008;190(5):1341–8.
90. Burrel M, Reig M, Forner A, et al. Survival of patients with hepatocellular carcinoma treated by transarterial chemoembolisation (TACE) using Drug Eluting Beads. Implications for clinical practice and trial design. J Hepatol 2012; 56(6):1330–5.
91. Nicolini D, Svegliati-Baroni G, Candelari R, et al. Doxorubicin-eluting bead vs conventional transcatheter arterial chemoembolization for hepatocellular carcinoma before liver transplantation. World J Gastroenterol 2013;19(34):5622–32.
92. Riaz A, Lewandowski RJ, Kulik LM, et al. Complications following radioembolization with Yttrium-90 microspheres: a comprehensive literature review. J Vasc Interv Radiol 2009;20(9):1121–30.

93. Lam M, Louie JD, Iagaru AH, et al. Safety of repeated Yttrium-90 radioemboliza-tion. Cardiovasc Intervent Radiol 2013;36(5):1320–8.
94. Ng SSM, Yu SCH, Lai PBS, et al. Biliary complications associated with selective internal radiation (SIR) therapy for unresectable liver malignancies. Dig Dis Sci 2008;53(10):2813–7.
95. Salem R, Mazzaferro V, Sangro B. Yttrium 90 radioembolization for the treatment of hepatocellular carcinoma: biological lessons, current challenges, and clinical perspectives. Hepatology 2013;58(6):2188–97.
96. Abdelfattah MR, Al-sebayel M, Broering D, et al. Radioembolization using Yttrium-90 microspheres as bridging and downstaging treatment for unresect-able hepatocellular carcinoma before liver transplantation: initial single-center experience. Transplant Proc 2015;47(2):408–11.
97. Saborido BP, Meneu JC, Moreno E, et al. Is transarterial chemoembolization necessary before liver transplantation for hepatocellular carcinoma? Am J Surg 2005;190(3):383–7.
98. Frangakis C, Geschwind JF, Kim D, et al. Chemoembolization decreases drop-Off risk of hepatocellular carcinoma patients on the liver transplant list. Cardio-vasc Intervent Radiol 2011;34(6):1254–61.
99. Tsochatzis E, Garcovich M, Marelli L, et al. Transarterial embolization as neo-adjuvant therapy pretransplantation in patients with hepatocellular carcinoma. Liver Int 2013;33(6):944–9.
100. Nicolini D, Svegliati-Baroni G, Candelari R, et al. Doxorubicin-eluting bead vs conventional transcatheter arterial chemoembolization for hepatocellular carci-noma before liver transplantation. World J Gastroenterol 2013;19(34):5622–32.
101. Sala M, Fuster J, Llovet JM, et al. High pathological risk of recurrence after sur-gical resection for hepatocellular carcinoma: an indication for salvage liver transplantation. Liver Transpl 2004;10(10):1294–300.
102. Earl TM, Chapman WC. Hepatocellular carcinoma: resection versus transplanta-tionansplantation. Semin Liver Dis 2013;33(3):282–92.
103. Majno PE, Sarasin FP, Mentha G, et al. Primary liver resection and salvage trans-plantation or primary liver transplantation in patients with single, small hepato-cellular carcinoma and preserved liver function: an outcome-oriented decision analysis. Hepatology 2000;31(4):899–906.
104. Del Gaudio M, Ercolani G, Ravaioli M, et al. Liver transplantation for recurrent hepatocellular carcinoma on cirrhosis after liver resection: University of bologna experience. Am J Transplant 2008;8(6):1177–85.
105. Liu F, Wei YG, Wang WT, et al. Salvage liver transplantation for recurrent hepa-tocellular carcinoma within UCSF criteria after liver resection. PLoS One 2012; 7(11):e48932.
106. Hwang S, Lee SG, Moon DB, et al. Salvage living donor liver transplantation af-ter prior liver resection for hepatocellular carcinoma. Liver Transpl 2007;13(5): 741–6.
107. Kaido T, Mori A, Ogura Y, et al. Living donor liver transplantation for recurrent hepatocellular carcinoma after liver resection. Surgery 2012;151(1):55–60.

Coagulopathy Before and After Liver Transplantation

From the Hepatic to the Systemic Circulatory Systems

Jonathan G. Stine, MD, MSc, Patrick G. Northup, MD, MHS*

KEYWORDS

- End-stage liver disease • Hypercoagulable state • Thromboembolic disease
- Coagulation • Hemostasis

KEY POINTS

- The hemostatic environment in patients with cirrhosis is a delicate balance between pro-hemostatic and antihemostatic factors.
- In general, there is a lack of effective laboratory measures of the coagulation cascade, platelet function, and thrombolysis in patients with cirrhosis.
- Contrary to prior widespread belief, patients with cirrhosis are predisposed to pulmonary embolus (PE), deep vein thrombosis (DVT), and portal vein thrombosis (PVT) in the pre-transplantation setting.
- The pretransplantation hypercoagulable milieu seems to extend for at least several months post-transplantation and may result in venous thromboembolism (VTE) or intra-cardiac thrombosis, portal vein thrombosis, or hepatic artery thrombosis (HAT).
- The optimal anticoagulation regimen both for prevention of and therapy for pathologic thrombosis in cirrhosis has yet to be established but early reports suggest a potential role for low-molecular-weight heparins (LMWHs) and the direct-acting anticoagulants.

INTRODUCTION

The research field of hemostasis in chronic liver disease is ever-expanding yet poorly understood. Although the majority of clinical research focuses on PVT and relevant patient-centered outcomes, interpreting the delicate homeostasis between prohemo-stasis and antihemostasis in patients with cirrhosis is an issue that clinicians face on a

Disclosure Statement: The authors have nothing to disclose.
Funding: This work was supported in part by the American Association for the Study of Liver Diseases and an Advanced/Transplant Hepatology Fellowship award.
Center for the Study of Coagulation Disorders in Liver Disease, Division of Gastroenterology and Hepatology, Department of Medicine, University of Virginia, 1215 JPA and Lee Street, Charlottesville, VA 22908, USA
* Corresponding author. Division of Gastroenterology and Hepatology, University of Virginia, JPA and Lee Street, MSB 2145, PO Box 800708, Charlottesville, VA 22908-0708.
E-mail address: northup@virginia.edu

Clin Liver Dis 21 (2017) 253–274
http://dx.doi.org/10.1016/j.cld.2016.12.003
1089-3261/17/© 2016 Elsevier Inc. All rights reserved.

liver.theclinics.com

daily basis in an attempt to assess for both bleeding and clotting risk. Despite this risk assessment being a well-established practice, conventional laboratory testing has proved unreliable, making this assessment one of the more challenging arenas of caring for patients with chronic liver disease. Historically, patients with cirrhosis were thought to have coagulopathy, as defined by elevations in conventional laboratory tests, such as the prothrombin time (PT) and PT–international normalized ratio (INR). This coagulopathy was thought to be protective from a hypercoagulable state and even predisposed patients with cirrhosis to spontaneous bleeding events. It is now known that conventional laboratory tests, such as PT and PT-INR, do not accurately predict thrombotic or bleeding risk in patients with cirrhosis[1,2]; specifically, PT-INR does not predict risk of VTE in hospitalized patients with cirrhosis.[3,4] Furthermore, measures of other components of the hemostatic system are not widely available, further limiting assessment of prohemostasis and antihemostasis in patients with cirrhosis.

Hemostasis can be broken down into primary, secondary, and tertiary components.[5] Primary hemostasis is defined by platelet activation and formation of a platelet plug. Secondary hemostasis involves the activation of the coagulation cascade by tissue factor and platelet factors, ultimately leading to thrombin activation and deposition of fibrin in an attempt to stabilize the platelet plug formed by primary hemostasis. Tertiary hemostasis occurs when the clot is dissolved through fibrinolysis mediated by tissue plasminogen activator and plasminogen.

Thrombosis and bleeding risk in patients with cirrhosis is due to a complex interaction of hypercoagulability, stasis in the form of reduced portal vein velocity, and vessel wall injury leading to endothelial dysfunction in the setting of circulating endotoxemia.[6,7] In terms of hypercoagulability, abnormalities in primary hemostasis, including elevated levels of von Willebrand factor and low levels of ADAMTS13,[8,9] reinforce a prohemostatic environment. Decreased levels of protein C and protein S, antithrombin III, and heparin cofactor II in addition to elevated levels of factor VIII also shift the equilibrium in favor of baseline thrombosis.[8,10] Interpretations of independent levels of anticoagulant protein C, protein S, and antithrombin III, however, are wrought with error in the setting of DVT or PVT due to activation of the coagulation system and artificially low circulating levels.[11] Low levels of plasminogen are found in patients with cirrhosis and affect the fibrinolytic system promoting an environment rich for clotting.[10,12] In addition, patients with chronic liver disease may have concurrent hypercoagulable disorders, including the presence of the antiphospholipid antibody syndrome, factor V Leiden mutation, prothrombin G20210A mutation, Janus kinase 2 (JAK2) mutation, or methylenetetrahydrofolate reductase C677T mutation.[13–15] These mutations are found more commonly in patients with PVT than in those without.[13] Several reports have suggested that bacterial lipopolysaccharide may predispose patients with cirrhosis to clotting because this gut-derived endotoxin translocation into the systemic circulation has been associated both with increased thrombin production through increased tissue factor activity[6,16,17] and increased release of von Willebrand factor from endothelial cells.[18] An endotoxin gradient has been described between the portosystemic and peripheral circulation systems, with the greatest values found in the portal circulation when directly measured in patients with cirrhosis.[6]

In summation, cirrhosis patients have a rebalanced hemostatic system with simultaneous changes in both their prohemostatic and antihemostatic pathways that is precarious at best and often tipped one way or another by infection, invasive procedures, hospitalization, and renal failure.[19] It is possible to have both bleeding and thrombosis in sequential fashion in a short time frame.

PITFALLS AND CAVEATS OF DIAGNOSTIC TESTING: PREDICTING THROMBOTIC AND BLEEDING RISK

In general, conventional laboratory testing is unreliable in determining thrombotic or bleeding risk in patients with chronic liver disease. Bleeding time (BT), an indirect measure of platelet function and primary hemostasis, may be prolonged in patients with cirrhosis and may be affected not only by thrombocytopenia[20] but also the prominent vasodilation due to nitric oxide in patients with portal hypertension.[21] BT correlates with the severity of liver disease and is the most prolonged in patients with Child-Pugh-Turcotte (CPT) class C disease[20]; BT is inversely proportional to fibrinogen. BT may be decreased with the administration of desmopressin, which enhances platelet aggregation[22]; however, routine administration in treating esophageal variceal bleeding has not led to decreased bleeding rates or better treatment outcomes.[23] Unfortunately, BT is a widely variable assay due to much interobserver variability, therefore limiting the effective clinical use of this test, and has not been correlated with procedural bleeding risk.[24] The authors do not recommend routinely obtaining this for evaluation of bleeding or clotting risk.

PT helps measure the extrinsic coagulation pathway and includes functional assessment of factors II (prothrombin), V, VII, IX, and X as well as tissue factor and fibrinogen. These coagulation factors are vitamin K dependent and, therefore, affected by both dietary and nutritional factors as well as the administration of concurrent vitamin K antagonists (VKAs). PT was initially designed to assist in the diagnosis and treatment of patients with hemophilia whereas INR was developed to monitor patients on VKA therapy ensuring a narrow therapeutic window. These tests were never intended to be used to assess thrombotic risk in patients with cirrhosis.[25] It is known that in cirrhosis there is an imbalance between prohemostatic protein C, antithrombin, tissue factor pathway inhibitor, and antihemostatics. Knowing that PT-INR only measures procoagulant activity,[25] it is not surprising that PT or PT-INR does not accurately predict thrombotic or bleeding risk in patients with cirrhosis.[1,2] Furthermore, PT correlates poorly with postprocedure bleeding in patients with cirrhosis undergoing invasive procedures, including central venous catheter placement, liver biopsy, polypectomy, transjugular intrahepatic portosystemic shunt, bone marrow biopsy, cholecystectomy, and splenectomy.[26,27] For these reasons, the authors recommend that PT and PT-INR not be the only factors of bleeding risk assessment in patients with cirrhosis; rather, concomitant incorporation of both fibrinogen levels as well as a dynamic measure of whole clot formation should be considered.

Thromboelastography (TEG) and rotational thromboelastometry (ROTEM) are both older technologies that can now be applied to cirrhosis physiology. Both of these assays provide a global measurement of hemostasis and clot stability based on a combination of clot initiation time, maximal clot strength, rate of change in clot strength, and rate of clot decline with lysis. TEG measures the degree of torque on a central pin while clotting whole blood is rotated in a cylinder at a constant rate; torque increases with clot formation and decreases with fibrinolysis and clot breakdown.[28] TEG can be performed either as a point-of-care test or within 3 hours of obtaining a whole blood sample due to advances with citrated medium and recalcified blood, increasing its clinical utility.[29] This has been adapted in cirrhosis patients and is widely used to guide fibrinolytic therapy and transfusion of deficient factors during liver transplantation, effectively preventing the necessity for protocol transfusions.[30–32] TEG values have been found to be normal in patients with compensated cirrhosis[33]; however, they then become abnormal in the setting of decompensating events, such as bleeding or infection.[33] TEG is superior to PT-INR or platelet count when used to estimate rebleeding risk from gastroesophageal varices.[33]

ROTEM is a slightly different technology and requires a rotating pin with a stationary cup of whole blood.[34] ROTEM has been applied to patients with cirrhosis and PVT.[34] TEG and ROTEM are limited in that they are not widely available at all medical centers and their exact standardized role in predicting bleeding or clotting risk in patients with cirrhosis has yet to be determined. Although most investigators agree that TEG or ROTEM is superior to the traditional laboratory measures, such as PT-INR, BT, or platelet count risk, the authors are unaware of any studies comparing this dynamic testing to the more commonly used static testing to determine the primary clotting risk. Thrombin generation assays, although not readily available today, are anticipated to be available in the near future and may provide a more effective tool for assessing the hemostatic system in patients with cirrhosis.[35]

PRETRANSPLANT VENOUS THROMBOEMBOLIC DISEASE

Based on large national registry data, patients with end-stage liver disease seem at increased risk not only for VTE, including both PE and DVT, but also for short-term mortality.[36,37] Depending on definition and population at risk, incidence rates of VTE range from 0.5% to 8.2% and seem even more common in the setting of other advanced medical comorbidities, including congestive heart failure or chronic kidney disease or a higher Charlson comorbidity index.[1,3,4,38–41] In the largest study to date based on a national registry of more than 500,000 Danish hospitalized patients, the relative risk for unprovoked VTE in hospitalized patients with liver disease in the absence of cirrhosis is 1.89 (95% CI, 1.73–2.03) and 1.74 (95% CI, 1.54–1.95) for those patients with cirrhosis.[26] The clinical importance of this cannot be understated as 30-day mortality risk is more than 2-times greater for cirrhosis patients with DVT compared with noncirrhosis patients despite similar rates of anticoagulation prescription[37]; 30-day mortality from PE alone was even greater, with 35% in patients with cirrhosis versus 16% in those without cirrhosis.[37]

Although established risk factors for VTE for any hospitalized patient apply to patients with cirrhosis, hypoalbuminemia has been associated with increased rates of VTE, because low levels of albumin can be viewed as a surrogate for severity of liver disease and degree of portal hypertension.[1,38] Dabbagh and colleagues[4] and Aldawood and colleagues[3] found similar rates of VTE when stratifying by CPT score, questioning the role of liver disease severity in VTE risk. Hypoalbuminemia may also be approximated as a surrogate for malnutrition, which has been associated with increased rates of VTE in patients with cirrhosis.[41] A study by Wu and Nguyen[40] found that VTE rates in cirrhosis patients ages less than 45 years were significantly higher; however, the investigators found similar rates between compensated and decompensated liver disease.

Historically, there has been reluctance for prescribing medical DVT prophylaxis to patients with cirrhosis with utilization rates that are reported as low as 24%.[3] This practice is traditionally not based on data or outcomes, because a study of 235 hospitalized patients found that the use of thromboprophylaxis in decompensated cirrhosis patients was not associated with high rates of gastrointestinal bleeding or death[42]; 9 (2.5%) cases of gastrointestinal bleeding were documented in this population.[42] The 2012 CHEST guidelines[43] recommend use of antihemostatic thromboprophylaxis with LMWH, low-dose unfractionated heparin (UFH), or fondaparinux in all acutely ill hospitalized medical patients at increased risk of thrombosis, which includes patients with chronic liver disease. In 2010, Barber and colleagues[44] established the Padua Prediction Score to stratify acutely ill medical patients for risk of VTE (**Table 1**). A Padua Prediction Score of greater than or equal to 4 indicates a hospitalized patient is at increased risk of VTE. In a retrospective cohort of 163 hospitalized patients with cirrhosis, 8.6% of

Table 1
Padua Prediction Score predicts risk of venous thromboembolism in acutely ill hospitalized medical patients (including those with cirrhosis)

Risk Factor	Score
Active cancer ≤180 d	3
Previous VTE (excluding superficial thrombosis)	3
Reduced mobility	3
Inherited or acquired thrombophilic condition	3
Trauma/surgery ≤30 d	2
Age ≥70 y	1
CHF and/or respiratory failure	1
Acute MI or ischemic CVA	1
Acute infection and/or rheumatologic condition	1
Obesity (BMI >30 kg/m^2)	1
Hormonal treatment	1

A score ≥4 indicates increased risk of VTE.

Abbreviations: BMI, body mass index; CHF, congestive heart failure; CVA, cerebrovascular accident; MI, myocardial infarction.

Data from Barbar S, Noventa F, Rossetto V, et al. A risk assessment model for the identification of hospitalized medical patients at risk for venous thromboembolism: the Padua Prediction Score. J Thromb Haemost 2010;8(11):2450–7.

whom had VTE and 11% PVT, Bogari and colleagues[45] found a mean Padua Prediction Score of 5.8 in patients with VTE compared with those without VTE (mean 2.1). This mean score is greater than the Padua Prediction Score for other severe medical illnesses, including hospitalized medical patients with sepsis (mean 4.9 ± 2.3),[46] and bears attention when considering appropriate chemical thromboprophylaxis, for which the dosing and interval of administration remain controversial. This prescribing is guided by premarketing pharmacokinetics in the absence of robust clinical data demonstrating a clear methodology for thromboprophylaxis in patients with cirrhosis.

PRETRANSPLANT PORTAL VEIN THROMBOSIS IN PATIENTS WITH CIRRHOSIS

Pretransplant PVT and thrombosis of the splanchnic venous system are common occurrences.[47–49] Classified into 1 of 4 grades by the percentage of vascular occlusion and extent of vessels involved (**Table 2**),[50] prevalence rates may be as high as 30% at

Table 2
Grading of portal vein thrombosis

Grade	Description
1	<50% PV occlusion ± minimal SMV extension
2	>50% PV occlusion ± minimal SMV extension
3	Complete PV occlusion + complete proximal SMV occlusion; distal SMV is nonoccluded
4	Complete occlusion of the PV, proximal and distal SMV

Abbreviations: PV, portal vein; SMV, superior mesenteric vein.

From Yerdel MA, Gunson B, Mirza D, et al. Portal vein thrombosis in adults undergoing liver transplantation: risk factors, screening, management, and outcome. Transplantation 2000;69(9):1875; with permission.

the time of liver transplantation,[47–49,51] and PVT presents challenges to the transplant team when creating the venous anastomosis often after mechanical thrombectomy in the operating room.[52–54] The risk of intestinal infarction is greatly increased in grade III or grade IV acute PVT owing to the degree of extension into the superior mesenteric vein.[55,56] Although multiple studies have demonstrated that PVT is associated with worse outcomes both in patients with cirrhosis undergoing liver transplantation and in the nontransplant population,[57–63] a recent European multicenter prospective series of 1243 adult patients with cirrhosis published by Nery and colleagues[64] argues that PVT may be a reflection of worsening portal hypertension and not an independent predictor of outcome; however, in their intention-to-treat analysis, the investigators included 101 subjects with partial PVT (17 complete PVT), 70% of which spontaneously resolved or had a false-positive result on initial Doppler examination, which may introduce bias toward the null. A post hoc analysis limited to just those subjects with PVT throughout the entire study would be of interest.

The development of pretransplantation PVT in patients with cirrhosis is influenced by dysfunctional endothelial cell activation resultant from fibrosis in the setting of impaired portal vein flow.[7,57] Sluggish and turbulent blood flow through the portal system leads to an increased amount of time that blood remains in the venous system and presumptively impaired thrombin degradation and/or removal.[7] Flow in the portal vein is inversely proportional to the degree of hepatic impairment because the slowest rates of flow are found in CPT class C subjects[65] and, when examining this subset of at-risk patients, is associated with increased mortality.[66] Although only one report, by Zocco and colleagues,[7] has thoroughly examined the threshold for increased PVT risk as defined by portal vein flow, the precise cutoff where risk increases has yet to be firmly established. Although evaluation of portal vein flow is limited by inherent measurement error and imprecision, a cutoff of portal vein flow less than 15 cm/s seems to place patients at increased risk of future PVT within 12 months. Whether or not a patient is prescribed a nonselective β-blocker is theoretically important as well, because appropriate pulse reduction has been described to lead to decreases in portal vein flow, and there is a developing body of literature suggesting that patients with CPT class C liver disease should not be prescribed this class of medication.[67,68] Splenectomy or portosystemic shunting, including the presence of splenorenal shunts, also may increase the risk of PVT.[47]

Although universal testing for inherited or acquired hypercoagulable disorders remains controversial, patients with PVT have an inherited thrombophilia in as many as 5.6% of cases,[69] and screening for factor V Leiden mutation, prothrombin G20210A mutation, or methylenetetrahydrofolate reductase C677T mutation may be considered (**Box 1**).[13–15,55] The JAK2 V617F mutation is also found in

---

Box 1
Recommended testing for inherited or acquired hypercoagulable states in cirrhosis patients with portal vein thrombosis

Hypercoagulable factor

Factor V Leiden mutation

Prothrombin G20210A mutation

Methylenetetrahydrofolate reductase C677T mutation

JAK2

Antiphospholipid antibody syndrome

Data from Refs.[13–15,55]

increased prevalence in patients with cirrhosis and PVT, with rates approximating 10%.[70]

In addition to slow portal vein velocity and inherited or acquired thrombophilia, several other well-described risk factors for PVT in patients with cirrhosis have been established, including previous PVT, the presence of hepatocellular carcinoma, severity of liver disease, and age,[71] the latter two of which may be a phenomenon associated with portal vein flow because flow is inversely proportional to age and directly related to CPT score.[65]

Pretransplantation PVT has been independently associated with post–liver transplantation HAT and resultant early graft loss, based on large cross-sectional US-based registry data, suggesting a continuation of the pretransplantation hypercoagulable milieu for several months after transplantation of the new graft.[62]

NONALCOHOLIC STEATOHEPATITIS

Patients with cirrhosis attributable to nonalcoholic steatohepatitis (NASH) seem at increased risk for thrombotic complications, including both PVT prior to liver transplantation[72] and PE/DVT, when adjusting for comorbid conditions, including diabetes and obesity.[73] Patients with nonalcoholic fatty liver disease (NAFLD) also seem at increased risk for VTE even in the absence of cirrhosis.[73] Although the exact mechanism for this prothrombotic state remains indeterminate, chronic inflammation from NASH is known to lead to both necroapoptosis and oxidative injury through lipid deposition as well as endothelial cell activation.[74–77] Ultimately this poorly understood disease state may lead to activation of the coagulation system and imbalances in primary and secondary hemostasis and perhaps thrombolysis.[78,79] Increased platelet activation has been observed in patients with NAFLD as have elevated levels of von Willebrand factor.[79] Furthermore, mean platelet volume, which can be used as a surrogate of platelet activation, is directly correlated to both the presence of simple steatosis and to NASH.[80] Hypercoagulability in NASH is manifested through increased levels of factor VIII as well as fibrinogen.[78,79] Levels of both antithrombin and protein C are decreased in NASH, with the more severe prothrombotic imbalance seen in patients with NASH cirrhosis compared with other causes of liver disease.[78,79] Patients with NASH in the absence of cirrhosis also manifest this procoagulant imbalance.[78] Plasminogen activator inhibitor-1 levels are elevated in NAFLD whereas tissue-activating factor antigen and tissue plasminogen activator are decreased, ultimately resulting in a state of hypofibrinolysis.[79] Plasminogen activator inhibitor-1 correlates histologically with increasing severity of hepatocyte ballooning, lobular inflammation, and both steatosis and fibrosis.[81] Plasminogen activator inhibitor-1 inhibits breakdown of fibrin-based clots and, therefore, elevated levels promote thrombotic risk both in the macrovascular system and locally, resulting in tissue ischemia due to the intrahepatic thrombi, which has the potential to accelerate liver disease progression through stellate cell activation and fibrogenesis.[81] A series by Papatheodoris and colleagues[82] found that the presence of at least one thrombotic risk factor was associated with an approximately 2-fold fibrosis stage increase in NASH patients, confirming earlier observational reports correlating thrombotic risk factors to the extent of hepatic fibrosis.[83]

Despite this large body of work suggesting a hypercoagulable state existing in patients with NASH and NASH cirrhosis, a recent report by Potze and colleagues[84] challenges this thinking because the investigators found that, in general, hemostatic profiles were comparable between noncirrhotic biopsy-proved NAFLD and controls without NAFLD, with several exceptions. NAFLD patients had increased plasminogen activator inhibitor-1 levels levels, less fibrinolysis, and a greater degree of prothrombotic structure to the fibrin clot; however, these prohemostatic features were also found in obese controls, leading the investigators to conclude that prothrombotic risk was a reflection of obesity rather than NAFLD.[84] More study in this high-risk population seems warranted at this time.

THERAPEUTIC ANTICOAGULATION IN CIRRHOSIS

Anticoagulation studies in patients with cirrhosis are divided between those investigating prophylaxis of VTE or PVT versus treatment of PVT. Although the majority of the prophylaxis literature is in acutely ill hospitalized medical patients, an early study by Vivarelli and colleagues[85] studied surgical patients with cirrhosis and found statistically similar rates of surgical bleeding when comparing those who received thromboprophylaxis with LMWH after hepatic resection of hepatocellular carcinoma to those who did not receive thromboprophylaxis. A thought-provoking and controversial trial was published in 2012 by Villa and colleagues[86] and compared 70 subjects with cirrhosis at high risk for PVT at a single European center who were randomized to LMWH 4000 IU/d versus standard of care in an unblinded fashion. The primary endpoint of PVT was reached in 8.8% of cases prescribed LMWH compared with 27.7% of controls ($P<.001$) and, although the study was terminated at 48 weeks, the effect persisted through follow-up at 5 years.[86] Additionally, the investigators demonstrated fewer hepatic decompensating events in the LMWH arm (11.7% vs 59.4%, $P<.001$) and, unexpectedly, a significant all-cause survival benefit,[86] perhaps in part due to prevention of microthombosis and resultant localized ischemic tissue injury, thus inhibiting stellate cell activation and effectively preventing worsening fibrosis.[48] Although this study has been criticized for a lack of placebo control and possible selection bias, it is nonetheless thought provoking as is the lack of major bleeding experienced in the LMWH prevention group. More recent studies have found incidence rates of bleeding with LMWH or UFH in prophylactic doses ranging from 2% to 8% in cirrhosis patients.[42,87] **Table 3** summarizes the available literature on PVT and VTE prevention in patients with cirrhosis.

The index PVT treatment trial was published in 2005 by Francoz and colleagues.[63] Using either LMWH or VKA for a mean duration of 8.1 months, the investigators enrolled 19 subjects with PVT and compared them to 10 PVT subjects who did not receive treatment; 42% of subjects achieved some degree of treatment response with either partial or complete recanalization of the portal vein and in the absence of significant gastroesophageal variceal bleeding.[63] Several other studies[88–91] have built on this work and, using similar doses of LMWH or VKA, found even better treatment responses, ranging from 60% to 82%, with complete responses as high as 75%. Senzolo and colleagues[90] found that none of the 21 subjects enrolled in their study with untreated PVT had any regression in their thrombosis. Rates of major bleeding are variable with treatment doses of anticoagulation and range from 4% to 20%[88–91]; however, rates of gastroesophageal variceal bleeding are in general low when varices are treated endoscopically or medically prior to initiation of anticoagulation therapy (0%–11%). Cui and colleagues[92] published a single-center Chinese experience with 65 patients randomized to different therapeutic doses of LMWH (1 mg/kg every 12 hours or 1.5 mg/kg daily) where 78.5% (n = 51) responded to treatment with either complete or partial recanalization within 6 months of starting therapy. No variceal hemorrhage was noted; however, higher rates of nonvariceal bleeding (6.4%–23.5%) were found most predominantly in the daily dosing group. A recent meta-analysis of observational anticoagulation treatment trials published by Qi and colleagues[93] demonstrated a pooled bleeding rate of 3.3% for LMWH or VKA (95% CI, 1.1%–6.7%) when used for the treatment of PVT. This rate is similar to the bleeding rate for LMWH use in acutely ill medical patients (**Table 4**).[94]

Table 3
Primary thromboprophylaxis of portal vein thrombosis or venous thromboembolism in patients with cirrhosis

Study Publication Year	Anticoagulation Therapy	Study Design	Endpoint	Cases	Controls	Complete or Partial Response	Complications from Bleeding
Shatzel et al,[87] 2015	LMWH UFH	Retrospective cohort	VTE	N = 296 treated medical inpatients	N = 304 untreated medical inpatients	N/A	All bleeding (8.1% vs 5.5%, $P = .3$)
Intagliata et al,[42] 2014	LMWH UFH	Retrospective	VTE	N = 355 medical inpatients	N/A	N/A	2.5% GI bleeding
Villa et al,[86] 2012	LMWH 4000 IU/d	Prospective, randomized (nonblinded)	PVT	No PVT, prevention study (n = 40)	Untreated patients (n = 36)	De novo PVT (8.8% cases, 27.7% controls) Hepatic decompensation (11.7% cases vs 59.4% controls) Survival (60.0% vs 40.0%)	5% EV bleeding (n = 2 cases), 1 EV bleed control
Bechmann et al,[136] 2011	LMWH 40 mg/d (n = 75) Or LMWH 1 mg/kg/BID (n = 9)	Prospective cohort	PVT	No PVT (n = 84)	N/A	De novo PVT 0.0%	8.3% major bleeding (n = 7) 6.0% EV bleeding (n = 5)
Vivarelli et al,[85] 2010	LMWH	Retrospective cohort	VTE	N = 157 surgical inpatients	N = 72 surgical inpatients	N/A	3.2% vs 1.4% surgical bleeding, $P = .4$

Abbreviations: BID, twice-daily dosing; EV, esophageal varices; GI, gastrointestinal.

Table 4
Anticoagulation treatment studies in cirrhosis patients with portal vein thrombosis

Study Publication Year	Anticoagulation Therapy	Study Design	Cases	Controls	Duration of Treatment	Complete or Partial Response	Complications from Bleeding
Intagliata et al,[95] 2016	DOAC (n = 12) VKA or LMWH (n = 6)	Retrospective	PVT (n = 18)	N/A	DOAC mean 267 d LMWH/VKA mean 478 d	Unknown	7.7% (n = 2 ICH, n = 1 RP bleed) major bleeding for entire cohort (n = 39) 5.1% GI bleeding for entire cohort (n = 39)
Chen et al,[137] 2016	VKA	Retrospective	PVT (n = 30)	PVT, untreated (n = 36)	Median 7.6 mo	68.2% (n = 15) partial or complete 25% (n = 9) for untreated controls	13.3% GI bleeding (n = 4) 13.3% minor bleeding (n = 1 epistaxis, n = 3 gingival)
Ageno et al,[138] 2015	LMWH VKA	Prospective	PVT (n = 167)	N/A	Mean 13.9 mo	Unknown	13.2% major bleeding (n = 22)
Cui et al,[92] 2015	LMWH 1.5 mg/kg/d LMWH 1 mg/kg BID	Randomized, Prospective, unblinded	PVT (n = 65) HBV only	N/A	6 mo	78.4% (n = 51) partial or complete	23.5% bleeding with 1.5 mg/kg/d dose[a] 6.4% bleeding with 1 mg/kg BID dose[a]
Naeshiro et al,[139] 2015	Danaparoid 2500 units/d[c]	Retrospective	PVT (n = 26)	N/A	2 wk	76.9% (n = 16 partial, n = 4 complete)	None
Dell'Era et al,[140] 2014	LMWH	Retrospective	PVT (n = 10)	N/A	Unknown	Unknown	Unknown

Study	Anticoagulation	Study type	PVT	Control	Duration	Recanalization	Bleeding
Werner et al,[88] 2013	VKA	Retrospective	PVT (n = 28)		Mean 302 d	82.1% (n = 11 complete, n = 12 partial)	4% (n = 1)[a]
Delgado et al,[89] 2012	LMWH (n = 21) VKA (n = 8) LMWH transitioned to VKA (n = 21)	Retrospective	PVT (n = 55)	N/A	Median 6.8 mo	60.0% (n = 25 complete, n = 8 partial)	20% major bleeding (n = 11) 10.9% EV bleeding (n = 6) 3.6% GI bleeding (n = 2)
Senzolo et al,[90] 2012	Nadroparin 95 IU/kg/d	Prospective	PVT (n = 35)	Untreated PVT (n = 21)	6 mo	60.0% (n = 12 complete, n = 9 partial) 0.0% for untreated controls	11.4% major bleeding (n = 4) 2.9% EV bleeding (n = 1)[b] 2.9% ICH (n = 1)
Amitrano et al,[91] 2010	LMWH 200 IU/kg/d	Prospective	PVT (n = 28)	N/A	>6 mo	82.1% (n = 21 complete, n = 2 partial)	7.1% major bleeding, all non-EV GI
Francoz et al,[63] 2005	LMWH VKA	Prospective	PVT (n = 19)	Untreated PVT (n = 10)	Mean 8.1 mo	42.1% (n = 8) partial or complete	5.3% EV bleeding (n = 1)

Abbreviations: BID, twice-daily dosing; DOAC, apixiban and rivaroxaban; EV, esophageal varices; GI, gastrointestinal; HBV, hepatitis B virus; ICH, intracranial hemorrhage; RP, retroperitoneal.

[a] No gastroesophageal variceal bleeding.

[b] Higher rates of gastroesophageal variceal bleeding in the no treatment control group (n = 5; 23.8%).

[c] If antithrombin III activity decreased by less than 70%, antithrombin III 1500 U/d given for 3 days intravenously.

In North America, there is widespread use of the new direct oral anticoagulants (DOACs), including factor Xa inhibitors apixiban and rivaroxaban, in cardiovascular and hematologic disease, with favorable safety and efficacy profiles. Extension into the realm of cirrhosis seems inevitable. A recent series of 39 patients with cirrhosis found similar rates of bleeding (5%) when comparing DOAC use to treat PVT to the more traditional VKAs or LMWH.[95] No episodes of drug-induced liver injury were observed and the investigators concluded that DOACs had an acceptable safety profile when used in patients with CPT class A or B cirrhosis.[95] Safety and efficacy data in CPT class C disease are still not available and the US package inserts for these agents have variable warnings against use in CPT class B or class C cirrhosis patients. The widespread use of DOACs is further limited by a lack of currently available reversal agents because only idarucizumab is approved by the Food and Drug Administration for reversal of dabigatran.[96,97] Phase II and phase III trials investigating andexanet alfa for factor Xa inhibitor reversal and ciraparantag for direct thrombin inhibitor, factor Xa inhibitor, and heparin reversal are under way.[96,98] In lieu of a reversal agent, prothrombin complex concentrates may be considered because multiple small studies have shown administration of this product to normalize PT.[99,100] LMWH does not have a reversal agent; however, this does not limit its widespread use for thromboprophylaxis or treatment of VTE, perhaps in part due to the shorter half-life of this medication, and several groups have recommended we view the DOACs similar to LMWH in this regard.[95,97]

INTRAOPERATIVE AND POST–LIVER TRANSPLANTATION THROMBOSIS
Intraoperative Thromboembolic Events

Intraoperative thromboembolic events occur mainly as acute PE or intracardiac right atrial thrombosis.[101–103] Intraoperative thrombosis is rare, complicating 1% to 1.5% of liver transplantations; however, associated mortality is high, with rates between 50% and 82%, and thrombosis typically occur immediately after graft reperfusion. Potential risk factors include antifibrinolytics, air embolism, utilization of venous-venous bypass, pulmonary artery catheter use, octreotide administration, and hepatitis B immune globulin.

Venous Thromboembolic Disease

Major surgery is a well-established risk factor for the development of DVT. Incidence rates after general surgical procedures without DVT prophylaxis range from 15% to 40%.[104] Rates of DVT after liver transplantation, taking into account all cases both with and without DVT prophylaxis (including both mechanical and pharmacologic), have been reported as high as 9%, with PE occurring even less commonly with incidence rates approximating 1%.[105–108] Mechanical prophylaxis alone, however, does not seem sufficient because postoperative DVT rates can be even greater.[108] Most DVTs do not occur in the immediate postoperative time frame because one single-center series of 314 liver transplant recipients over a 7-year period reported a median postoperative day of diagnosis of 21.[108] Risk factors for postoperative VTE include preoperative factors (end-stage renal disease, diabetes, and history of prior DVT/PE), intraoperative factors (increased transfusions of cryoprecipitate or fresh frozen plasma and factor VII), and postoperative factors (elevated INR, bleeding, renal failure, and prolonged mechanical ventilation).[107–109] In general, liver transplant surgery guidelines regarding VTE prophylaxis are lacking from both safety and efficacy standpoints; however, given the accepted bleeding rates of approximately 1% after major surgery, including abdominal surgery and partial hepatectomy, the rates of postoperative VTE are significantly greater than postoperative bleeding with chemical thromboprophyalxis.[110] Despite this, other investigators have argued that the bleeding risk is too great for universal VTE chemical thromboprophylaxis after liver transplantation and that this should be reserved for high-risk patients where prevention of post-transplantation vascular issues, including PVT and/or HAT, are of concern.[111]

Portal Vein Thrombosis

Incidence rates of post-transplantation PVT, although generally lower than that for HAT, have been reported to be as high as 2.5%.[112,113] Post-transplantation PVT is associated with a very high mortality rate, ranging from 65% to 75%. Pretransplantation PVT, living donor liver transplant recipients, and hypercoagulable states, including pretransplantation Budd-Chiari syndrome, pediatric liver transplant recipients, and postoperative portal vein stenosis, have all been reported in association with post-transplantation PVT.[112,113]

Hepatic Artery Thrombosis

HAT is an uncommon complication, with incidence rates between 1% and 5% after liver transplantation.[15,62,114] HAT is associated with deleterious clinical ramifications, including graft loss and increased recipient mortality.[15,62,114] Surgical risk factors for HAT are well established and include prolonged donor organ cold ischemia time (CIT); surgical technique, including the use of aortic jump grafts; a delay in reperfusion; and variant donor or recipient anatomy (eg, replaced hepatic artery).[115,116] Other issues affecting vascular reconstruction, including utilization of vascular patches, increase HAT risk. Specifically, use of a gastroduodenal artery patch is associated with a 5.2% incidence of HAT, a donor splenic artery patch 7.4%, and an aortic patch 13.5%.[117] Donor risk index, the most widely used scoring system to evaluate donor risk and assist the transplant team in decision making regarding graft allocation, is also directly proportional to the risk of post-transplantation HAT.[62,118] HAT has also been described in recipients who underwent prior liver transplantation or were diagnosed with inherited thrombophilia, primary sclerosing cholangitis or acute intermittent porphyria pretransplantation, or new onset of diabetes post-transplantation.[119–125] Pretransplantation recipient PVT has also been associated with increased risk of early graft loss from HAT,[62] in many cases leading to retransplantation, sometimes urgently.[118]

Intraoperative Doppler ultrasound monitoring of hepatic artery flow may be helpful in predicting which transplant recipients have subsequent increased risk of HAT because lower blood flow rates have been associated with increased early HAT; although the exact threshold predicting the greatest risk has yet to be established, flow rates between 100 mL/min and 200 mL/min are the minimum recommended velocities in the operating room.[126,127]

The role for aspirin use to prevent post-transplantation HAT remains controversial because reports supporting both a decreased incidence[128] and no significant difference[129] in early HAT have surfaced; however, a series by Vivarelli and colleagues[130] demonstrated significant reduction (0.6% in the aspirin group vs 3.6% nonaspirin group) in late HAT (>90 days post-transplantation) in high-risk recipients. Historically, other investigators have considered administration of fresh-frozen plasma to restore protein C levels as a way to prevent HAT; however, reports of increased HAT in the pediatric population have limited its widespread use, perhaps in part due to the large volume of fresh-frozen plasma required to correct protein C levels.[131,132] Heparin use to prevent HAT has also been considered; however, it remains largely an empiric and center-specific therapy, with limited used in deceased donor liver transplantation.[133]

Treatment of early HAT typically requires surgical revision and direct thrombolysis or retransplantations because endovascular treatment by interventional radiologists has been largely unsuccessful owing to failed responses to thrombolysis or an inability of a guide wire to safely cross the arterial thrombosis.[134] In a single-center US experience of 17 transplant recipients with mean postoperative diagnosis of early HAT at seven days, surgical administration of urokinase at a dose of 50,000 U to 100,000 U directly into the hepatic artery led to restoration of hepatic artery flow in 88% of recipients with only one reoperation for bleeding.[135] Long-term outcomes were promising because 65% of these recipients recovered to have normal liver function by a mean time frame of 15 months and only 35% experienced biliary complications. Alteplase is now the preferred agent because urokinase is no longer available in the United States.

SUMMARY

Navigating the delicate rebalance between prohemostatic and antihemostatic factors in patients with cirrhosis is a challenge clinicians face on a daily basis. Often, the balance is shifted toward one or the other by common situations facing patients with cirrhosis, including invasive procedures, such as paracenteses or surgical procedures, and blood flow alterations, often precipitated by medications, changes in vascular status, infection, inflammation, and/or malignancy. In general, PT-INR should not be used in the routine assessment of either bleeding or thrombotic risk. Rather, the authors favor using a combination of fibrinogen levels, dynamic testing with TEG or ROTEM, and/or thrombin generation assays when available. Patients with cirrhosis are predisposed to PE, DVT, and PVT in the pretransplantation setting. VTE or PVT in cirrhosis patients is associated with significant morbidity and mortality and treatment with anticoagulation should not be withheld unless there is a strong contraindication. Furthermore, all hospitalized patients with cirrhosis, regardless of if they are medical or surgical patients, should receive chemical thromboprophylaxis unless there is a compelling reason not to do so, as in the general medicine population. The role of prophylactic anticoagulation for PVT in outpatients with compensated liver disease remains debatable; however, current data are intriguing in terms of not only preventing PVT but also improving patient-centered outcomes of decreased hepatic decompensation and lower mortality rates. Future prospective study in larger patient populations with more rigorous methodology is needed to confirm these findings prior to the widespread adoption of this clinical practice, and consideration should be given to the risks of anticoagulation in liver transplant candidates who often do not know when they will be receiving an organ offer, making the timing of the last dose prior to transplantation difficult to anticipate.

This pretransplantation hypercoagulable milieu seems to extend for at least several months post-transplantation because intraoperative PE or right atrial thrombosis directly after reperfusion, delayed PE or DVT, PVT, or early and late HAT are all well described and, although rare, are associated with significant morbidity and high mortality rates. Patients with NAFLD and inherited thrombophilia are unique populations where an individualized approach to anticoagulation is often required. To date, the optimal anticoagulation regimen both for prevention of and therapy for clotting in cirrhosis has yet to be established but early reports suggest a potential role for LMWH and the newer DOACs.

REFERENCES

1. Northup PG, McMahon MM, Ruhl AP, et al. Coagulopathy does not fully protect hospitalized cirrhosis patients from peripheral venous thromboembolism. The Am J Gastroenterol 2006;101(7):1524–8 [quiz: 1680].

2. Caldwell SH, Hoffman M, Lisman T, et al. Coagulation disorders and hemostasis in liver disease: pathophysiology and critical assessment of current management. Hepatology 2006;44(4):1039–46.

3. Aldawood A, Arabi Y, Aljumah A, et al. The incidence of venous thromboembolism and practice of deep venous thrombosis prophylaxis in hospitalized cirrhotic patients. Thromb J 2011;9(1):1.

4. Dabbagh O, Oza A, Prakash S, et al. Coagulopathy does not protect against venous thromboembolism in hospitalized patients with chronic liver disease. Chest 2010;137(5):1145–9.

5. Gale AJ. Continuing education course #2: current understanding of hemostasis. Toxicologic Pathol 2011;39(1):273–80.

6. Violi F, Ferro D, Basili S, et al. Ongoing prothrombotic state in the portal circulation of cirrhotic patients. Thromb Haemost 1997;77(1):44–7.

7. Zocco MA, Di Stasio E, De Cristofaro R, et al. Thrombotic risk factors in patients with liver cirrhosis: correlation with MELD scoring system and portal vein thrombosis development. J Hepatol 2009;51(4):682–9.

8. Lisman T, Bongers TN, Adelmeijer J, et al. Elevated levels of von Willebrand Factor in cirrhosis support platelet adhesion despite reduced functional capacity. Hepatology 2006;44(1):53–61.

9. Arshad F, Lisman T, Porte RJ. Hypercoagulability as a contributor to thrombotic complications in the liver transplant recipient. Liver Int 2013;33(6):820–7.

10. Tripodi A, Mannucci PM. The coagulopathy of chronic liver disease. N Engl J Med 2011;365(2):147–56.

11. Qi X, Chen H, Han G. Effect of antithrombin, protein C and protein S on portal vein thrombosis in liver cirrhosis: a meta-analysis. Am J Med Sci 2013;346(1): 38–44.

12. Stein SF, Harker LA. Kinetic and functional studies of platelets, fibrinogen, and plasminogen in patients with hepatic cirrhosis. J Lab Clin Med 1982;99(2): 217–30.

13. Amitrano L, Brancaccio V, Guardascione MA, et al. Inherited coagulation disorders in cirrhotic patients with portal vein thrombosis. Hepatology 2000;31(2): 345–8.

14. Violi F, Ferro D, Basili S, et al. Relation between lupus anticoagulant and splanchnic venous thrombosis in cirrhosis of the liver. BMJ 1994;309(6949): 239–40.

15. Ayala R, Martinez-Lopez J, Cedena T, et al. Recipient and donor thrombophilia and the risk of portal venous thrombosis and hepatic artery thrombosis in liver recipients. BMC Gastroenterol 2011;11:130.

16. Lumsden AB, Henderson JM, Kutner MH. Endotoxin levels measured by a chromogenic assay in portal, hepatic and peripheral venous blood in patients with cirrhosis. Hepatology 1988;8(2):232–6.

17. Nolan JP. The role of intestinal endotoxin in liver injury: a long and evolving history. Hepatology 2010;52(5):1829–35.

18. Ferro D, Quintarelli C, Lattuada A, et al. High plasma levels of von Willebrand factor as a marker of endothelial perturbation in cirrhosis: relationship to endotoxemia. Hepatology 1996;23(6):1377–83.

19. Lisman T, Porte RJ. Rebalanced hemostasis in patients with liver disease: evidence and clinical consequences. Blood 2010;116(6):878–85.

20. Violi F, Leo R, Vezza E, et al. Bleeding time in patients with cirrhosis: relation with degree of liver failure and clotting abnormalities. C.A.L.C. Group. Coagulation Abnormalities in Cirrhosis Study Group. J Hepatol 1994;20(4):531–6.

21. Laffi G, Marra F. Complications of cirrhosis: is endothelium guilty? J Hepatol 1999;30(3):532–5.
22. Cattaneo M, Tenconi PM, Alberca I, et al. Subcutaneous desmopressin (DDAVP) shortens the prolonged bleeding time in patients with liver cirrhosis. Thromb Haemost 1990;64(3):358–60.
23. de Franchis R, Arcidiacono PG, Carpinelli L, et al. Randomized controlled trial of desmopressin plus terlipressin vs. terlipressin alone for the treatment of acute variceal hemorrhage in cirrhotic patients: a multicenter, double-blind study. New Italian Endoscopic Club. Hepatology 1993;18(5):1102–7.
24. Lehman CM, Blaylock RC, Alexander DP, et al. Discontinuation of the bleeding time test without detectable adverse clinical impact. Clin Chem 2001;47(7): 1204–11.
25. Tripodi A, Caldwell SH, Hoffman M, et al. Review article: the prothrombin time test as a measure of bleeding risk and prognosis in liver disease. Aliment Pharmacol Ther 2007;26(2):141–8.
26. Ewe K. Bleeding after liver biopsy does not correlate with indices of peripheral coagulation. Dig Dis Sci 1981;26(5):388–93.
27. Shah A, Amarapurkar D, Dharod M, et al. Coagulopathy in cirrhosis: a prospective study to correlate conventional tests of coagulation and bleeding following invasive procedures in cirrhotics. Indian J Gastroenterol 2015;34(5):359–64.
28. Mallett SV, Cox DJ. Thrombelastography. Br J Anaesth 1992;69(3):307–13.
29. Mancuso A, Fung K, Cox D, et al. Assessment of blood coagulation in severe liver disease using thromboelastography: use of citrate storage versus native blood. Blood Coagul Fibrinolysis 2003;14(2):211–6.
30. Kang Y. Coagulation and liver transplantation. Transpl Proc 1993;25(2):2001–5.
31. Owen CA Jr, Rettke SR, Bowie EJ, et al. Hemostatic evaluation of patients undergoing liver transplantation. Mayo Clinic Proc 1987;62(9):761–72.
32. Krzanicki D, Sugavanam A, Mallett S. Intraoperative hypercoagulability during liver transplantation as demonstrated by thromboelastography. Liver Transpl 2013;19(8):852–61.
33. Chau TN, Chan YW, Patch D, et al. Thrombelastographic changes and early re-bleeding in cirrhotic patients with variceal bleeding. Gut 1998;43(2):267–71.
34. Rossetto V, Spiezia L, Senzolo M, et al. Whole blood rotation thromboelastometry (ROTEM(R)) profiles in subjects with non-neoplastic portal vein thrombosis. Thromb Res 2013;132(2):e131–4.
35. Potze W, Adelmeijer J, Porte RJ, et al. Preserved clot formation detected by the thrombodynamics analyzer in patients with cirrhosis. Thromb Res 2015;135(5): 1012–6.
36. Sogaard KK, Horvath-Puho E, Gronbaek H, et al. Risk of venous thromboembolism in patients with liver disease: a nationwide population-based case-control study. Am J Gastroenterol 2009;104(1):96–101.
37. Sogaard KK, Horvath-Puho E, Montomoli J, et al. Cirrhosis is associated with an increased 30-day mortality after venous thromboembolism. Clin translational Gastroenterol 2015;6:e97.
38. Gulley D, Teal E, Suvannasankha A, et al. Deep vein thrombosis and pulmonary embolism in cirrhosis patients. Dig Dis Sci 2008;53(11):3012–7.
39. Garcia-Fuster MJ, Abdilla N, Fabia MJ, et al. Venous thromboembolism and liver cirrhosis. Rev Esp Enferm Dig 2008;100(5):259–62 [in Spanish].
40. Wu H, Nguyen GC. Liver cirrhosis is associated with venous thromboembolism among hospitalized patients in a nationwide US study. Clin Gastroenterol Hepatol 2010;8(9):800–5.

41. Ali M, Ananthakrishnan AN, McGinley EL, et al. Deep vein thrombosis and pulmonary embolism in hospitalized patients with cirrhosis: a nationwide analysis. Dig Dis Sci 2011;56(7):2152–9.
42. Intagliata NM, Henry ZH, Shah N, et al. Prophylactic anticoagulation for venous thromboembolism in hospitalized cirrhosis patients is not associated with high rates of gastrointestinal bleeding. Liver Int 2014;34(1):26–32.
43. Kahn SR, Lim W, Dunn AS, et al. Prevention of VTE in nonsurgical patients: antithrombotic therapy and prevention of thrombosis, 9th ed: American College of Chest Physicians evidence-based clinical practice guidelines. Chest 2012; 141(2 Suppl):e195S–226S.
44. Barbar S, Noventa F, Rossetto V, et al. A risk assessment model for the identification of hospitalized medical patients at risk for venous thromboembolism: the Padua Prediction Score. J Thromb Haemost 2010;8(11):2450–7.
45. Bogari H, Patanwala AE, Cosgrove R, et al. Risk-assessment and pharmacological prophylaxis of venous thromboembolism in hospitalized patients with chronic liver disease. Thromb Res 2014;134(6):1220–3.
46. Vardi M, Ghanem-Zoubi NO, Zidan R, et al. Venous thromboembolism and the utility of the Padua Prediction Score in patients with sepsis admitted to internal medicine departments. J Thromb Haemost 2013;11(3):467–73.
47. DeLeve LD, Valla DC, Garcia-Tsao G. Vascular disorders of the liver. Hepatology 2009;49(5):1729–64.
48. Wanless IR, Wong F, Blendis LM, et al. Hepatic and portal vein thrombosis in cirrhosis: possible role in development of parenchymal extinction and portal hypertension. Hepatology (Baltimore, Md) 1995;21(5):1238–47.
49. Okuda K, Ohnishi K, Kimura K, et al. Incidence of portal vein thrombosis in liver cirrhosis. An angiographic study in 708 patients. Gastroenterology 1985;89(2): 279–86.
50. Yerdel MA, Gunson B, Mirza D, et al. Portal vein thrombosis in adults undergoing liver transplantation: risk factors, screening, management, and outcome. Transplantation 2000;69(9):1873–81.
51. Fimognari FL, De Santis A, Piccheri C, et al. Evaluation of D-dimer and factor VIII in cirrhotic patients with asymptomatic portal venous thrombosis. J Lab Clin Med 2005;146(4):238–43.
52. Cavallari A, Vivarelli M, Bellusci R, et al. Treatment of vascular complications following liver transplantation: multidisciplinary approach. Hepato-gastroenterology 2001;48(37):179–83.
53. Settmacher U, Nussler NC, Glanemann M, et al. Venous complications after orthotopic liver transplantation. Clin Transplant 2000;14(3):235–41.
54. Lendoire J, Raffin G, Cejas N, et al. Liver transplantation in adult patients with portal vein thrombosis: risk factors, management and outcome. HPB 2007; 9(5):352–6.
55. Amitrano L, Guardascione MA, Brancaccio V, et al. Risk factors and clinical presentation of portal vein thrombosis in patients with liver cirrhosis. J Hepatol 2004;40(5):736–41.
56. Tsochatzis EA, Senzolo M, Germani G, et al. Systematic review: portal vein thrombosis in cirrhosis. Aliment Pharmacol Ther 2010;31(3):366–74.
57. Englesbe MJ, Kubus J, Muhammad W, et al. Portal vein thrombosis and survival in patients with cirrhosis. Liver Transplant 2010;16(1):83–90.
58. Rodriguez-Castro KI, Porte RJ, Nadal E, et al. Management of nonneoplastic portal vein thrombosis in the setting of liver transplantation: a systematic review. Transplantation 2012;94(11):1145–53.

59. Hibi T, Nishida S, Levi DM, et al. When and why portal vein thrombosis matters in liver transplantation: a critical audit of 174 cases. Ann Surg 2014;259(4):760–6.

60. Ponziani FR, Zocco MA, Senzolo M, et al. Portal vein thrombosis and liver transplantation: implications for waiting list period, surgical approach, early and late follow-up. Transplant Rev (Orlando) 2014;28(2):92–101.

61. Stine JG. Portal vein thrombosis, mortality and hepatic decompensation in patients with cirrhosis: a meta-analysis. World J Hepatol 2015;7(27):2774–80.

62. Stine JG. Pre-transplant portal vein thrombosis is an independent risk factor for graft loss due to hepatic artery thrombosis in liver transplant recipients. HPB 2015;18(3):279–86.

63. Francoz C, Belghiti J, Vilgrain V, et al. Splanchnic vein thrombosis in candidates for liver transplantation: usefulness of screening and anticoagulation. Gut 2005; 54(5):691–7.

64. Nery F, Chevret S, Condat B, et al. Causes and consequences of portal vein thrombosis in 1,243 patients with cirrhosis: results of a longitudinal study. Hepatology 2015;61(2):660–7.

65. Zironi G, Gaiani S, Fenyves D, et al. Value of measurement of mean portal flow velocity by Doppler flowmetry in the diagnosis of portal hypertension. J Hepatol 1992;16(3):298–303.

66. Zoli M, Iervese T, Merkel C, et al. Prognostic significance of portal hemodynamics in patients with compensated cirrhosis. J Hepatol 1993;17(1):56–61.

67. Zoli M, Marchesini G, Brunori A, et al. Portal venous flow in response to acute beta-blocker and vasodilatatory treatment in patients with liver cirrhosis. Hepatology 1986;6(6):1248–51.

68. Westaby D, Bihari DJ, Gimson AE, et al. Selective and non-selective beta receptor blockade in the reduction of portal pressure in patients with cirrhosis and portal hypertension. Gut 1984;25(2):121–4.

69. Qi X, De Stefano V, Wang J, et al. Prevalence of inherited antithrombin, protein C, and protein S deficiencies in portal vein system thrombosis and Budd-Chiari syndrome: a systematic review and meta-analysis of observational studies. J Gastroenterol Hepatol 2013;28(3):432–42.

70. Saugel B, Lee M, Feichtinger S, et al. Thrombophilic factor analysis in cirrhotic patients with portal vein thrombosis. J Thromb Thrombolysis 2015;40(1):54–60.

71. Violi F, Corazza RG, Caldwell SH, et al. Portal vein thrombosis relevance on liver cirrhosis: Italian venous thrombotic events registry. Intern Emerg Med 2016;30:30.

72. Stine JG, Shah NL, Argo CK, et al. Increased risk of portal vein thrombosis in patients with cirrhosis due to non-alcoholic steatohepatitis (NASH). Liver Transpl 2015;21(8):1016–21.

73. Di Minno MN, Tufano A, Rusolillo A, et al. High prevalence of nonalcoholic fatty liver in patients with idiopathic venous thromboembolism. World J Gastroenterol 2010;16(48):6119–22.

74. Targher G, Bertolini L, Rodella S, et al. NASH predicts plasma inflammatory biomarkers independently of visceral fat in men. Obesity (Silver Spring) 2008;16(6): 1394–9.

75. Targher G, Zoppini G, Moghetti P, et al. Disorders of coagulation and hemostasis in abdominal obesity: emerging role of fatty liver. Semin Thromb Hemost 2010; 36(1):41–8.

76. Argo CK, Caldwell SH. Epidemiology and natural history of non-alcoholic steatohepatitis. Clin Liver Dis 2009;13(4):511–31.

77. Cigolini M, Targher G, Agostino G, et al. Liver steatosis and its relation to plasma haemostatic factors in apparently healthy men–role of the metabolic syndrome. Thromb Haemost 1996;76(1):69–73.
78. Tripodi A, Fracanzani AL, Primignani M, et al. Procoagulant imbalance in patients with nonalcoholic fatty liver disease. J Hepatol 2014;61(1):148–54.
79. Potze W, Siddiqui MS, Sanyal AJ. Vascular disease in patients with nonalcoholic fatty liver disease. Semin Thromb Hemost 2015;41(5):488–93.
80. Alkhouri N, Kistangari G, Campbell C, et al. Mean platelet volume as a marker of increased cardiovascular risk in patients with nonalcoholic steatohepatitis. Hepatology 2012;55(1):331.
81. Verrijken A, Francque S, Mertens I, et al. Prothrombotic factors in histologically proven nonalcoholic fatty liver disease and nonalcoholic steatohepatitis. Hepatology 2013;59(1):121–9.
82. Papatheodoridis GV, Chrysanthos N, Cholongitas E, et al. Thrombotic risk factors and liver histologic lesions in non-alcoholic fatty liver disease. J Hepatol 2009;51(5):931–8.
83. Assy N, Bekirov I, Mejritsky Y, et al. Association between thrombotic risk factors and extent of fibrosis in patients with non-alcoholic fatty liver diseases. World J Gastroenterol 2005;11(37):5834–9.
84. Potze W, Siddiqui MS, Boyett SL, et al. Preserved hemostatic status in patients with non-alcoholic fatty liver disease. J Hepatol 2016;65(5):980–7.
85. Vivarelli M, Zanello M, Zanfi C, et al. Prophylaxis for venous thromboembolism after resection of hepatocellular carcinoma on cirrhosis: is it necessary? World J Gastroenterol 2010;16(17):2146–50.
86. Villa E, Camma C, Marietta M, et al. Enoxaparin prevents portal vein thrombosis and liver decompensation in patients with advanced cirrhosis. Gastroenterology 2012;143(5):1253–60.e1-4.
87. Shatzel J, Dulai PS, Harbin D, et al. Safety and efficacy of pharmacological thromboprophylaxis for hospitalized patients with cirrhosis: a single-center retrospective cohort study. J Thromb Haemost 2015;13(7):1245–53.
88. Werner KT, Sando S, Carey EJ, et al. Portal vein thrombosis in patients with end stage liver disease awaiting liver transplantation: outcome of anticoagulation. Dig Dis Sci 2013;58(6):1776–80.
89. Delgado MG, Seijo S, Yepes I, et al. Efficacy and safety of anticoagulation on patients with cirrhosis and portal vein thrombosis. Clin Gastroenterol Hepatol 2012;10(7):776–83.
90. Senzolo M, M Sartori T, Rossetto V, et al. Prospective evaluation of anticoagulation and transjugular intrahepatic portosystemic shunt for the management of portal vein thrombosis in cirrhosis. Liver Int 2012;32(6):919–27.
91. Amitrano L, Guardascione MA, Menchise A, et al. Safety and efficacy of anticoagulation therapy with low molecular weight heparin for portal vein thrombosis in patients with liver cirrhosis. J Clin Gastroenterol 2010;44(6):448–51.
92. Cui SB, Shu RH, Yan SP, et al. Efficacy and safety of anticoagulation therapy with different doses of enoxaparin for portal vein thrombosis in cirrhotic patients with hepatitis B. Eur J Gastroenterol Hepatol 2015;27(8):914–9.
93. Qi X, De Stefano V, Li H, et al. Anticoagulation for the treatment of portal vein thrombosis in liver cirrhosis: a systematic review and meta-analysis of observational studies. Eur J Intern Med 2015;26(1):23–9.
94. Samama MM, Cohen AT, Darmon JY, et al. A comparison of enoxaparin with placebo for the prevention of venous thromboembolism in acutely ill medical

patients. Prophylaxis in Medical Patients with Enoxaparin Study Group. N Engl J Med 1999;341(11):793–800.

95. Intagliata NM, Henry ZH, Maitland H, et al. Direct oral anticoagulants in cirrhosis patients pose similar risks of bleeding when compared to traditional anticoagulation. Dig Dis Sci 2016;61(6):1721–7.

96. Rogers KC, Shelton MP, Finks S. Reversal agents for direct oral anticoagulants: understanding new and upcoming options. Cardiol Rev 2016;24(6):310–5.

97. Hu TY, Vaidya VR, Asirvatham SJ. Reversing anticoagulant effects of novel oral anticoagulants: role of ciraparantag, andexanet alfa, and idarucizumab. Vasc Health Risk Manag 2016;12:35–44.

98. Siegal DM, Curnutte JT, Connolly SJ, et al. Andexanet alfa for the reversal of factor xa inhibitor activity. N Engl J Med 2015;373(25):2413–24.

99. Eerenberg ES, Kamphuisen PW, Sijpkens MK, et al. Reversal of rivaroxaban and dabigatran by prothrombin complex concentrate: a randomized, placebo-controlled, crossover study in healthy subjects. Circulation 2011;124(14):1573–9.

100. Levi M, Moore KT, Castillejos CF, et al. Comparison of three-factor and four-factor prothrombin complex concentrates regarding reversal of the anticoagulant effects of rivaroxaban in healthy volunteers. J Thromb Haemost 2014; 12(9):1428–36.

101. Ellenberger C, Mentha G, Giostra E, et al. Cardiovascular collapse due to massive pulmonary thromboembolism during orthotopic liver transplantation. J Clin Anesth 2006;18(5):367–71.

102. Gologorsky E, De Wolf AM, Scott V, et al. Intracardiac thrombus formation and pulmonary thromboembolism immediately after graft reperfusion in 7 patients undergoing liver transplantation. Liver Transpl 2001;7(9):783–9.

103. Warnaar N, Molenaar IQ, Colquhoun SD, et al. Intraoperative pulmonary embolism and intracardiac thrombosis complicating liver transplantation: a systematic review. J Thromb Haemost 2008;6(2):297–302.

104. Hirsh J, Hoak J. Management of deep vein thrombosis and pulmonary embolism. A statement for healthcare professionals. council on thrombosis (in consultation with the council on cardiovascular radiology), American Heart Association. Circulation 1996;93(12):2212–45.

105. Ishitani M, Angle J, Bickston S, et al. Liver transplantation: incidence and management of deep venous thrombosis and pulmonary emboli. Transpl Proc 1997; 29(7):2861–3.

106. Cherian TP, Chiu K, Gunson B, et al. Pulmonary thromboembolism in liver transplantation: a retrospective review of the first 25 years. Transpl Int 2010;23(11): 1113–9.

107. Salami A, Qureshi W, Kuriakose P, et al. Frequency and predictors of venous thromboembolism in orthotopic liver transplant recipients: a single-center retrospective review. Transpl Proc 2013;45(1):315–9.

108. Annamalai A, Kim I, Sundaram V, et al. Incidence and risk factors of deep vein thrombosis after liver transplantation. Transpl Proc 2014;46(10):3564–9.

109. Emuakhagbon V, Philips P, Agopian V, et al. Incidence and risk factors for deep venous thrombosis and pulmonary embolus after liver transplantation. Am J Surg 2016;211(4):768–71.

110. Tzeng CW, Katz MH, Fleming JB, et al. Risk of venous thromboembolism outweighs post-hepatectomy bleeding complications: analysis of 5651 National Surgical Quality Improvement Program patients. HPB 2012;14(8):506–13.

111. Mukerji AN, Karachristos A, Maloo M, et al. Do postliver transplant patients need thromboprophylactic anticoagulation? Clin Appl Thrombosis/Hemostasis 2014; 20(7):673–7.

112. You S, He XS, Hu AB, et al. The analysis of portal vein thrombosis following orthotopic liver transplantation. Zhonghua Wai Ke Za Zhi 2008;46(3):176–8 [in Chinese].

113. Khalaf H. Vascular complications after deceased and living donor liver transplantation: a single-center experience. Transpl Proc 2010;42(3):865–70.

114. Iida T, Kaido T, Yagi S, et al. Hepatic arterial complications in adult living donor liver transplant recipients: a single-center experience of 673 cases. Clin Transplant 2014;28(9):1025–30.

115. Cescon M, Zanello M, Grazi GL, et al. Impact of very advanced donor age on hepatic artery thrombosis after liver transplantation. Transplantation 2011; 92(4):439–45.

116. Warner P, Fusai G, Glantzounis GK, et al. Risk factors associated with early hepatic artery thrombosis after orthotopic liver transplantation - univariable and multivariable analysis. Transpl Int 2011;24(4):401–8.

117. Mourad MM, Liossis C, Gunson BK, et al. Etiology and management of hepatic artery thrombosis after adult liver transplantation. Liver Transpl 2014;20(6): 713–23.

118. Sharma R, Kashyap R, Jain A, et al. Surgical complications following liver transplantation in patients with portal vein thrombosis–a single-center perspective. J Gastrointest Surg 2010;14(3):520–7.

119. Vivarelli M, Cucchetti A, La Barba G, et al. Ischemic arterial complications after liver transplantation in the adult: multivariate analysis of risk factors. Arch Surg 2004;139(10):1069–74.

120. Oh CK, Pelletier SJ, Sawyer RG, et al. Uni- and multi-variate analysis of risk factors for early and late hepatic artery thrombosis after liver transplantation. Transplantation 2001;71(6):767–72.

121. Dunn TB, Linden MA, Vercellotti GM, et al. Factor V Leiden and hepatic artery thrombosis after liver transplantation. Clin Transplant 2006;20(1):132–5.

122. Mas VR, Fisher RA, Maluf DG, et al. Hepatic artery thrombosis after liver transplantation and genetic factors: prothrombin G20210A polymorphism. Transplantation 2003;76(1):247–9.

123. Dowman JK, Gunson BK, Mirza DF, et al. Liver transplantation for acute intermittent porphyria is complicated by a high rate of hepatic artery thrombosis. Liver Transpl 2012;18(2):195–200.

124. Graziadei IW, Wiesner RH, Marotta PJ, et al. Long-term results of patients undergoing liver transplantation for primary sclerosing cholangitis. Hepatology 1999; 30(5):1121–7.

125. Moon JI, Barbeito R, Faradji RN, et al. Negative impact of new-onset diabetes mellitus on patient and graft survival after liver transplantation: long-term follow up. Transplantation 2006;82(12):1625–8.

126. Marin-Gomez LM, Bernal-Bellido C, Alamo-Martinez JM, et al. Intraoperative hepatic artery blood flow predicts early hepatic artery thrombosis after liver transplantation. Transpl Proc 2012;44(7):2078–81.

127. Muller SA, Schmied BM, Mehrabi A, et al. Feasibility and effectiveness of a new algorithm in preventing hepatic artery thrombosis after liver transplantation. J Gastrointest Surg 2009;13(4):702–12.

128. Shay R, Taber D, Pilch N, et al. Early aspirin therapy may reduce hepatic artery thrombosis in liver transplantation. Transpl Proc 2013;45(1):330–4.

129. Wolf DC, Freni MA, Boccagni P, et al. Low-dose aspirin therapy is associated with few side effects but does not prevent hepatic artery thrombosis in liver transplant recipients. Liver Transplant Surg 1997;3(6):598–603.
130. Vivarelli M, La Barba G, Cucchetti A, et al. Can antiplatelet prophylaxis reduce the incidence of hepatic artery thrombosis after liver transplantation? Liver Transpl 2007;13(5):651–4.
131. Hatano E, Terajima H, Yabe S, et al. Hepatic artery thrombosis in living related liver transplantation. Transplantation 1997;64(10):1443–6.
132. Hashikura Y, Kawasaki S, Okumura N, et al. Prevention of hepatic artery thrombosis in pediatric liver transplantation. Transplantation 1995;60(10):1109–12.
133. Sugawara Y, Kaneko J, Akamatsu N, et al. Anticoagulant therapy against hepatic artery thrombosis in living donor liver transplantation. Transpl Proc 2002; 34(8):3325–6.
134. Saad WE, Dasgupta N, Lippert AJ, et al. Extrahepatic pseudoaneurysms and ruptures of the hepatic artery in liver transplant recipients: endovascular management and a new iatrogenic etiology. Cardiovasc Intervent Radiol 2013; 36(1):118–27.
135. Pinna AD, Smith CV, Furukawa H, et al. Urgent revascularization of liver allografts after early hepatic artery thrombosis. Transplantation 1996;62(11): 1584–7.
136. Bechmann LP, Sichau M, Wichert M, et al. Low-molecular-weight heparin in patients with advanced cirrhosis. Liver Int 2011;31(1):75–82.
137. Chen H, Liu L, Qi X, et al. Efficacy and safety of anticoagulation in more advanced portal vein thrombosis in patients with liver cirrhosis. Eur J Gastroenterol Hepatol 2016;28(1):82–9.
138. Ageno W, Riva N, Schulman S, et al. Long-term clinical outcomes of splanchnic vein thrombosis: results of an international registry. JAMA Intern Med 2015; 175(9):1474–80.
139. Naeshiro N, Aikata H, Hyogo H, et al. Efficacy and safety of the anticoagulant drug, danaparoid sodium, in the treatment of portal vein thrombosis in patients with liver cirrhosis. Hepatol Res 2015;45(6):656–62.
140. Dell'Era A, Iannuzzi F, Fabris FM, et al. Impact of portal vein thrombosis on the efficacy of endoscopic variceal band ligation. Dig Liver Dis 2014;46(2):152–6.

Model for End-Stage Liver Disease–Sodium Score

The Evolution in the Prioritization of Liver Transplantation

Victor Ilich Machicao, MD

KEYWORDS

- Organ allocation • MELD score • MELD sodium score • Liver transplantation
- Waiting-list mortality • Hepatocellular carcinoma • Liver cirrhosis
- Mathematical model

KEY POINTS

- The model for end-stage liver disease (MELD) -based allocation system implemented in 2002 was the first step toward prioritizing liver transplantation for the patients with the highest risk of mortality.
- The incorporation of sodium to the MELD score has made the model stronger in predicting mortality among liver transplant candidates.
- The current allocation system for patients with hepatocellular carcinoma still allows outcome disparity compared with patients without hepatocellular carcinoma.

HISTORICAL PERSPECTIVE: STARTING TO REGULATE LIVER TRANSPLANTATION

It has been more than 50 years since Starzl and colleagues[1] performed the first successful human liver transplantation (LT) in the United States. In the following years, LT gradually established its role as definitive therapy for patients with acute liver failure and end-stage liver disease, and later on for selected patients with hepatocellular carcinoma (HCC). Afterward, the limited availability of cadaveric organs became the main limiting factor for the wider use of LT. At the same time, the increased mortality seen among patients awaiting transplantation became an issue. A system of prioritization was critical in order to reconcile the disparity between supply and demand of organs for transplantation.

The author has nothing to disclose.
Division of Gastroenterology, Hepatology and Nutrition, McGovern Medical School, University of Texas Health Science Center at Houston, 6400 Fannin Street, MSB 4.234, Houston, TX 77030, USA
E-mail address: Victor.I.Machicao@uth.tmc.edu

Clin Liver Dis 21 (2017) 275–287
http://dx.doi.org/10.1016/j.cld.2016.12.014
1089-3261/17/Published by Elsevier Inc.

The first step to regulate organ allocation for LT came only 3 decades ago. It started with the US Congress passing the National Organ Transplant Act in 1984, which created the Organ Procurement and Transplantation Network (OPTN), as a public-private national nonprofit organization with expertise in organ transplantation and procurement. The OPTN is composed by all organ procurement organizations (OPO) and transplant centers nationwide, voluntary health organizations, and the general public. The immediate task upon creation of the OPTN was to establish a national list of individuals who need organ transplantation and to institute a national system to match organs and individuals included on the list. The United Network for Organ Sharing (UNOS) was incorporated as an independent, nonprofit organization in March 1984. UNOS has served as the OPTN since 1986, after receiving the initial contract to develop the requirements for the operation of the OPTN.

Before 1997, patients with end-stage liver disease were listed for LT by UNOS in each local OPO and were categorized mainly by their inpatient status. Patients requiring hospitalization in an intensive care unit (ICU) were given top priority, followed by hospitalized non-ICU patients, and finally ambulatory patients. Each category was then composed of a large number of patients, which were ranked among them by the waiting time accrued since the day they were placed on the LT waiting list. Therefore, the waiting list time became the most important variable defining priority for LT. Timely referral became fundamental for a patient's chance to receive LT. However, waiting time was a variable completely unrelated to the severity of the underlying liver disease. Patients referred for listing early in their natural history of disease for LT, particularly those with well-compensated cirrhosis, had the advantage of lower mortality risk, which allow them to accrue time on the LT list, compared to sicker patients with decompensated cirrhosis, who carried a higher mortality risk, which did not allow them to survive until an organ could be available. Patients with advanced cirrhosis required staying in the ICU or inpatient hospital status in order to get a reasonable chance of undergoing LT, which was an issue of contention at that time. Accumulating time on the waiting list was the critical measure to receive higher priority for LT at that time.

THE FIRST IMPROVEMENT: CREATION OF THE UNOS STATUS CLASSIFICATION

Child and Turcotte[2] described in 1964 the first classification system for the prediction of survival among patients with cirrhosis complicated by variceal bleeding undergoing portosystemic shunt surgery, which was based on 3 clinical variables: ascites, hepatic encephalopathy, and nutritional status, plus 2 laboratory values: serum bilirubin and albumin. This classification divided patients with cirrhosis into 3 categories, based on their mortality risk for major surgery. In 1973, Pugh and colleagues[3] modified the original Child-Turcotte classification, assigning a score ranging from 1 to 3 to each of the 5 variables and replacing nutritional status by prothrombin time (PT). The modified score was renamed the Child-Turcotte-Pugh (CTP) score. The CTP score was calculated by UNOS based on the severity of ascites, hepatic encephalopathy, PT/international normalized ratio (INR), serum bilirubin, and albumin. Although the CTP score was never prospectively validated, several subsequent studies demonstrated that the CTP score is useful in the prediction of survival among patients with cirrhosis.[4,5]

OPTN/UNOS modified the organ allocation criteria for LT in 1997. Each LT candidate was assigned a status code, corresponding to the degree of medical urgency. For the first time in solid organ transplantation, a medical scoring system to assess disease severity, the CTP score, was incorporated in the definition of these categories.

Therefore, LT candidates were classified into 4 mutually exclusive categories for organ allocation, which were called UNOS status 1, 2A, 2B, and 3 in decreasing order of transplant priority. This classification system was based on the patient's hospital inpatient status, CTP score, and the presence of complications of end-stage liver disease. The highest priority group (status 1) comprised the small number of patients diagnosed with fulminant liver failure, and imminent risk of death without urgent LT. This category included also acute decompensated Wilson disease and primary graft nonfunction or acute hepatic artery thrombosis diagnosed within 7 days of LT. Status 2A patients required a CTP score ≥10 (Child-Pugh class C), ICU stay, life expectancy without LT of less than 7 days, in addition to the presence of at least one of the following complications of cirrhosis: documented unresponsive active variceal hemorrhage, hepatorenal syndrome, severe hepatic encephalopathy (stage III-IV), refractory ascites, or hepatic hydrothorax. Status 2B required a CTP score ≥10 (Child-Pugh class C), or CTP ≥7 (Child-Pugh class B or C), plus the presence of at least one of the following complications of cirrhosis: documented unresponsive active variceal hemorrhage, hepatorenal syndrome, spontaneous bacterial peritonitis, refractory ascites, or hepatic hydrothorax. Status 3 patients required a CTP score ≥7 (Child-Pugh class B or C), under continuous medical care.[6]

REDEFINING PRIORITY FOR TRANSPLANTATION: THE FINAL RULE

The 1997 UNOS status classification for transplant priority, although an improvement, was neglecting patients with decompensated cirrhosis who were not requiring ICU care. Several drawbacks were identified with the use of the CTP score, including the fact that relied on subjective data to assess the severity of hepatic encephalopathy and ascites. The most critical issue was the fact that within each status category the tiebreaker for priority was still time on the waiting list, rather than the numerical CTP score.

Inequities were still perceived despite the OPTN/UNOS improvements in organ allocation.[7] Geographic disparities were not affected by the changes implemented. The standard practice of retaining organs within each OPO, the variable efficiency among different OPOs to identify and properly consent potential donors, and the significant variation in the size of different OPOs were the most important factors contributing to these inequalities. Within certain large OPOs, there was competition among different transplant centers for a limited organ supply, whereas in smaller OPOs, a single center could get LT for patients with well compensated cirrhosis with a shorter waiting time.

The principles of organ allocation policies and procedures were redefined by the Final Rule on the OPTN, published in April of 1998 by the US Department of Health and Human Services with the goal to "assure that allocation of scarce organs be based on common medical criteria, not accidents of geography."[8] This document emphasized the concept of organ allocation among transplant candidates defined by medical urgency, while minimizing the role of waiting list time. It also recorded the ultimate goal of equalizing waiting times among different areas of the country. Most importantly, the Final Rule outlined solid principles for organ allocation, but did not issue any specific guidelines for their implementation. The Final Rule faced initial resistance by the transplant community, particularly concerned about potential limitation of access to transplantation, closure of small transplant programs, and decrease in organ donation. In October 1998, the US Congress suspended the implementation of the Final Rule. The Institute of Medicine (IOM) was invited to examine the national organ allocation policies and establish the impact of the Final Rule on solid organ transplantation.

The report of the IOM Committee on Organ Procurement and Transplantation was published in 1999 and recommended the discontinuation of the use of waiting list time for organ allocation, particularly for patients listed as status 2B and 3. The IOM suggested also the development of an objective scoring system based on medical characteristics for disease prognosis, which could provide a more equitable allocation of organs. In addition, the IOM suggested the establishment of uniform organ allocation areas, defined by a population base of more than 9 million people, in order to eliminate geographic disparities.[9]

A MATHEMATICAL FORMULA HELP SOLVING THE LIVER ALLOCATION PROBLEM

The Mayo End-Stage Liver Disease model was originally derived from a cohort of patients with cirrhosis as a tool to predict short-term survival (3 months) after undergoing transjugular intrahepatic portosystemic shunt (TIPS).[10] Its original name reflected the affiliation of the investigators that developed this mathematical model. The formula used for calculation required the addition of the logarithmic expression of 3 laboratory values: serum creatinine, bilirubin, and INR, which reflect the degree of liver dysfunction, and the underlying cause of chronic liver disease for additional adjustment.

Later on, the same group of investigators modified and renamed the scoring as the "Model for End-Stage Liver Disease" (MELD), and the cause of liver disease was excluded from the calculation. The MELD score, as it was called, was validated as an accurate predictor of short-term survival in ambulatory patients with cirrhosis, with or without cholestasis, hospitalized patients with cirrhosis, and in a historical cohort of patients diagnosed with cirrhosis a decade earlier.[11] The presence of cirrhosis complications, including ascites, hepatic encephalopathy, variceal bleeding, and spontaneous bacterial peritonitis, did not affect the predictive value of the MELD score.[12]

The validity of the MELD model was determined using the c-statistic or concordance statistic, which is commonly used in evaluating prognostic models. The c-statistic ranges from 0 to 1, with a value of 1 corresponding to perfect discrimination, whereas 0.5 would be the result of chance alone. A c-statistic of 0.8 to 0.9 indicates excellent accuracy, whereas a c-statistic of 0.7 indicates a useful test model.[13] Numerous studies published later have confirmed the superiority of the MELD score compared with the CTP score predicting short-term mortality, including patients with end-stage liver disease listed for transplantation.[14–16] Several other retrospective cohorts have at least demonstrated comparable value of MELD and CTP scores for the prediction of short-term mortality in cirrhosis.[17–19]

One of the advantages of the MELD model is the fact that relies merely on objective laboratory parameters, which are measured in a continuous scale. These laboratory values are easily available and reproducible. Most importantly, its main strength lies in its validity as a mathematical model to predict mortality in patients with cirrhosis. The MELD score became the best option available for the determination of disease severity in order to allocate donor organs to the sickest patient first.

OPTN/UNOS modified for the second time the system of organ allocation for LT, in order to fulfill the Final Rule recommendation. The MELD score replaced the CTP-based organ-sharing system starting on February 27, 2002. The status 1 category was maintained, retaining top priority for patients with acute liver failure. The policy change by OPTN/UNOS required several adjustments regarding the MELD calculation. The upper limit of serum creatinine was capped at 4 mg/dL, particularly for patients on chronic hemodialysis, and the lower limit for serum creatinine, bilirubin, and INR were fixed at 1, to avoid negative values in the formula. In its final UNOS version, the MELD score ranged between 6 and 40.

LIVER ORGAN ALLOCATION IMPROVES WITH THE MELD IMPLEMENTATION

Within 1 year after the MELD score was implemented, there was a 12% reduction in the number of new LT candidate registrations in the UNOS Database, mainly among candidates with MELD score less than 10.[20] Likewise, there was a 10.2% increase in the rate of cadaveric LT, which was attributable to an increase in organ availability and also to the effect of MELD implementation, and the median time to transplantation was reduced by more than 200 days.[21] Most notably, the use of the MELD score for organ allocation led to an almost 3.5% reduction of the mortality in the waiting list, likely related to better prediction of short-term mortality in the patients listed for LT when compared with the pre-MELD era.[22] This reduction of mortality happened only among patients with chronic liver disease, but not among patients with acute liver failure, a group not affected by the MELD implementation.[23] Recent data have corroborated the described original observations, showing that 5 years after MELD-based allocation, the number of LT candidates has decreased by 3.4%, whereas the annual dropout rate has remained stable, and a higher proportion of candidates underwent transplantation within 30 days of listing.[24] Therefore, the MELD-based allocation system has been a fundamental change leading to more rational use of cadaveric organs in the United States.

One of the main criticisms at the time of MELD implementation was the fact that the new allocation system, which provided LT priority to patients with a high risk of mortality without transplantation, could result in higher post-LT mortality. However, data collected early after implementation revealed that despite an increase in the average MELD from 17 to 21 at the time of transplantation, the 1-year patient and graft survival remained stable.[20,24] Moreover, data collected 5 years after the MELD system for allocation was approved showed improvement in the adjusted 1-year patient and graft survival, from 1998 to 2007.[24,25]

The change in the MELD score over time (ΔMELD) was proposed as a tiebreaker for patients in the LT waiting list with identical MELD scores. In a retrospective series, the ΔMELD was a better predictor of mortality than the baseline MELD.[26] A larger retrospective study found that current MELD provides better prediction of mortality than the ΔMELD.[27] This later study confirmed that ΔMELD may just capture the dying process among the sicker patients that get frequent MELD assessments before death. Likewise, it contributed indirectly to validate the role of serial MELD score measurements to reassess liver disease severity after patient is listed for LT.

IMPROVING THE PREDICTION OF SURVIVAL WITH ADDING SODIUM TO THE CALCULATION

Hypervolemic hyponatremia is a complication of decompensated cirrhosis, characterized by a low serum sodium concentration in patients with an expanded extracellular volume, commonly with ascites. The pathophysiology of the hyponatremia is related to increased secretion of antidiuretic hormone (ADH), as a compensatory mechanism to the circulatory dysfunction present in cirrhosis. ADH causes impairment of solute-free water excretion in the renal collecting tube. Hyponatremia has long been associated with late complications of decompensated cirrhosis, including refractory ascites and hepatorenal syndrome.[28,29] In a recent prospective study, a prevalence of serum sodium level ≤130 mEq/L or ≤125 mEq/L has been described in 21.6% and 5.7% of patients with cirrhosis, respectively.[29]

The first report of a relative weakness of the MELD score as predictor of mortality was identified early after its implementation, showing limited prognostic accuracy among cirrhotic patients with ascites and low serum sodium concentration.[30] Subsequently, a single-center retrospective study showed that serum sodium less than 126 mEq/L at listing or while listed for LT was a strong independent predictor of mortality.[31] The addition of serum sodium to the MELD improved its predictive accuracy, particularly for patients with low MELD scores.[30–32]

The first mathematical score incorporating sodium into the MELD formula was developed from a database of patients with end-stage liver disease listed for LT at 6 US transplant centers.[33] This model for end-stage liver disease-sodium (MELD-Na) score modified the MELD formula only among patients with serum sodium between 120 and 135 mEq/L. An MELD-Na score of 20, 30, and 40 was associated with 6%, 16%, and 37% risk of death within 6 months of transplant listing, respectively. The MELD-Na showed better correlation with 6-month mortality than MELD score and affected 27% of patients listed for LT. A validation of the MELD-Na score in a large cohort of Chinese patients with hepatitis B cirrhosis was later published, showing better prediction of mortality compared with MELD score.[34] Another retrospective study found that MELD and serum sodium were strong independent predictors of mortality at 3 and 12 months among LT candidates with end-stage liver disease.[35] A reduction of 1 mEq/L of the serum sodium less than 135 was associated with a 12% decrease in 3-month survival. In the same study, the MELD-Na score was found to be similar to MELD at the prediction of 3- and 12-month survival, but the sample size of the study was not large enough to test the superiority of the MELD-Na.

Other models incorporating serum sodium have been proposed as alternatives to the MELD score. The Model for End-Stage Liver Disease to Sodium (MESO) index was developed in Taiwan to predict 3-month mortality and has limited use.[36] The integrated MELD score (iMELD), a European variation of the MELD formula, which integrates serum sodium and age of the recipient, was also proposed for the prediction of 12-month survival after TIPS placement.[37] The United Kingdom has incorporated a formula including sodium for organ allocation, labeled as the UK End-Stage Liver Disease model (UKELD), which includes INR, serum creatinine, bilirubin, and sodium for calculation.[38] The UKELD score was developed and validated in a prospective cohort of patients listed for LT in the UK, showing better prediction value than MELD and MELD-Na.[39] A UKELD score of greater than 49 predicts a greater than 9% 1-year mortality, which is considered the minimum criteria for listing in the UK.

The OPTN/UNOS database was used to measure the effect of MELD and serum sodium as predictors of mortality among US patients on a waiting list for LT. As a result, the formula for the calculation of MELD-Na was modified and validated as a multivariate survival model to predict mortality at 90 days after registration.[40] A 7% reduction in waiting-list mortality could have been achieved using the new version of the MELD-Na score. This study confirmed in a large population the importance of MELD and serum sodium as predictors of survival among LT candidates. The new version of the MELD-Na score has also performed better as predictor of 6-month survival than MELD in a single-center retrospective series of patients with cirrhosis that underwent TIPS.[41]

Since the MELD was implemented in 2002, the proportion of LT candidates with serum creatinine ≥ 2.0 mg/dL increased from 7.9% in April 1999 to 10% in December 2004.[42] Similarly, the number of simultaneous liver kidney transplants also increased from 2.6% in 2001 to 5.2% in 2004. Based on the UNOS data collected from the Scientific Registry of Transplant Recipients (SRTR), a group of investigators from the University of Michigan proposed an update on the original MELD formula as a way to mitigate the relative contribution of the serum creatinine in the MELD calculation. This updated MELD (uMELD) assigned a lower weight to creatinine and INR and increased the weight to bilirubin. The uMELD predicted better than MELD waiting list mortality.[43] More recently, another model was developed and validated based on UNOS data that include updated coefficients and amended upper and lower limit bounds and included serum sodium.[44] This new score was labeled as Refit MELD-Na, had a modest but significant gain in discrimination, and could affect up to 12% of patients.

Three new MELD models, the MELD-Na, iMELD, and MESO, were compared against MELD for prediction of survival in a Chinese cohort of patients with cirrhosis. The MELD-Na and iMELD were superior for prediction of 3- and 6-month mortality.[45] Similarly, a single-center Italian cohort was used to compare 6 different versions of MELD, showing the iMELD and MELD-Na both were superior to MELD, modified CTP, UKELD, and uMELD.[46] In a single-center experience from China, the new version of the MELD-Na and CTP were superior to MELD for prediction of 90-day mortality in candidates for surgery.[47] In a Brazilian single-center study, the iMELD and new version of the MELD-Na were superior to MELD for estimation of 3- and 6-month mortality.[48,49]

OPTN/UNOS approved the addition of sodium into the MELD score calculation starting on January 2016, using a modified version of the MELD-Na formula for any patient with an initial MELD greater than 11. The formula increases the MELD score for patients with serum sodium below 137 mEq/dL. Patients with sodium below 125 mEq/dL do not get any additional MELD increase.

ADDRESSING GEOGRAPHIC DISPARITIES: DISTRIBUTION OF ORGANS

The MELD implementation had no significant effect on the geographic disparities regarding organ allocation, which were previously identified by the IOM report. The average MELD at time of transplantation is quite variable depending on the specific UNOS region.[50] Similarly, within each UNOS region, there exists variability between the donor service areas (DSA) that conform a specific region. There is a 10-point range in average MELD score at time of transplantation, among different DSAs within the United States.[51] The risk of death for patients listed for LT is higher in 2 specific UNOS regions, after controlling for the effect of MELD score.[50] Different referral patterns for transplantation and regional variations in the medical care of the patients may be responsible for this observed variability.

In the first 2 years after MELD implementation, 24% of LT recipients were listed with an MELD score less than 15 just before transplantation.[50] Retrospective data analysis of the SRTR database showed a higher post-LT mortality among recipients listed with MELD less than 15 just before LT, compared with the mortality without LT for candidates with MELD less than 15 that remained on the LT list.[52] This finding challenged the concept of expected survival benefit offered by LT. Moreover, almost 20% of LT were performed in candidates with an MELD of less than 15 at that time. Subsequently, in 2005, OPTN/UNOS implemented the "Regional Share 15" policy to restrict LT for local candidates within a specific DSA with MELD less than 15, who become only eligible for LT after all candidates with MELD ≥15 within the corresponding UNOS region have been exhausted.

UNOS region 1 adopted a policy of region-wide sharing of cadaveric livers for UNOS status 1 recipients, achieving lower mortality risk while waiting for a transplant and with a shorter waiting time to transplantation.[53] As a result, in December 2010, OPTN/UNOS implemented full regional sharing of adult donor livers for all status 1A and status 1B patients in order to maximize organ offers for the sickest patients on the LT list.

The most recent changes in the distribution of organs were applied by OPTN/UNOS on June 2013. The first modification has been an extension of the regional sharing of organs to a national level, for candidates with an MELD score of at least 15 (National Share 15). The second change in distribution policy has been the regional sharing of livers for candidates with an MELD score of at least 35 (Share 35). One year after the change in allocation policy, the median waiting time for candidates with a MELD score of at least 35 decreased dramatically from 14 months in 2012 to 1.4 months in 2013.[54] Two years after the approval of Share 35 policy, a greater percentage of patients with MELD ≥35 underwent LT, without change in overall cold ischemia time.[55]

MODEL FOR END-STAGE LIVER DISEASE EXCEPTIONS: THE CASE FOR HEPATOCELLULAR CARCINOMA

The most significant limitation of the MELD score system has been its inability to properly prioritize for transplantation patients with the concomitant diagnosis of HCC. The candidates with HCC commonly have relatively low MELD scores at time of diagnosis, that underestimate their urgency for transplantation before progression of tumor beyond that amenable to LT.

At the same time of MELD implementation in 2002, an MELD exception system was also designed for patients carrying the diagnosis of HCC. The patients with HCC stage I or II were entitled to MELD exception points. Strict size criteria (Milan criteria) based on available literature were used, which included either a single lesion less than 5 cm in maximum diameter or up to 3 lesions with a maximum diameter of any lesion of 3 cm.[56] Stage I tumors (<2 cm size) were granted an MELD score of 24, and stage II lesions were granted an MELD score of 29. An increase in MELD was granted every 3 months, provided tumor remains within Milan criteria for LT. With the original MELD exception system, HCC patients had better access to the LT donor pool compared with non-HCC patients as evidenced by their lower dropout from the waiting list.[57] Several modifications to the original MELD score exception assigned to HCC patients were issued in order to reduce this advantage. In April 2003, OPTN/UNOS reduced the inital MELD scores for exception to 20 for stage I HCC, and 24 for stage II HCC. The MELD exception priority for stage I lesions was later on eliminated in 2004.[58] The initial MELD exception score for stage II HCC was reduced to 22 in March 2005.

Analysis of the SRTR database in 2008 showed that after the MELD allocation system was approved, there was a 6-fold increase in the proportion of patients undergoing LT with HCC. Poor survival after LT was associated with high α-fetoprotein, large tumors (≥3 cm), or MELD ≥20.[59] The most recent changes to the MELD exception system for HCC have included delaying the MELD exception score of 22 to be applied 6 months after listing and to incorporate a capping MELD of 34.[60]

MODEL FOR END-STAGE LIVER DISEASE EXCEPTION: PULMONARY COMPLICATIONS OF CIRRHOSIS

OPTN/UNOS grants MELD exceptions to LT candidates with cirrhosis and pulmonary complications carrying a higher risk of mortality, not accounted for by the MELD formula. The 2 recognized pulmonary complications are hepatopulmonary syndrome (HPS) and portopulmonary hypertension (POPH). In the case of HPS, the presence of clinical evidence of pulmonary hypertension, documentation of intrapulmonary shunt, and a partial pressure of oxygen in arterial blood (Pao_2) of ≤60 mm Hg are required for MELD exception, in the absence of clinical evidence of underlying primary pulmonary disease. Then, HPS patients get an MELD score of 22 (equivalent to 15% 3-month mortality) assigned upon application, with allowance for an increase in MELD points equivalent to 10% increase in mortality every 3 months, provided Pao_2 remains less than 60 mm Hg. For POPH, the basic requirement is the documentation of initial mean pulmonary artery pressure (MPAP) $\geq$35 mm Hg, transpulmonary gradient of 12 mm Hg, and pulmonary vascular resistance (PVR) >400 dyn/s/cm^{-5}, which are consistent with at least moderate pulmonary hypertension. However, upon initiation of medical therapy for pulmonary hypertension, the MPAP must be reduced to less than 35 mm Hg and PVR less than 400 dyn/s/cm^{-5}. POPH patients meeting the above-mentioned criteria get an MELD score of 22 (equivalent to 15% 3-month mortality) assigned upon application, with allowance for an increase in MELD points equivalent to 10% mortality every 3 months, provided MPAP remains less than 35 mm Hg and PVR less than 400 dyn/s/cm^{-5}.

OTHER MODEL FOR END-STAGE LIVER DISEASE EXCEPTIONS

Rare metabolic conditions, which benefit from LT, are also eligible for MELD exception by OPTN/UNOS, because intrinsic MELD would never increase due to the underlying disease, which has no effect on the intrinsic function of the liver. These conditions include familial amyloid polyneuropathy, cystic fibrosis, and primary hyperoxaluria. The requirement for MELD exception for each condition is disease specific and out of the scope of this review. The diagnosis of hilar cholangiocarcinoma could be eligible for MELD exception, but requires each transplant center to get a written protocol for patient care submitted to the Liver and Intestinal Organ Transplantation Committee, including patient selection criteria, administration of neoadjuvant therapy before LT, operative staging to exclude regional lymph node involvement, and peritoneal metastases. A malignant-appearing biliary stricture on cholangiography is required plus one of the following: carbohydrate antigen 19-9 greater than 100 U/mL, or biopsy or cytology showing malignancy and/or aneuploidy. If any mass is identified by cross-sectional imaging study should be less than 3 cm in diameter, the patient must be considered surgically unresectable either due to technical reasons or severity of liver disease.

OPTN/UNOS has also provided guidance, which can be used by regional review boards for MELD exception in patients with neuroendocrine tumors, polycystic liver disease, and primary sclerosing cholangitis. However, these MELD exceptions are not considered standard OPTN policy, and therefore, are not mandatory.

SUMMARY

The criteria used for prioritization of LT in the United States have evolved over time. The concept of favoring LT for the patients with the highest risk of mortality due to liver disease has been the widely accepted criteria. The greatest change in the liver allocation system has been the adoption of the MELD scoring system as a surrogate marker of the severity of chronic liver disease. Following the implementation of MELD score for organ allocation by OPTN/UNOS, waiting time has lost significance as a factor affecting prioritization. The MELD score calculation was later modified to reflect the contribution of hyponatremia in the estimation of the mortality risk. The MELD score does not capture accurately the risk of mortality while waiting for LT for specific conditions, particularly for HCC. Therefore, the arbitrary assignment of MELD points has been used, with adjustments made over time to avoid the preferential prioritization for HCC patients.

REFERENCES

1. Starzl TE, Marchioro TL, Vonkaulla KN, et al. Homotransplantation of the liver in humans. Surg Gynecol Obstet 1963;117:659–76.
2. Child GC II, Turcotte JG. Surgery and portal hypertension. In: Child GC II, editor. The liver and portal hypertension. Philadelphia: Saunders; 1964. p. 50–8.
3. Pugh RN, Murray-Lyon IM, Dawson JL, et al. Transection of the oesophagus for bleeding esophageal varices. Br J Surg 1973;60:646–9.
4. Christensen E, Schlichting P, Fauerholdt L, et al. Prognostic value of Child-Turcotte criteria in medically treated cirrhosis. Hepatology 1984;4:430–5.
5. Infante-Rivard C, Esnaola S, Villeneuve JP. Clinical and statistical validity of conventional prognostic factors in predicting short-term survival among cirrhotics. Hepatology 1987;7:660–4.
6. Lucey MR, Brown KA, Everson GT, et al. Minimal criteria for placement of adults on the liver transplant waiting list: a report of a national conference organized by the American Society of Transplant Physicians and the American Association for the Study of Liver Diseases. Liver Transpl Surg 1997;3:628–37.
7. Freeman R, Edwards E. Liver transplant waiting time does not correlated with waiting time list mortality. Liver Transpl 2000;6:543–52.
8. U.S. Department of Health and Human Services. Organ Procurement and Transplantation Network-HRSA. Final Rule. Fed Regist 1998;63:635–44.
9. Institute of Medicine. Organ Procurement and Transplantation: assessing current policies and the potential imapct of the DHHS Final Rule. Washington, DC: The National Academies Press; 1999.
10. Malinchoc M, Kamath PS, Gordon FD, et al. A model to predict poor survival in patients undergoing transjugular intrahepatic portosystemic shunts. Hepatology 2000;31:864–71.
11. Kamath PS, Wiesner RH, Malinchoc M, et al. A model to predict survival in patients with end-stage liver disease. Hepatology 2001;33:464–70.
12. Botta F, Giannini E, Romagnoli P, et al. MELD scoring system is useful for predicting prognosis in patients with liver cirrhosis and is correlated with residual liver function: a European study. Gut 2003;52:134–9.
13. Hanley JA, McNeil BJ. A method of comparing the areas under receiving operating characteristic curves derived from the same cases. Radiology 1983;148: 839–43.
14. Wiesner R, Edwards E, Freeman R, et al. Model for end-stage liver disease (MELD) and allocation of donor livers. Gastroenterology 2003;124:91–6.
15. Huo TI, Wu JC, Lin HC, et al. Evaluation of the increase in model for end-stage liver disease (DeltaMELD) score over time as a prognostic predictor in patients with advanced cirrhosis: risk factor analysis and comparison with initial MELD and Child-Turcotte-Pugh score. J Hepatol 2005;42:826–32.
16. Salerno F, Merli M, Cazzaniga M, et al. MELD score is better than Child-Pugh score in predicting 3-month survival of patients undergoing transjugular intrahepatic portosystemic shunt. J Hepatol 2002;36:494–500.
17. Said A, Williams J, Holden J, et al. Model for end stage liver disease score predicts mortality across a broad spectrum of liver disease. J Hepatol 2004;40: 897–903.
18. Angermayr B, Cejna M, Karnel F, et al. Child-Pugh versus MELD score in predicting survival in patients undergoing transjugular intrahepatic portosystemic shunt. Gut 2003;52:879–85.

19. Schepke M, Roth F, Fimmers R, et al. Comparison of MELD, Child-Pugh and Emory model for the prediction of survival in patients undergoing transjugular intrahepatic portosystemic shunt. Am J Gastroenterol 2003;98:1167–74.

20. Freeman RB, Wiesner RH, Edwards E, et al. Results of the first year of the new liver allocation plan. Liver Transpl 2004;10:7–15.

21. Wiesner R, Lake JR, Freeman RB, et al. Model for end-stage liver disease (MELD) exception guidelines. Liver Transpl 2006;12:S85–8.

22. Brown RS, Rush SH, Rosen HR, et al. Liver and intestine transplantation. Am J Transplant 2004;4(Suppl9):81–92.

23. Freeman RB, Harper A, Edwards EB. Excellent liver transplant survival rates under the MELD/PELD system. Transplant Proc 2005;37:585–8.

24. Tuluvath PJ, Guidinger MK, Funk JJ, et al. Liver transplantation in the United States, 1999-2008. Am J Transplant 2010;10:1003–19.

25. Kanwal F, Dulai GS, Spiegel BM, et al. A comparison of liver transplantation outcomes in the pre- vs. post-MELD eras. Aliment Pharmacol Ther 2005;21:169–77.

26. Merion RM, Wolfe RA, Dykstra DM, et al. Longitudinal assessment of mortality risk among candidates for liver transplantation. Liver Transpl 2003;9:12–8.

27. Bambha K, Kim WR, Kremers WK, et al. Predicting survival among patients listed for liver transplantation: an assessment of serial MELD measurements. Am J Transplant 2004;4:1798–804.

28. Arroyo V, Rodés J, Gutierrez-Lizárraga MA, et al. Prognostic value of spontaneous hyponatremia in cirrhosis with ascites. Am J Dig Dis 1976;21:249–56.

29. Angeli P, Wong F, Watson H, et al. Hyponatremia in cirrhosis: results of a patient population survey. Hepatology 2006;44:1532–42.

30. Heuman DM, Abou-Assi SG, Habib A, et al. Persistent ascites and low serum sodium identify patients with cirrhosis and low MELD scores who are at high risk for early death. Hepatology 2004;40:802–10.

31. Biggins SW, Rodriguez HJ, Bacchetti P, et al. Serum sodium predicts mortality in patients listed for liver transplantation. Hepatology 2005;41:32–9.

32. Ruf AE, Kremers WK, Chavez LL, et al. Addition of serum sodium into the MELD score predicts waiting list mortality better than MELD alone. Liver Transpl 2005; 11:336–43.

33. Biggins SW, Kim WR, Terrault NA, et al. Evidence-based incorporation of serum sodium concentration into MELD. Gastroenterology 2006;130:1652–60.

34. Wong VW, Chim AM, Wong GL, et al. Performance of the new MELD-Na score in predicting 3-month and 1-year mortality in Chinese patients with chronic hepatitis B. Liver Transpl 2007;13:1228–35.

35. Londoño MC, Cárdenas A, Guevara M, et al. MELD score and serum sodium in the prediction of survival of patients with cirrhosis awaiting liver transplantation. Gut 2007;56:1283–90.

36. Huo TI, Wang YW, Yang YY, et al. Model for end-stage liver disease score to serum sodium ratio index as a prognostic predictor and its correlation with portal pressure in patients with liver cirrhosis. Liver Int 2007;27:498–506.

37. Luca A, Angermayr B, Bertolini G, et al. An integrated MELD model including serum sodium and age improves the prediction of early mortality in patients with cirrhosis. Liver Transpl 2007;13:1174–80.

38. Neuberger J, Gimson A, Davies M, et al. Selection of patients for liver transplantation and allocation of donated livers in the UK. Gut 2008;57:252–7.

39. Barber K, Madden S, Allen J, et al. Elective liver transplant list mortality: development of a United Kingdom end-stage liver disease score. Transplantation 2011; 92:469–76.

40. Kim WR, Biggins SW, Kremers WK, et al. Hyponatremia and mortality among patients on the liver-transplant waiting list. N Engl J Med 2008;359:1018–26.
41. Guy J, Sumsouk M, Shiboski S, et al. New model for end-stage liver disease improves prognostic capability, after transjugular intrahepatic portosystemic shunt. Clin Gastroenterol Hepatol 2009;7:1236–40.
42. Gonwa TA, McBride MA, Anderson K, et al. Continued influence of preoperative renal function on outcome of orthotopic liver transplant (OLTX) in the US: where will MELD lead us? Am J Transplant 2006;6:2651–9.
43. Sharma P, Schaubel DE, Sima CS, et al. Re-weighting the model for end stage liver disease score components. Gastroenterology 2008;135:1575–81.
44. Leise MD, Kim WR, Kremers WK, et al. A revised model for end-stage liver disease prediction of mortality among patients awaiting liver transplantation. Gastroenterology 2011;140:1952–60.
45. Biggins SW. Use of serum sodium for liver transplant graft allocation: a decade in the making, now is it ready for primetime? Liver Transpl 2015;21:279–81.
46. Huo TI, Lin HC, Hus SC, et al. Comparison of four model for end-stage liver disease-based prognostic systems for cirrhosis. Liver Transpl 2008;14:837–44.
47. Biselli M, Gitto S, Gramenzi A, et al. Six score systems to evaluate candidates with advanced cirrhosis for orthotopic liver transplant: which is the winner? Liver Transpl 2010;16:964–73.
48. Cho HC, Jung NY, Sinn DH, et al. Mortality after surgery in patients with liver cirrhosis: comparison of Child-Turcotte-Pugh score, MELD and MELDNa score. Eur J Gastroenterol Hepatol 2011;23:51–9.
49. Marroni CP, de Mello Brandão AB, Hennigen AW, et al. MELD scores with incorporation of serum sodium and death prediction in cirrhotic patients on the waiting list for liver transplantation: a single center experience in Southern Brazil. Clin Transplant 2012;26:E395–401.
50. Roberts JP, Dykstra DM, Goodrich NP, et al. Geographic differences in event rates by model for end-stage liver disease risk. Am J Transplant 2006;6:2470–5.
51. Yeh H, Smoot E, Schoenfeld DA, et al. Geographic inequity in access to liver transplantation. Transplantation 2011;91:479–86.
52. Merion RM, Schaubel DE, Dykstra DM, et al. The survival benefit of liver transplantation. Am J Transplant 2005;5:307–13.
53. Humar A, Khwaja K, Glessing B, et al. Regionwide sharing for status 1 liver patients—beneficial impact on waiting time and pre- and posttransplant survival. Liver Transpl 2004;10:661–5.
54. Kim WR, Lake JR, Smith JM, et al. OPTN/SRTR 2013 annual data report: liver. Am J Transplant 2015;15(Suppl2):1–28.
55. Edwards EB, Harper AM, Hirose R, et al. The impact of broader regional sharing of livers: 2-year results of "Share35". Liver Transpl 2016;22:399–409.
56. Mazzaferro V, Regalia E, Doci R, et al. Liver transplantation for the treatment of small hepatocellular carcinomas in patients with cirrhosis. N Engl J Med 1996;334:693–9.
57. Washburn K, Edwards E, Harper A, et al. Hepatocellular carcinoma patients are advantaged in the current liver transplant allocation system. Am J Transplant 2010;10:1652–7.
58. Pomfret EA, Washburn K, Wald C, et al. Report of a national conference on liver allocation in patients with hepatocellular carcinoma in the United States. Liver Transpl 2010;16:262–78.

59. Ioannou GN, Perkins JD, Carithers RL. Liver transplantation for hepatocellular carcinoma: impact of the MELD allocation system and predictors of survival. Gastroenterology 2008;134:1342–51.

60. Heimback JK, Hirose R, Stock PG, et al. Delayed hepatocellular carcinoma model for end-stage liver disease exception improves disparity in access to liver transplant in the United States. Hepatology 2015;61:1643–50.

Extended Criteria Donors in Liver Transplantation

Irine Vodkin, MD*, Alexander Kuo, MD

KEYWORDS

- Extended criteria donor • Liver transplantation • Donation after cardiac death
- Disease transmission • Centers for Disease Control and Prevention high-risk donors

KEY POINTS

- Donor age is associated with inferior transplant outcomes; however, excellent results can be achieved with careful attention to both donor and recipient factors, such as avoiding use of older donors in recipients with hepatitis C virus (HCV), minimizing cold ischemia time (CIT), avoiding use in recipients with high Model for End-Stage Liver Disease (MELD) scores, and avoiding use of donor grafts with greater than 30% steatosis.
- Macrovesicular steatosis greater than 30% is associated with increased graft loss; however, excellent outcomes can be achieved by minimizing CIT to fewer than 8 hours, selecting recipients with lower MELD scores less than 25, and potentially using defatting protocols to recondition donor livers.
- The availability of highly effective, well-tolerated, direct-acting antiviral agents for HCV may make it feasible to consider transplanting livers from HCV+ donors into HCV− recipients in the future.
- Use of DCD livers is associated with higher rates of ischemic cholangiopathy (IC) and graft loss; however, outcomes can be improved with careful recipient selection and possibly with ex vivo machine perfusion of the donor liver.

INTRODUCTION

Mortality rates on the liver transplant waiting list are increasing.[1] The shortage of organs has resulted in higher utilization of extended criteria donors (ECDs), with centers pushing the limits of what is acceptable for transplantation. Donor quality is more appropriately represented as a continuum of risk, and careful selection and matching of ECD grafts with recipients may lead to excellent outcomes.[2] Although there is no precise definition for what constitutes an ECD liver, frequently cited characteristics are listed in **Box 1**. This review focuses discussion on donor age, steatosis, donation after cardiac death (DCD), and donors with increased risk of disease transmission.

Disclosures: The authors have nothing to disclose.
Division of Gastroenterology and Hepatology, University of California, San Diego, 200 West Arbor Drive M/C 8413, San Diego, CA, USA
* Corresponding author.
E-mail address: ivodkin@ucsd.edu

> **Box 1**
> **Definition of extended criteria donors**
>
> Advanced age
>
> Macrovesicular steatosis
>
> DCD
>
> Organ dysfunction at procurement
>   ICU stay greater than 7 days
>   Hypernatremia greater than 165
>   Bilirubin greater than 3
>   Elevated aspartate aminotransferase/alanine aminotransferase
>   Vasopressor use
>
> Cause of death: anoxia, cerebrovascular accident
>
> Disease transmission
>   HBcAb+
>   HBsAg+
>   Hepatitis C virus
>   CDC high-risk donors
>   HIV positive
>   Extrahepatic malignancy
>
> CIT greater than 12 hours

DONOR AGE

Over the past 2 decades, the use of older donors has increased significantly and centers are stretching the limits of donor age. In the United States, 8% of donors were age 65 and older in 2014.[1] A similar trend is observed in Europe, where 29% of donors were older than 60% and 11% of donors were older than 65.[3]

The liver seems to age slowly and changes are not reflected in routine laboratory testing. There is a decline in hepatobiliary function, however, with reduction in hepatic and bile flow and moderate reduction in cytochrome P450 content.[4] On the ultrastructure level, there is pseudocapillarization of the sinusoidal endothelium with thickening and defenestration, which restricts the availability of oxygen and other substances.[5] Telomeres shorten, growth regulatory gene expression is reduced, and the rate of DNA repair is diminished along with a decreased ability to respond to oxidative stress.[6] The hepatocyte volume decreases with fewer larger hepatocytes,[7] which can diminish the mass of functional hepatocytes even when the total organ mass is unchanged.

Changes associated with aging may decrease the regenerative capacity of the transplanted liver and make it more susceptible to ischemia/reperfusion injury, particularly with increasing CIT. The increased prevalence of steatosis in older livers can further delay graft function.[5,8–10] There are also reports of higher rates of hepatic artery thrombosis[11,12] and ischemic-type biliary complications.[13–15] Although there is heterogeneity in the cutoff that defines an older donor (anywhere from over 40 to over 80), numerous studies have shown that older donors are associated with increased mortality and graft loss.[16–20] Feng and colleagues,[21] in defining the donor risk index, found that the relative risk associated with each decade of increasing donor age rose with each decade starting at age 40, with age over 60 the strongest risk factor for graft failure.

Donor age seems to be an even more powerful determinant for graft loss in patients with HCV infection.[20,22,23] Wali and colleagues[24] found a fibrosis rate of 0.6 U/y in recipients with donors younger than 40 compared with 2.7 U/y with donors over age 50. The latter group had a progression to cirrhosis as short as 2.2 years. In a large database study of European liver transplant recipients, Mutimer and colleagues[25] compared the impact of donor age on graft and patient survival for 4736 recipients with HCV-related liver disease and 5406 recipients with alcohol-related liver disease (ALD). Survival was similar for donors younger than age 40. For donors older than 50, HCV recipient survival was significantly inferior to ALD recipient survival. For donors older than 60, recipients with ALD had a 16.7% 5-year graft survival advantage over recipients with HCV.[25] Accordingly, both the International Liver Transplantation Society Expert Panel Consensus conference and the Paris consensus conference advise against the use of older donors, particularly over age 50, in HCV-positive recipients.[2,26]

Although donor age can have a detrimental effect on graft survival and mortality, there is mounting evidence that using older donors, even beyond age 80, can have excellent outcomes.[27–31] Cescon and colleagues[28] achieved a 5-year graft survival rate of 81% with highly selected octogenarian donors when these donor livers were transplanted to recipients with a MELD score of less than 24. Donors were excluded based on strict criteria, including macrovesicular steatosis greater than 30% and arterial wall thickening greater than 60%. Biopsy was relied on significantly in deciding to use these grafts. Kim and colleagues[29] achieved improved 5-year graft survival when eliminating the following risk factors for donors over age 65: HCV and MELD greater than 20 in the recipient, glucose greater than 200 mg/dL at the time of liver recovery, and skin incision to aortic cross-clamp time greater than 40 minutes in the donor surgery. The 5-year graft survival rates for having 0, 1, 2, 3, or 4 risk factors were 100%, 82.0%, 81.7%, 39.3%, and 25.0%, respectively ($P<.05$).[29] In addition to careful donor and recipient selection, minimizing CIT is a key strategy for improving outcomes with older donors. Optimal liver function is achieved by keeping CIT to 8 hours or less.[2,15] Finally, for recipients with HCV, the recent availability of well-tolerated, highly potent, direct-acting antiviral agents to eradicate HCV before and after transplant is changing the established thinking regarding the use of older donors for this population.

DONOR STEATOSIS

Nonalcoholic fatty liver disease (NAFLD) may affect up to 30% of the population in Western countries and up to 70% to 80% of obese individuals.[32,33] Traditional risk factors for NAFLD include obesity, diabetes, hyperlipidemia, and the metabolic syndrome. Already, 1 in 5 Americans has a body mass index above 30 kg/m^2 and this incidence may double by 2025.[34] Other metabolic risk factors are also on the rise, which inevitably reflects on steatosis rates in the pool of both deceased and living donors.

Steatosis lowers mitochondrial membrane potential and causes deterioration in mitochondrial function. Kupffer cell activity is increased and the sinusoidal lining is disrupted and narrowed. These changes enhance cell damage during cold ischemia and potentiate ischemia/reperfusion injury.[35,36] In animal models, defatting protocols can reverse the incidence of hepatocyte damage seen during reperfusion.[35,37] The amount of steatosis can be graded based on histology as mild (<30%), moderate (30%–60%), or severe (>60%). The type of steatosis exerts a differential effect on transplant outcomes. In macrovesicular steatosis, hepatocytes contain a single fat vacuole displacing the nucleus to the periphery of the cell. In microvesicular steatosis, hepatocytes contain numerous, small, fatty inclusions, which do not cause nuclear displacement.[38,39] The latter imparts significantly less risk for reperfusion injury and has not been associated with poor early graft function.[38,40]

Determining the presence and grade of macrosteatosis is a key step in evaluating the suitability of an organ for transplant. The Paris consensus meeting concluded that mild steatosis has minimal impact on post-transplant outcomes as long as CIT is kept short, ideally less than 8 hours.[2] Higher degrees of steatosis have been associated with primary nonfunction, graft failure, early renal failure, and biliary complications.[40–42] In a study using United Network for Organ Sharing (UNOS)/Organ Procurement and Transplantation Network (OPTN) registry data, Spitzer and colleagues[42] found that macrovesicular steatosis is an independent risk factor for graft survival, with recipients of livers with greater than 30% steatosis having a 71% increased adjusted risk of 1-year graft failure ($P = .007$).

Although livers with severe steatosis have generally been discarded, there is growing interest in using increasingly steatotic organs.[43–45] Dutkowski and colleagues[45] found acceptable outcomes using livers with greater than 30% macrosteatosis with a balance of risk score of 9 or less. To achieve such a score, the recipient had to have a MELD less than 25, along with favorable donor and recipient age and low CIT.[45] Chavin and colleagues[44] saw good outcomes with moderate and severe steatosis when they excluded higher-risk donors based on age greater than 60, presence of diabetes, vasopressor use, greater than 48 hours' intensive care unit stay, and elevated liver function tests. Wong and colleagues[43] also had good outcomes in low risk donors with an average MELD of 20 by keeping CIT to approximately 6 hours.

Given the clinical importance of excluding moderate and severe steatosis, studies have evaluated the effectiveness of determining less than 30% steatosis by pretransplant imaging and surgical assessment compared with the gold standard: histologic evaluation by a trained liver pathologist. In a study by Ahn and colleagues[46] of 492 living donors without evidence of steatosis on ultrasound, only 0.8% had moderate and 0% had severe steatosis on liver biopsy. Cucchetti and colleagues[47] found that the combination of body mass index, elevated alanine aminotransferase (ALT), presence of diabetes mellitus type 2, and heavy alcohol use coupled with ultrasonography identified greater than 30% with area under the receiver operating characteristic curve (AUROC) of 0.86 (95% CI, 0.81–0.91). Lee and colleagues[48] used noncontrast CT to determine greater than 30% steatosis in living donors with AUROC of 0.93 (95% CI, 0.82–1.00). Unfortunately, imaging and key historical details may not be available at the time of procurement. Surgeons may suspect significant steatosis based on texture criteria, such as degree of yellow hue when blanched, degree of firmness, blunted edges, and absence of scratch marks. Texture criteria had an accuracy of 86.2% for predicting greater than 30% steatosis, but direct estimation of steatosis percent was less accurate at 75.5%.[49] Histologic assessment is still the best way to determine the actual volume of macrovesicular steatosis. Even this technique is limited, however, by sampling error, freezing artifact (underestimates macrovesicular steatosis compared with permanent section), and expertise of a local pathologist. In a study by Lo and colleagues,[50] local pathologists were able to accurately identify macrovesicular steatosis greater than 20%, but increasing fat content led to more variation. Underestimation of macrovesicular steatosis occurred in only 4% of cases but did affect clinical outcome. On the other hand, using frozen sections and local expertise is likely to limit CIT, which could improve outcomes.

DONORS AFTER CARDIAC DEATH

DCD is based on cardiopulmonary rather than neurologic criteria for death. It currently accounts for 5% to 6% of liver transplants in the United States[1] and up to 20% in the United Kingdom.[51] Such donors have inadequate organ perfusion first during progression to circulatory arrest and subsequently during 5 minutes of pulseless arrest. The period of hypoperfusion from the time of arrest to either cold flush or regional perfusion is termed warm ischemia time (WIT)[52] and represents an additional injury phase inherent to this form of organ donation.

Numerous studies show worse outcomes with DCD donors compared with donors after brain death (DBD).[21,53–57] The most consistently reported complication leading to graft loss in DCD transplantation is ischemic cholangiopathy (IC).[54,57,58] Feng and colleagues[21] found that DCD status was associated with a 51% higher risk of graft failure compared with DBD. In a OPTN/UNOS study, Uemura and colleagues[55] showed significantly worse 1-year and 5-year graft survival rates in 1164 non–HCV-infected recipients of DCD versus DBD organs. In a meta-analysis of 11 studies with 489 DCD donors, Jay and colleagues[59] found higher odds of 1-year patient mortality (OR 1.6; 95% CI, 1.04–2.5) and graft failure (OR 2.1; 95% CI, 1.5–2.8) for recipients of DCD versus DBD organs.

Despite these results, excellent outcomes with DCD grafts are possible with risk modification. In a database study of 1567 DCD donors, Mathur and colleagues[60] identified WIT greater than or equal to 35 minutes and donor age greater than or equal to 50 as risks for graft failure. Each hour increase in CIT was associated with 6% higher graft failure rate (hazard ratio [HR] 1.06; $P<.001$). A large single-center study by de Vera and colleagues[57] found that WIT greater than 20 minutes, CIT greater than 8 hours, and donor age greater than 60 were associated with poorer outcomes. Chan and colleagues[58] found that CIT greater than or equal to 9 hours and donor age greater than 50 predicted IC. Both studies, by Mathur and colleagues[60] and Chan and colleagues,[58] found that donor weight greater than 100 kg predicted worse outcomes.[58,60] It is hypothesized that high donor weight may be associated with inadequate flushing of smaller arterioles with preservation solution, thus leading to more IC. Recipients who seem to benefit most from DCD donors have a MELD at least greater than 20 or have HCC without MELD exception points.[57,59] There have been mixed results in recipients with HCV, with some studies showing worse outcomes[53,60,61] and more rapid HCV recurrence.[62] Some investigators, however, have shown comparable survival in HCV recipients with DCD versus DBD grafts,[63,64] with improvement in outcomes particularly in recent years.[55]

Centers that have implemented strict donor and recipient selection criteria report decreased rates of biliary complications and both graft and patient survival comparable to those seen in DBD donors.[61,65,66] There is also interest in improving the viability of both DCD and steatotic grafts through ex vivo machine perfusion. Hypothermia during static cold storage causes sinusoidal constriction. Machine perfusion circuits are able to maintain continuous circulation, thereby allowing the preservation solution better penetration into the microcirculation.[67] The optimal circuit, duration, and temperature of the preservation solutions are still being determined.[67–69]

CENTERS FOR DISEASE CONTROL AND PREVENTION HIGH-RISK DONORS

The prevalence rates of human immunodeficiency virus (HIV) and HCV in the general population of donors are 0.1% and 0.5%, respectively. The Centers for Disease Control and Prevention (CDC) identified a set of high-risk behaviors and criteria that may increase the risk of these infections to 3.5% for HIV and 18.2% for HCV.[70,71] Between January 2009 and December 2011, there were 10 HCV transmissions, 4 HBV transmissions, and 1 HIV transmission from solid organ transplants.[72]

Infections can be identified by serologic testing. There can be a significant lag time, however, between infection and the generation of antibodies. Antibodies to HIV may be produced between 2 weeks and 12 weeks after exposure. For HCV, antibodies can be detected 4 weeks and 10 weeks after infection with greater than 97% detection by 6 months.[73] The period between exposure and the generation of antibodies (the window period) can result in unintentional transmission of infection through organ donation, particularly in high-risk groups. Testing aimed at detecting the virus, however, can significantly decrease the window period. As a result, the CDC now recommends HCV nucleic acid testing (NAT) for all decreased donors and HIV NAT for those meeting at least 1 CDC high-risk criterion.[72] In a study estimating the risk of HIV and HCV transmission using potential donor serologic data from 17 organ procurement organizations in the United States, the use of routine NAT testing for HCV was estimated to decrease the risk of HCV transmission in normal risk donors from 1 in 5000 to 1 in 50,000. The risk of HCV transmission in high-risk donors was decreased from 1 in 1000 to 1 in 10,000.[71] Although the routine use of NAT testing for HIV and HCV can decrease the window period and potentially reduce disease transmission, this benefit is somewhat tempered by the possibility of rejecting acceptable donor organs due to false-positive NAT testing.

VIRAL HEPATITIS C

Hepatitis C virus antibody–positive (HCV+) donors made up 3.9% of US donors in 2012.[1] It is estimated that 20% of these donors have cleared the infection and are not viremic[74] but RNA and genotype status are frequently unknown at the time of procurement. Because transplantation of viremic organs guarantees de novo infection, they are transplanted nearly exclusively into HCV viremic recipients.

Survival in HCV+ recipients transplanted with HCV+ compared with HCV– donors seems equivalent.[74–76] Ballarin and colleagues[76] found no statistically significant difference in cumulative 1-year and 5- year survival rates in patients with HCV cirrhosis receiving HCV+ versus HCV– organs. Northup and colleagues[74] found that mean survival in HCV+ recipients was 9.8 years compared with 10.6 years in HCV+ versus HCV– donors. The HR was equivalent for both groups after adjustment for other factors affecting post-transplant survival.

Transplantation with HCV+ donors may lead to more advanced fibrosis, but this seems dependent on certain risk factors. Lai and colleagues[77] evaluated 99 patients with HCV who received HCV+ grafts. HCV+ grafts were older, with higher donor risk index. Transplantation with these grafts was associated with a 58% increased risk of advanced fibrosis (95% CI, 1.05–2.36; $P = .03$). This increased risk of fibrosis was only seen, however, when donors were greater than 45 years old.[77] In the aforementioned study by Ballarin and colleagues,[76] increased risk of fibrosis progression was seen with HCV+ grafts that had F1 fibrosis but not those with F0 fibrosis. With the increasing availability of direct-acting antiviral agents, early treatment of HCV positive patients likely decreases the risk of fibrosis progression. With the advent of the pangenotypic agents, there should also be less concern about the acquisition of a second or more unfavorable genotype.

VIRAL HEPATITIS B
Hepatitis B Core Antibody–Positive Donors

The prevalence of hepatitis B core antibody (HBcAb) positivity varies geographically. Rates reported among liver donors are 4.8% in the United States,[1] 12% in Spain, and more than 50% in China.[78] HBcAb+ donors can contain intrahepatic covalently closed circular DNA (cccDNA) as well as occult infection with positive serum HBV DNA.[79] After transplantation, recipients of HBcAb+ livers are at risk for de novo or recurrent HBV infection.

Transplantation of HBcAb+ donors to hepatitis B surface antigen (HBsAg)+ recipients seems to have the best outcomes. A meta-analysis by Cholangitas and colleagues[78] found recurrent HBV infection in 11% of HBsAg+ recipients compared with de novo HBV infection of 19% of HBsAg− recipients. The latter group could be subdivided into HBcAb+/HBsAb+ and HBV-naïve cases, with 15% versus 28% de novo HBV without and 3% versus 12% with antiviral prophylaxis, respectively.[78] Similarly, a meta-analysis by Skagen and colleagues[80] evaluated de novo hepatitis in HBsAg− patients, finding the highest rates for HBV naïve patients (58% vs 11% with antiviral prophylaxis). Antiviral prophylaxis strategies typically used are HBV immune globulin (HBIG), an oral nucleos(t)ide analogue (to date, most studies with lamivudine) or a combination of the 2.[78,80] HBIG alone seemed inferior compared with the other 2 strategies.

Most studies report good post-transplant survival, although some have shown this is limited to HBsAg+ recipients.[81–83] Angelico and colleagues[82] showed significantly lower survival when using HBcAb+ donors in HBsAg− recipients ($P = .0007$), but only 1 case of graft loss occurred secondary to de novo hepatitis. The investigators hypothesized that HBcAb positivity may be a surrogate for decreased donor quality.

Hepatitis B Surface Antigen–Positive Donors

Recently, there has been increasing interest in using HBsAg+ donors in liver transplantation.[84–86] The largest study to date by Yu and colleagues compared outcomes from 42 HBsAg+ donors to 327 HBsAg− donors. Post-transplant antiviral regimens included either HBIG in combination with an oral antiviral agent (entecavir or adefovir added onto lamivudine) or an oral antiviral agent alone. Mean follow-up times for recipients with HBsAg+ compared with HBsAg− grafts were 13.9 ± 11.2 versus 19.1 ± 11.8 months, respectively. The investigators found no difference in post-transplant complications between the 2 groups, with similar graft survival. There were no HBV flares detected during follow-up.[86] More data are needed before this practice is widely adopted but early results seem promising.

HUMAN IMMUNODEFICIENCY VIRUS

Liver disease has become the second leading cause of non–AIDS-related deaths, accounting for approximately 7% to 14% of all deaths in patients with HIV infection.[87,88] HIV+ patients awaiting liver transplantation experience higher waiting list mortality compared with HIV− patients with similar MELD scores.[89] Liver transplantation with HIV− donors has shown acceptable outcomes.[90] Transplantation of HIV+ organs has been barred since 1988. With the passage of the HIV Organ Policy Equity (HOPE) Act in 2013, however, HIV is no longer considered an absolute contraindication to organ donation.[91] This may represent a pool of approximately 500 to 600 donors per year, which could attenuate the increased waiting list mortality for HIV+ patients.[92] The minimal data that exist in this field are from South Africa, with 27 cases reported to date in HIV+ donors used for kidney transplantation. All patients were able to maintain an undetectable HIV viral load after transplantation.[93] The generalizability of this data is unclear. In particular, transmitted drug resistance in South Africa is less than 5% compared with 10% to 18% in the United States, which could have a significant impact on virologic control and necessitate the use of more complex regimens. Another concern is HIV superinfection, especially with a potentially large inoculum from the donor liver.[92] With the publication of the Final HIV HOPE Act research protocol, data for HIV+ liver donation are on the horizon.[94]

SUMMARY

ECD grafts are thought to be of lower than average quality, associated with poor post-transplant outcomes or an increase in disease transmission. Grafts, however, which have been traditionally thought of as suboptimal or even marginal, can be used safely through careful selection of both donor and recipient risks. Patients with HCV benefit from the introduction of direct-acting antiviral agents. Defatting and machine perfusion strategies may salvage more steatotic and non–heart-beating donor grafts in the future. Developing strategies for the continued expansion of the acceptable ECD pool are crucial to combating the shortage of organs.

REFERENCES

1. Kim WR, Lake JR, Smith JM, et al. Liver. Am J Transplant 2016;16:69–98.
2. Durand F, Renz JF, Alkofer B, et al. Report of the Paris consensus meeting on expanded criteria donors in liver transplantation. Liver Transpl 2008;14: 1694–707.
3. Adam R, Karam V, Delvart V, et al. Evolution of indications and results of liver transplantation in Europe. A report from the European Liver Transplant Registry (ELTR). J Hepatol 2012;57:675–88.
4. Zeeh J, Platt D. The aging liver: structural and functional changes and their consequences for drug treatment in old age. Gerontology 2002;48:121–7.
5. Briceno J, Marchal T, Padillo J, et al. Influence of marginal donors on liver preservation injury. Transplantation 2002;74:522–6.
6. Schmucker DL. Age-related changes in liver structure and function: implications for disease. Exp Gerontol 2005;40:650–9.
7. Wakabayashi H, Nishiyama Y, Ushiyama T, et al. Evaluation of the effect of age on functioning hepatocyte mass and liver blood flow using liver scintigraphy in preoperative estimations for surgical patients: comparison with CT volumetry. J Surg Res 2002;106:246–53.
8. Washburn WK, Johnson LB, Lewis WD, et al. Graft function and outcome of older (> or = 60 years) donor livers. Transplantation 1996;61:1062–6.
9. Jimenez Romero C, Moreno Gonzalez E, Colina Ruiz F, et al. Use of octogenarian livers safely expands the donor pool. Transplantation 1999;68:572–5.
10. Ploeg RJ, D'Alessandro AM, Knechtle SJ, et al. Risk factors for primary dysfunction after liver transplantation–a multivariate analysis. Transplantation 1993;55: 807–13.
11. Stewart ZA, Locke JE, Segev DL, et al. Increased risk of graft loss from hepatic artery thrombosis after liver transplantation with older donors. Liver Transpl 2009; 15:1688–95.
12. Grazi GL, Cescon M, Ravaioli M, et al. A revised consideration on the use of very aged donors for liver transplantation. Am J Transplant 2001;1:61–8.
13. Serrano MT, Garcia-Gil A, Arenas J, et al. Outcome of liver transplantation using donors older than 60 years of age. Clin Transplant 2010;24:543–9.
14. Ghinolfi D, De Simone P, Lai Q, et al. Risk analysis of ischemic-type biliary lesions after liver transplant using octogenarian donors. Liver Transpl 2016;22:588–98.
15. Chapman WC, Vachharajani N, Collins KM, et al. Donor age-based analysis of liver transplantation outcomes: short- and long-term outcomes are similar regardless of donor age. J Am Coll Surg 2015;221:59–69.
16. Schemmer P, Nickkholgh A, Hinz U, et al. Extended donor criteria have no negative impact on early outcome after liver transplantation: a single-center multivariate analysis. Transplant Proc 2007;39:529–34.

17. Singhal A, Sezginsoy B, Ghuloom AE, et al. Orthotopic liver transplant using allografts from geriatric population in the United States: is there any age limit? Exp Clin Transplant 2010;8:196–201.

18. Busquets J, Xiol X, Figueras J, et al. The impact of donor age on liver transplantation: influence of donor age on early liver function and on subsequent patient and graft survival. Transplantation 2001;71:1765–71.

19. Moore DE, Feurer ID, Speroff T, et al. Impact of donor, technical, and recipient risk factors on survival and quality of life after liver transplantation. Arch Surg 2005; 140:273–7.

20. Lake JR, Shorr JS, Steffen BJ, et al. Differential effects of donor age in liver transplant recipients infected with hepatitis B, hepatitis C and without viral hepatitis. Am J Transplant 2005;5:549–57.

21. Feng S, Goodrich NP, Bragg-Gresham JL, et al. Characteristics associated with liver graft failure: the concept of a donor risk index. Am J Transplant 2006;6: 783–90.

22. Nardo B, Masetti M, Urbani L, et al. Liver transplantation from donors aged 80 years and over: pushing the limit. Am J Transplant 2004;4:1139–47.

23. Uemura T, Nikkel LE, Hollenbeak CS, et al. How can we utilize livers from advanced aged donors for liver transplantation for hepatitis C? Transpl Int 2012;25:671–9.

24. Wali M, Harrison RF, Gow PJ, et al. Advancing donor liver age and rapid fibrosis progression following transplantation for hepatitis C. Gut 2002;51:248–52.

25. Mutimer DJ, Gunson B, Chen J, et al. Impact of donor age and year of transplantation on graft and patient survival following liver transplantation for hepatitis C virus. Transplantation 2006;81:7–14.

26. Wiesner RH, Sorrell M, Villamil F, et al. Report of the first International Liver Transplantation Society expert panel consensus conference on liver transplantation and hepatitis C. Liver Transpl 2003;9:S1–9.

27. Ghinolfi D, Marti J, De Simone P, et al. Use of octogenarian donors for liver transplantation: a survival analysis. Am J Transplant 2014;14:2062–71.

28. Cescon M, Grazi GL, Cucchetti A, et al. Improving the outcome of liver transplantation with very old donors with updated selection and management criteria. Liver Transpl 2008;14:672–9.

29. Kim DY, Moon J, Island ER, et al. Liver transplantation using elderly donors: a risk factor analysis. Clin Transplant 2011;25:270–6.

30. Gastaca M, Valdivieso A, Pijoan J, et al. Donors older than 70 years in liver transplantation. Transplant Proc 2005;37:3851–4.

31. Jimenez-Romero C, Clemares-Lama M, Manrique-Municio A, et al. Long-term results using old liver grafts for transplantation: sexagenerian versus liver donors older than 70 years. World J Surg 2013;37:2211–21.

32. Chalasani N, Younossi Z, Lavine JE, et al. The diagnosis and management of non-alcoholic fatty liver disease: practice guideline by the American Association for the Study of Liver Diseases, American College of Gastroenterology, and the American Gastroenterological Association. Hepatology 2012;55:2005–23.

33. Vernon G, Baranova A, Younossi ZM. Systematic review: the epidemiology and natural history of non-alcoholic fatty liver disease and non-alcoholic steatohepatitis in adults. Aliment Pharmacol Ther 2011;34:274–85.

34. Mokdad AH, Ford ES, Bowman BA, et al. Prevalence of obesity, diabetes, and obesity-related health risk factors, 2001. JAMA 2003;289:76–9.

35. Berthiaume F, Barbe L, Mokuno Y, et al. Steatosis reversibly increases hepatocyte sensitivity to hypoxia-reoxygenation injury. J Surg Res 2009;152:54–60.

36. Fukumori T, Ohkohchi N, Tsukamoto S, et al. The mechanism of injury in a steatotic liver graft during cold preservation. Transplantation 1999;67:195–200.
37. Nativ NI, Yarmush G, So A, et al. Elevated sensitivity of macrosteatotic hepatocytes to hypoxia/reoxygenation stress is reversed by a novel defatting protocol. Liver Transpl 2014;20:1000–11.
38. Selzner N, Selzner M, Jochum W, et al. Mouse livers with macrosteatosis are more susceptible to normothermic ischemic injury than those with microsteatosis. J Hepatol 2006;44:694–701.
39. Sanyal AJ, American Gastroenterological Association. AGA technical review on nonalcoholic fatty liver disease. Gastroenterology 2002;123:1705–25.
40. de Graaf EL, Kench J, Dilworth P, et al. Grade of deceased donor liver macrovesicular steatosis impacts graft and recipient outcomes more than the Donor Risk Index. J Gastroenterol Hepatol 2012;27:540–6.
41. McCormack L, Petrowsky H, Jochum W, et al. Use of severely steatotic grafts in liver transplantation: a matched case-control study. Ann Surg 2007;246:940–6 [discussion: 946–8].
42. Spitzer AL, Lao OB, Dick AA, et al. The biopsied donor liver: incorporating macrosteatosis into high-risk donor assessment. Liver Transpl 2010;16:874–84.
43. Wong TC, Fung JY, Chok KS, et al. Excellent outcomes of liver transplantation using severely steatotic grafts from brain-dead donors. Liver Transpl 2016;22:226–36.
44. Chavin KD, Taber DJ, Norcross M, et al. Safe use of highly steatotic livers by utilizing a donor/recipient clinical algorithm. Clin Transplant 2013;27:732–41.
45. Dutkowski P, Schlegel A, Slankamenac K, et al. The use of fatty liver grafts in modern allocation systems: risk assessment by the balance of risk (BAR) score. Ann Surg 2012;256:861–8 [discussion: 868–9].
46. Ahn JS, Sinn DH, Gwak GY, et al. Steatosis among living liver donors without evidence of fatty liver on ultrasonography: potential implications for preoperative liver biopsy. Transplantation 2013;95:1404–9.
47. Cucchetti A, Vivarelli M, Ravaioli M, et al. Assessment of donor steatosis in liver transplantation: is it possible without liver biopsy? Clinical Transplantation 2009;23:519–24.
48. Lee SW, Park SH, Kim KW, et al. Unenhanced CT for assessment of macrovesicular hepatic steatosis in living liver donors: comparison of visual grading with liver attenuation index. Radiology 2007;244:479–85.
49. Yersiz H, Lee C, Kaldas FM, et al. Assessment of hepatic steatosis by transplant surgeon and expert pathologist: a prospective, double-blind evaluation of 201 donor livers. Liver Transpl 2013;19:437–49.
50. Lo IJ, Lefkowitch JH, Feirt N, et al. Utility of liver allograft biopsy obtained at procurement. Liver Transpl 2008;14:639–46.
51. Broomhead RH, Patel S, Fernando B, et al. Resource implications of expanding the use of donation after circulatory determination of death in liver transplantation. Liver Transpl 2012;18:771–8.
52. Morrissey PE, Monaco AP. Donation after circulatory death: current practices, ongoing challenges, and potential improvements. Transplantation 2014;97:258–64.
53. Nguyen JH, Bonatti H, Dickson RC, et al. Long-term outcomes of donation after cardiac death liver allografts from a single center. Clin Transplant 2009;23:168–73.

54. Skaro AI, Jay CL, Baker TB, et al. The impact of ischemic cholangiopathy in liver transplantation using donors after cardiac death: the untold story. Surgery 2009; 146:543–52 [discussion: 552–3].

55. Uemura T, Ramprasad V, Hollenbeak CS, et al. Liver transplantation for hepatitis C from donation after cardiac death donors: an analysis of OPTN/UNOS data. Am J Transplant 2012;12:984–91.

56. Jay CL, Lyuksemburg V, Ladner DP, et al. Ischemic cholangiopathy after controlled donation after cardiac death liver transplantation: a meta-analysis. Ann Surg 2011;253:259–64.

57. de Vera ME, Lopez-Solis R, Dvorchik I, et al. Liver transplantation using donation after cardiac death donors: long-term follow-up from a single center. Am J Transplant 2009;9:773–81.

58. Chan EY, Olson LC, Kisthard JA, et al. Ischemic cholangiopathy following liver transplantation from donation after cardiac death donors. Liver Transpl 2008; 14:604–10.

59. Jay CL, Skaro AI, Ladner DP, et al. Comparative effectiveness of donation after cardiac death versus donation after brain death liver transplantation: recognizing who can benefit. Liver Transpl 2012;18:630–40.

60. Mathur AK, Heimbach J, Steffick DE, et al. Donation after cardiac death liver transplantation: predictors of outcome. Am J Transplant 2010;10:2512–9.

61. Hong JC, Yersiz H, Kositamongkol P, et al. Liver transplantation using organ donation after cardiac death: a clinical predictive index for graft failure-free survival. Arch Surg 2011;146:1017–23.

62. Hernandez-Alejandro R, Croome KP, Quan D, et al. Increased risk of severe recurrence of hepatitis C virus in liver transplant recipients of donation after cardiac death allografts. Transplantation 2011;92:686–9.

63. Tao R, Ruppert K, Cruz RJ Jr, et al. Hepatitis C recurrence is not adversely affected by the use of donation after cardiac death liver allografts. Liver Transpl 2010;16:1288–95.

64. Taner CB, Bulatao IG, Keaveny AP, et al. Use of liver grafts from donation after cardiac death donors for recipients with hepatitis C virus. Liver Transpl 2011; 17:641–9.

65. Vanatta JM, Dean AG, Hathaway DK, et al. Liver transplant using donors after cardiac death: a single-center approach providing outcomes comparable to donation after brain death. Exp Clin Transplant 2013;11:154–63.

66. Mateo R, Cho Y, Singh G, et al. Risk factors for graft survival after liver transplantation from donation after cardiac death donors: an analysis of OPTN/UNOS data. Am J Transplant 2006;6:791–6.

67. Bae C, Henry SD, Guarrera JV. Is extracorporeal hypothermic machine perfusion of the liver better than the 'good old icebox'? Curr Opin Organ Transpl 2012;17: 137–42.

68. Dutkowski P, Schlegel A, de Oliveira M, et al. HOPE for human liver grafts obtained from donors after cardiac death. J Hepatol 2014;60:765–72.

69. Franchello A, Gilbo N, David E, et al. Ischemic preconditioning (IP) of the liver as a safe and protective technique against ischemia/reperfusion injury (IRI). Am J Transplant 2009;9:1629–39.

70. Guidelines for preventing transmission of human immunodeficiency virus through transplantation of human tissue and organs. Centers for Disease Control and Prevention. MMWR Recomm Rep 1994;43(RR-8):1–17.

71. Ellingson K, Seem D, Nowicki M, et al. Estimated risk of human immunodeficiency virus and hepatitis C virus infection among potential organ donors from 17 organ

procurement organizations in the United States. Am J Transplant 2011;11: 1201–8.

72. Seem DL, Lee I, Umscheid CA, et al. PHS guideline for reducing human immunodeficiency virus, hepatitis B virus, and hepatitis C virus transmission through organ transplantation. Public Health Rep 2013;128:247–343.

73. Centers for Disease Control and Prevention. Viral Hepatitis - Hepatitis C Information. Available at: http://www.cdc.gov/hepatitis/hcv/. Accessed August, 25 2016.

74. Northup PG, Argo CK, Nguyen DT, et al. Liver allografts from hepatitis C positive donors can offer good outcomes in hepatitis C positive recipients: a US National Transplant Registry analysis. Transpl Int 2010;23:1038–44.

75. Burr AT, Li Y, Tseng JF, et al. Survival after liver transplantation using hepatitis C virus-positive donor allografts: case-controlled analysis of the UNOS database. World J Surg 2011;35:1590–5.

76. Ballarin R, Cucchetti A, Spaggiari M, et al. Long-term follow-up and outcome of liver transplantation from anti-hepatitis C virus-positive donors: a European multicentric case-control study. Transplantation 2011;91:1265–72.

77. Lai JC, O'Leary JG, Trotter JF, et al. Risk of advanced fibrosis with grafts from hepatitis C antibody-positive donors: a multicenter cohort study. Liver Transpl 2012;18:532–8.

78. Cholongitas E, Papatheodoridis GV, Burroughs AK. Liver grafts from anti-hepatitis B core positive donors: a systematic review. J Hepatol 2010;52:272–9.

79. Cheung CK, Lo CM, Man K, et al. Occult hepatitis B virus infection of donor and recipient origin after liver transplantation despite nucleoside analogue prophylaxis. Liver Transpl 2010;16:1314–23.

80. Skagen CL, Jou JH, Said A. Risk of de novo hepatitis in liver recipients from hepatitis-B core antibody-positive grafts - a systematic analysis. Clin Transplant 2011;25:E243–9.

81. Yu L, Koepsell T, Manhart L, et al. Survival after orthotopic liver transplantation: the impact of antibody against hepatitis B core antigen in the donor. Liver Transpl 2009;15:1343–50.

82. Angelico M, Nardi A, Marianelli T, et al. Hepatitis B-core antibody positive donors in liver transplantation and their impact on graft survival: evidence from the Liver Match cohort study. J Hepatol 2013;58:715–23.

83. Joya-Vazquez PP, Dodson FS, Dvorchik I, et al. Impact of anti-hepatitis Bc-positive grafts on the outcome of liver transplantation for HBV-related cirrhosis. Transplantation 2002;73:1598–602.

84. Choi Y, Choi JY, Yi NJ, et al. Liver transplantation for HBsAg-positive recipients using grafts from HBsAg-positive deceased donors. Transpl Int 2013;26: 1173–83.

85. Loggi E, Micco L, Ercolani G, et al. Liver transplantation from hepatitis B surface antigen positive donors: a safe way to expand the donor pool. J Hepatol 2012;56: 579–85.

86. Yu S, Yu J, Zhang W, et al. Safe use of liver grafts from hepatitis B surface antigen positive donors in liver transplantation. J Hepatol 2014;61:809–15.

87. Antiretroviral Therapy Cohort Collaboration. Causes of death in HIV-1-infected patients treated with antiretroviral therapy, 1996-2006: collaborative analysis of 13 HIV cohort studies. Clin Infect Dis 2010;50:1387–96.

88. Weber R, Sabin CA, Friis-Moller N, et al. Liver-related deaths in persons infected with the human immunodeficiency virus: the D: a:D study. Arch Intern Med 2006; 166:1632–41.

89. Subramanian A, Sulkowski M, Barin B, et al. MELD score is an important predictor of pretransplantation mortality in HIV-infected liver transplant candidates. Gastroenterology 2010;138:159–64.
90. Miro JM, Montejo M, Castells L, et al. Outcome of HCV/HIV-coinfected liver transplant recipients: a prospective and multicenter cohort study. Am J Transplant 2012;12:1866–76.
91. Durand CM, Segev D, Sugarman J. Realizing HOPE: the ethics of organ transplantation from HIV-positive donors. Ann Intern Med 2016;165:138–42.
92. Boyarsky BJ, Hall EC, Singer AL, et al. Estimating the potential pool of HIV-infected deceased organ donors in the United States. Am J Transplant 2011; 11:1209–17.
93. Muller E, Barday Z, Mendelson M, et al. HIV-positive-to-HIV-positive kidney transplantation–results at 3 to 5 years. N Engl J Med 2015;372:613–20.
94. Department of Health and Human Services. Safeguards and research criteria for transplantation of organs infected with HIV. Available at: https://www.niaid.nih.gov/topics/transplant/research/Documents/HOPEactCriteria.pdf. Accessed August 28, 2016.

Challenges in Renal Failure Treatment Before Liver Transplant

 CrossMark

Fabrizio Fabrizi, MD*, Piergiorgio Messa, MD

KEYWORDS

- Acute kidney injury • Cirrhosis • Hepatorenal syndrome • Survival • Terlipressin
- Liver transplant

KEY POINTS

- Various causes of renal failure among cirrhotics exist and outcomes after liver transplantation (LT) are worse for patients with acute tubular necrosis than those with hepatorenal syndrome (HRS).
- HRS syndrome is still a frequent complication of cirrhosis and plays a detrimental role on survival before and after LT, compared with non-HRS patients.
- The diagnostic criteria of acute kidney injury for the diagnosis of HRS have been recently revised to allow prompt recognition of kidney disease and earlier treatment; studies are in progress to demonstrate the benefits of the revised classification.
- Treatment of HRS now includes surgery (transjugular intrahepatic portosystemic shunt), medical management (vasoconstrictors), and support therapy (renal replacement therapy or extracorporeal artificial liver).

INTRODUCTION

Patients on the waiting list for liver transplantation (LT) show usually cirrhosis and are prone to several complications, such as ascites, bacterial infections, gastrointestinal hemorrhage, hepatic encephalopathy, and renal failure.[1] Renal failure is an important complication in end-stage liver disease and it has been known for many years that it confers greater morbidity and mortality in patients awaiting LT compared with those patients without renal failure. In addition, cirrhotic patients have more complications and reduced survival after LT; serum creatinine after LT is an important predictor of post-LT survival. This is well acknowledged by the Model for End-Stage Liver Disease (MELD) score, which is now used by the United Network for Organ Sharing for

The authors have nothing to disclose.
Division of Nephrology, Maggiore Hospital, IRCCS Foundation, Pad. Croff, Via Commenda 15, 20122 Milano, Italy
* Corresponding author.
E-mail address: fabrizi@policlinico.mi.it

Clin Liver Dis 21 (2017) 303–319
http://dx.doi.org/10.1016/j.cld.2016.12.005
1089-3261/17/© 2016 Elsevier Inc. All rights reserved.

liver.theclinics.com

prioritizing allocation of LTs instead of the older Child-Pugh score; it includes serum creatinine, in addition to parameters of liver function. This article reviews the most important and recent data regarding renal failure treatment in patients with cirrhosis awaiting LT, with special emphasis on diagnosis and management of HRS, which is the most important complication of advanced cirrhosis.

RENAL FAILURE IN CIRRHOSIS: EPIDEMIOLOGY AND OUTCOME

It has been recently calculated that up to 19% of hospitalized patients with cirrhosis and ascites show acute kidney injury (AKI). Also, chronic kidney disease occurs in approximately 1% of all patients with cirrhosis.[2] Multiple causes of renal failure in patients having cirrhosis exist. In some cases, renal failure is related to etiological factors that also lead to renal failure in patients without liver disease, such as consistent dehydration, hemorrhagic or septic shock, or nonsteroidal anti-inflammatory drugs. Renal failure among patients with cirrhosis can be the consequence of a parenchymal disease, including membranous nephropathy, immunoglobulin A glomerulopathy, and cryoglobulinemic glomerulonephritis. In cirrhotics, prerenal failure (42%) and acute tubular necrosis (ATN) (38%) are the most common reasons for acute renal failure; postrenal acute kidney failure is much less frequent (about 0.3%).[3,4] Hepatorenal syndrome (HRS) is a prerenal renal failure without any identifiable kidney disease occurring in around 20% of patients with advanced liver disease.[3,4] The cumulative probability of HRS in patients was prospectively addressed by Gines and colleagues[5] in a large (n = 229) cohort of patients with cirrhosis and ascites; it was 18% after 1 year, rising to 39% at 5 years. The prevalence of HRS declined over recent years, probably a result of a better understanding of its pathogenesis and improved clinical management. Although multiple causes of renal failure in patients with cirrhosis exist, HRS is probably the most challenging to treat.

There is abundant evidence in the medical literature regarding the prognostic value of renal function parameters, particularly serum creatinine, in cirrhotic patients before LT. It is less clear whether the cause of renal failure is relevant to prognosis. This information may be important not only for clinical management of patients and classification of patients in therapeutic trials but also in decision-making in LT. Recent evidence promotes the notion that the cause of renal failure affects the outcome of renal failure. Martin-Llahi and colleagues[6] studied 562 subjects with cirrhosis and renal failure who were consecutively hospitalized at a single institution over 6 years. They found that 3-month probability survival was 73% for parenchymal nephropathies, 46% for hypovolemia-associated renal failure, and 15% for HRS. In a multivariate analysis adjusted for potentially confounding variables, cause of renal failure was independently associated with prognosis, together with the MELD score, serum sodium, and hepatic encephalopathy at time of diagnosis of renal failure. Another study by Nadim and colleagues[7] investigated the impact of AKI cause (ATN vs HRS) on survival and renal outcomes after LT. At 5 years, the incidence of chronic kidney disease (stage 4 or 5) was statistically higher in the ATN group versus the HRS group (56% vs 16%, P<.001). A multivariate analysis revealed that the presence of ATN at the time of LT was the only variable associated with higher mortality 1 year after LT (odds ratio 6.68, 95% CI 1.96–22.78, P<.001).[7]

HISTORICAL PERSPECTIVE

Frerichs[8] and Flint[9] were the first investigators to note an association among advanced liver disease, ascites, and oliguric renal failure in the absence of significant renal histologic changes. The term HRS was initially used in 1939 to report the occurrence of renal failure after biliary tract surgery.[10,11] Many years later, in a seminal article by Hecker and Sherlock,[12] the pathogenesis of HRS was unraveled. The investigators demonstrated the lack of major renal histologic changes despite the severity of kidney failure, linked the deterioration in renal function to impairment of the systemic circulation, and concluded that the underlying mechanism of kidney failure is peripheral arterial vasodilation. The functional nature of HRS was confirmed in the 1960s: kidneys obtained from patients who died with HRS could be transplanted in patients with renal failure of a different cause because these kidneys recovered their function after transplant.[13] Around the same time, it was observed that the intense renal vasoconstriction, which is usually observed with renal arteriography in patients with HRS, disappeared at postmortem vascular injection.[14]

In 1979, an international group of clinicians defined HRS as a progressive form of renal dysfunction occurring in patients with cirrhosis and other severe parenchymal liver diseases and having features of prerenal renal failure (low urine sodium concentration, hyperosmolar urine) but without any improvement after volume expansion.[15] In 1996, the International Club of Ascites (ICA) reported the optimal criteria to define HRS. HRS was defined as a syndrome occurring in patients with cirrhosis, portal hypertension, and advanced liver failure, characterized by impaired renal function with marked abnormalities in the arterial circulation and increased activity of endogenous vasoactive systems.[16] Two types of HRS can be distinguished; type 1, or acute HRS, and type 2, or chronic HRS. The 2 types of HRS substantially differ in prognosis because median survival of type 1 HRS averages 2 weeks, whereas type 2 HRS progresses gradually over weeks to months.

An update in the definition and diagnostic criteria for HRS was made by the ICA with a meeting held in San Francisco in 2006.[17] This came from an improved understanding of the pathophysiology of HRS, a better appreciation of the role of bacterial infections, and the development of effective drugs for patients with HRS, particularly those with type 1 HRS. It was recognized that HRS no longer has a fatal outcome without LT.

HEPATORENAL SYNDROME: CLINICAL PICTURE

HRS type 1 is characterized by a rapid progression of renal failure; therefore, the main clinical presentation is overt acute renal failure. By contrast, in patients with type 2 HRS the degree of the impairment of renal failure is less severe and more stable over time. As a consequence, refractory ascites is the most frequent clinical symptom. Several precipitating factors often induce the development of HRS type 1, including bacterial infections, gastrointestinal hemorrhage, and large-volume paracentesis without plasma expansion.[18] The most frequent bacterial infection is bacterial peritonitis but urinary tract infections and infection of the biliary or intestinal tract may also occur. In most cases, renal failure is transient and recovers after the resolution of the infection but in some cases an acute renal failure with the hallmarks of type 1 HRS can occur. HRS frequently develops in patients with advanced cirrhosis; thus, HRS patients show jaundice and other clinical signs of advanced liver disease, including spider nevi, palmar erythema, and finger clubbing. Additional clinical manifestations are ascites, hepatic encephalopathy, splenomegaly, and gastrointestinal bleeding. The urine output is lowered particularly in type 1 HRS, and low arterial blood pressure usually is present.

In contrast, HRS type 2 is not precipitated by acute events and is characterized by a slow progressive deterioration of renal failure related to the degree of portal hypertension. Type 2 HRS has a spontaneous onset in many patients with cirrhosis and ascites, and represents the real functional renal failure associated with cirrhosis. In addition, patients with type 2 HRS are predisposed to develop type 1 HRS following infections or other trigger events.

HEPATORENAL SYNDROME: PATHOPHYSIOLOGY

The pathophysiology of HRS is incompletely understood and various hypotheses linking the alterations of renal hemodynamics and ascites synthesis have been made. The most popular hypothesis is the arterial vasodilation hypothesis that has been suggested by Schrier and colleagues[19] in 1988. According to the arterial vasodilation hypothesis, HRS occurs as a consequence of a marked arterial vasodilation, mainly located in the splanchnic bed. Splanchnic arterial vasodilation results in effective arterial underfilling and is clinically expressed by arterial hypotension (**Fig. 1**). In the early stage of cirrhosis, the increase in heart rate and cardiac output compensates the reduction of the arterial effective volume. As the liver disease progresses, leading to a further impairment in portal hypertension and hepatic insufficiency, there is activation of the systemic endogenous vasoconstrictor systems (the sympathetic nervous system (SNS), the renin-angiotensin-aldosterone system (RAAS), and the nonosmotic synthesis of vasopressin). The activation of such systems explains some functional abnormalities at the kidney level, such as renal sodium retention (leading to ascites) and renal water retention (leading to hyponatremia). Thus, vasoconstriction in several vascular regions (eg, liver and brain) occurs. In the early stage of cirrhosis, a greater activity of systemic and renal vasodilators preserves renal perfusion despite activation of the RAAS and SNS. The most important renal vasodilators are kinins, nitric oxide, prostaglandins, and natriuretic peptides. In the late stages of cirrhosis, renal perfusion cannot be maintained because of extreme arterial underfilling giving lower activity of local vasodilators and maximal activation of vasoconstrictors; at this critical point, there is the onset of HRS.

Recent advances in the pathogenesis of HRS have focused on the cirrhotic cardiomyopathy that is currently considered a risk factor for the HRS onset. Specific cardiac changes have been included in the so-called cirrhotic cardiomyopathy, including lower systolic and diastolic responses to stress stimuli, enlargement of cardiac

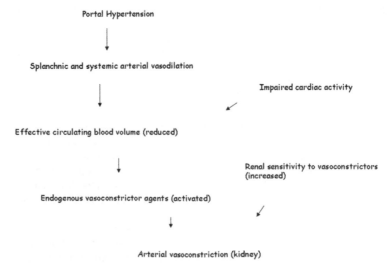

Portal Hypertension

Splanchnic and systemic arterial vasodilation

Impaired cardiac activity

Effective circulating blood volume (reduced)

Renal sensitivity to vasoconstrictors (increased)

Endogenous vasoconstrictor agents (activated)

Arterial vasoconstriction (kidney)

Fig. 1. Pathophysiology of HRS.

chambers, and abnormalities in the electrophysiological repolarisation.[20] Cirrhotic cardiomyopathy gives an inability to improve cardiac output during stress; thus, the cardiac output is unable to prevent a severe reduction of effective circulating blood volume due to splanchnic arterial vasodilatation. Cardiac dysfunction reverses 9 to 12 months after LT, suggesting that the diseased liver rather than the cause of liver disease is responsible for cardiac impairment. Inflammatory cytokines, nitric oxide, prostaglandins, and kallikrein have been also implicated in the pathogenesis of cirrhotic cardiomyopathy.

HEPATORENAL SYNDROME: DIAGNOSIS

The diagnosis of the HRS syndrome is based on exclusion because there are no specific diagnostic tests to distinguish between HRS and other reasons of renal failure that may occur in cirrhosis. According to the 2006 ICA criteria, type 1 HRS shows a rapid and progressive decline in renal function as measured by a doubling of the baseline serum creatinine to a level greater than 2.5 mg/dL or a 50% decline in the baseline creatinine clearance to a level less than 20 mL/min in less than 2 weeks. Type 2 HRS has an impairment in the renal function measured as a serum creatinine greater than 1.5 mg/dL but not meeting the criteria for the type 1 HRS. Type 2 HRS has a better prognosis; the most important clinical consequence of type 2 HRS is ascites with poor or no response to diuretics (a condition known as refractory ascites). The median survival of a patient with type 1 or type 2 HRS is about 2 weeks and 4 to 6 months, respectively. These survival rates are lower than that seen among patients with intact kidney function and ascites. Spontaneous recovery from HRS is infrequent unless there is a consistent improvement of liver function.

The criteria for diagnosing HRS have been recently reviewed; a major critical point is the novel definition of AKI (**Box 1**).[21] A new definition of AKI for the diagnosis of HRS has been proposed to help early identification of renal failure and implementation of prompt aggressive treatment. According to the 2006 consensus workshop of the ICA, serum creatinine greater than 1.5 mg/dL is a diagnostic criteria for HRS, and a time interval (2 weeks) should be considered over which serum creatinine must double to a value greater than 2.5 mg/dL for the diagnosis of type 1 HRS. Despite the widespread circulation of these ICA criteria, a serum creatinine cut-off of 1.5 mg/dL seems limited because it does not take into account the changes in serum creatinine that

---

Box 1
Diagnostic criteria for hepatorenal syndrome

- Cirrhosis with ascites

- Absence of shock

- No current or recent exposure to nephrotoxic drugs (eg, nonsteroidal anti-inflammatory drugs, aminoglycosides, iodinated contrast media)

- No macroscopic signs of structural kidney injury, defined as
  - No proteinuria (>500 mg/day)
  - No microscopic hematuria (>50 red blood cells per high power field)
  - Normal renal ultrasonography

- No improvement of serum creatinine after at least 2 days of diuretic withdrawal and volume expansion with albumin (1 gr per kg of body weight)

- Diagnosis of AKI (according to the criteria by International Club of Ascites)

occurred in the preceding days or weeks, which are needed to distinguish between acute or chronic kidney injury. In addition, a value of serum creatinine of 1.5 mg/dL often implies that the glomerular filtration rate is consistently depressed (<30 mL/min). It has been found that in patients with type 1 HRS, a higher serum creatinine at the beginning of treatment leads to a lower probability of response to vasoconstrictors (terlipressin) and albumin.[22] Thus, it has been suggested not to wait until the serum creatinine increases beyond 2.5 mg/dL before starting the treatment (**Box 2**). The potential advantage of this approach is an earlier treatment of patients with type 1 HRS, leading to a better outcome compared with the previous approach.

On the other hand, no published studies exist in which vasoconstrictor agents are used in the treatment of HRS with lower levels of serum creatinine. There is also need to change the definition of response to the pharmacologic treatment of HRS. Full response should be defined by return of serum creatinine to a value within 0.3 mg/dL of the baseline value. Partial responses should be defined by a regression of at least 1 AKI stage with a drop in the serum creatinine to greater than or equal to 0.3 mg/dL above the baseline value. On the grounds of the current data, it remains unclear whether the revised criteria improve the diagnosis of renal failure in cirrhosis in terms of prediction of morbidity and mortality. Another important pitfall of these criteria is that these do not rule out of the possibility of renal parenchymal damage such as tubular injury. Preliminary studies have found that the use of neutrophil gelatinase-associated lipocalin (NGAL) may be useful in the differential diagnosis of AKI in cirrhotics.[23] Urine biomarkers probably will become an important factor in making accurate differential diagnosis between HRS and ATN.[24]

Box 2
Diagnostic criteria for acute kidney injury in cirrhotics: revised criteria from International Club of Ascites

Baseline SCr

- It has been suggested to use a value of SCr obtained in the previous 3 months (when available)
- The value closest to the admission time to the hospital should be used (in patients with more than 1 value within the previous 3 months)
- The value on admission time to the hospital should be used as baseline (in patients without a previous SCr value)

Definition of AKI

- Increase in SCr greater than or equal to 0.3 mg/dL (≥26.5 μmol/L) within 48 hours or
- A percentage increase in SCr greater than or equal to 50% from baseline which is known, or presumed, to have occurred within the previous 7 days

Staging of AKI

Stage 1: Increase in SCr greater than or equal to 0.3 mg/dL (26.5 μmol/L) or an increase in SCr greater than or equal to 1.5-fold to 2-fold from baseline

Stage 2: Increase in SCr >2-fold to 3-fold from baseline

Stage 3: Increase of SCr >3-fold from baseline or SCr greater than or equal to 4.0 mg/dL (353.6 μmol/L) with an acute increase greater than 0.3 mg/dL (26.5 μmol/L) or initiation of RRT

Abbreviations: RRT, renal replacement therapy; SCr, serum creatinine.

OUTCOME OF PATIENTS WITH HEPATORENAL SYNDROME AND LIVER TRANSPLANT

The preferred treatment of HRS is LT but many patients die before LT because of the short survival associated with HRS and organ shortage. HRS should be treated before LT in an attempt to improve the renal function because evidence has shown that patients with HRS who receive LT have greater mortality than those without HRS. Patients with HRS before transplant are more likely to go to an intensive care unit (HRS vs non-HRS, 90% vs 33.4%, $P<.001$) and require dialysis (32.2% vs 1.5%, $P<.001$) than their counterparts without HRS.[25] Approximately 10% of patients with HRS will progress to end-stage renal disease during the postoperative period compared with 0.8% of recipients without HRS.[26]

Ruiz and colleagues[27] identified 130 patients with HRS who underwent LT over a 10-year period. A total of 13 patients developed type 1 HRS and 177 patients evolved with type 2 HRS (overall incidence of HRS: 9%). In the whole cohort, patient survival rates at 1, 3, and 5 years were 74%, 68%, and 62%, respectively. Survival was lower compared with non-HRS patients undergoing LT over the same study period ($P = .0001$). For patients presenting with type 2 HRS, 7 (6%) developed irreversible kidney failure post-transplant compared with 0.34% in the non-HRS population ($P<.001$).

PHARMACOLOGIC TREATMENT OF HEPATORENAL SYNDROME

Until 1999, the outcome of cirrhotic patients developing HRS was very poor with a mortality rate reaching 100% in some reports and a median survival time of 2 weeks from diagnosis. Evidence has been accumulated in the last 15 years showing that systemic vasoconstrictors for the treatment of type 1 or type 2 HRS have truly changed the outcome of these patients. Systemic vasoconstrictors for the treatment of HRS include vasopressin,[28] vasopressin analogs (ornipressin),[29,30] somatostatin analogs (octreotide),[31,32] and alpha-1 adrenergic receptor agonists such as midodrine[33,34] and noradrenaline.[35–37] Terlipressin is the most widely investigated drug in the treatment of HRS. It was first licensed for the management of acute variceal bleeding and has a much greater activity on vascular than on renal vasopressin receptors. Vascular receptors are expressed on vascular smooth muscle cells in the splanchnic circulation. Terlipressin is not currently available in the United States and Canada. The rationale for the administration of terlipressin is to counteract the extreme splanchnic arterial vasodilation in patients with HRS, resulting in an improvement of circulatory function (ie, increase in the effective arterial blood volume), which leads to a suppression of the activity of the vasoconstrictor systems with subsequent increase of renal perfusion and glomerular filtration rate.

RATIONALE OF THERAPY FOR HEPATORENAL SYNDROME

The impact of treatment of HRS before LT on the outcome after LT has been addressed by Restuccia and colleagues.[38] The outcome of subjects with HRS ($n = 9$) treated with vasopressin analogues before LT was compared with that of a contemporary control group of subjects without HRS ($n = 27$) matched by age, staging of liver disease, and immunosuppression. Three-year survival probability did not change between the 2 groups, 100% versus 83%, $P = .15$. No differences were found between the 2 groups with respect to the incidence of impaired renal function after LT, 22% (2/9) versus 30% (8/27) within the first 6 months after transplant. Severe infections (22% vs 33%), acute rejection (33% vs 41%), and transfusion requirement (11 ± 3 vs 10 ± 2 units) were not significantly different between the 2 groups. The length of the stay in intensive care facilities and the total duration of the hospitalization were similar between the 2 groups, 6 plus or minus 1 versus 8.1 and 27 plus or minus 4 versus 31 plus or minus 4, respectively (P = not significant, for both).

THERAPY FOR HEPATORENAL SYNDROME: VASOCONSTRICTORS (OBSERVATIONAL STUDIES)

Many studies have examined the efficacy and safety of terlipressin for the treatment of HRS but most studies had small size and uncontrolled design.[39–55] Fabrizi and colleagues[39] previously evaluated terlipressin for the treatment of HRS by a pooled analysis of uncontrolled studies. The primary outcome (as a measure of efficacy) was the rate of responder patients (ie, patients who had reversal of HRS after terlipressin). The secondary outcomes included the rate of responders who had recurrence of HRS after terlipressin withdrawal. Complete reversal of HRS was defined by a decrease of serum creatinine with a final value less than 1.5 mg/dL. Ten clinical studies (n = 154 unique subjects) were enrolled. The pooled rate of responders after terlipressin therapy was 0.52 (95% CI 0.42–0.61), according to a random-effects model. The rate of responder subjects who had recurrence of HRS after terlipressin withdrawal was 0.55 (95% CI 0.40–0.69) but evidence on this point was given in only a few studies (n = 6).[39]

Two small series (n = 6 subjects overall) have been recently published on long-term treatment (terlipressin plus albumin) of patients with recurring type 1 HRS who are in the waiting list for LT.[56,57] Therapy with terlipressin plus albumin usually lasts from a few days to 2 weeks, whereas in these patients terlipressin and albumin was effective as a bridge to LT over a period from 60 days to 8 months. No major side-effects were noted during terlipressin use. The outcome after LT was excellent in 4 subjects because they did not develop chronic kidney disease or require renal replacement therapy (RRT) after LT.[56,57]

According to the authors' systematic review, the overall estimate of the rate of patients showing side-effects and drop-outs during terlipressin therapy was 0.25% (95% CI 0.18–0.32) and 0%. Patients with HRS are prone to develop complications because they show severe dysfunction in various organs in addition to liver and kidney. Terlipressin is probably safer than other vasoconstrictor agents (ie, ornipressin) but adverse effects during terlipressin therapy had been noted.[58] Thus, a careful selection of patients and close clinical surveillance during terlipressin therapy are required. Contraindications to terlipressin therapy include a history of coronary artery disease, cardiomyopathies, cardiac arrhythmias, cerebrovascular disease, chronic obstructive pulmonary disease, arterial hypertension, and obliterative arterial disease of the lower limbs. The safety of terlipressin therapy reported by various investigators was probably related to the efforts made to exclude patients with contraindications to treatment.

An important question is the prediction of response to terlipressin treatment. The most important predictors of response to terlipressin and of survival are the baseline serum creatinine and bilirubin, and an increase in mean arterial pressure (MAP) of greater than or equal to 5 mm Hg at day 3 of treatment.[59–61] Patients who most likely will benefit from terlipressin have earlier onset of renal failure (serum creatinine <3 mg/dL). It has been estimated that the cut-off level of serum bilirubin that best predicted response to treatment was 10 mg/dL. Predictive factors of response in various studies among subjects with HRS included baseline Child-Pugh and MELD scores. Interestingly, a Child-Pugh score above 13 is predictive of a lack of beneficial effect of terlipressin on renal function. Younger age seems to be another independent predictive factor of improved renal function in response to terlipressin.[50]

THERAPY FOR HEPATORENAL SYNDROME: VASOCONSTRICTORS (RANDOMIZED, CONTROLLED TRIALS)

More convincing evidence on the efficacy and safety of terlipressin has been provided by some randomized controlled trials (RCTs). Systematic review of the literature with meta-analyses of RCTs comparing terlipressin versus placebo on renal function and survival among patients with HRS have been recently reported. The authors identified 5 studies ($n = 419$ unique subjects), the pooled odds ratio of the rate of reversal of HRS was 4.71 (95% CI 1.81–12.2, $P = .0001$) (Fig. 2).[62–67] The publication bias assessment (ie, the number of void or negative trials necessary to render the meta-analysis meaningless) was 22. The test of funnel plot asymmetry was 2.66 (95% CI 0.04–5.28, $P = .05$).

In their systematic review of RCTs on vasoconstrictor drugs for HRS ($n = 376$ subjects), the Cochrane Hepato-Biliary Group observed that vasoconstrictor drugs lowered mortality compared with no intervention at 15 days only (relative risk [RR] 0.60, 95% CI 0.37–0.97).[68] The occurrence of a link between terlipressin therapy and survival over the short-term only may explained by taking account that the prognosis in the HRS population mostly depends on the degree of liver failure. A consistent impairment of liver function is a poor predictor for the response to terlipressin but also for their overall survival.

A recent RCT has compared efficacy and safety of terlipressin given by continuous intravenous administration versus intravenous boluses in the treatment of type 1 HRS. A large group ($n = 78$) of HRS subjects was recruited. The rate of response to treatment, including both complete and partial response, was not different between the 2 groups, 76.5% versus 64.8% $P = NS$. The mean daily effective dose of terlipressin was lower in the first (continuous intravenous administration) than in the second (intravenous boluses) group (2.23 ± 0.65 vs 3.51 ± 1.77 mg/day, $P>.05$). The rate of adverse events was lower in the first (35.3%) than in the second group (35.3% vs 62.2%, $P<.025$). The conclusion of the investigators was that terlipressin is effective at doses lower than those required for intravenous bolus administration. In addition, terlipressin given by continuous intravenous infusion is better tolerated than intravenous boluses in the treatment of type 1 HRS.[69]

THERAPY FOR HEPATORENAL SYNDROME: ARTERIAL BLOOD PRESSURE AND VASOCONSTRICTORS

Although the aim of vasoconstrictor therapy in HRS is specifically to optimize renal hemodynamics, this effect is typically achieved with a concomitant increase in systemic

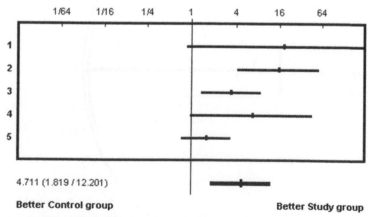

Fig. 2. Terlipressin versus placebo for HRS: Forrest plot.

blood pressure. A pooled analysis of 21 clinical studies ($n = 501$ subjects) revealed that an increase in MAP is strongly associated with a decline in serum creatinine (rho $= -0.76$, $P<.001$).[70] On average, for every 1-mm Hg increase in MAP, a 0.12 mg/dL decline in serum creatinine is expected; every 8.6 mm Hg increase in MAP is associated with a 1.0 mg/dL decline in serum creatinine. The investigators suggested that, independent of which vasoconstrictor is chosen, targeting a systematic rise in MAP of around 10 to 15 mm Hg during vasoconstrictor therapy may lead to more favorable kidney outcomes. Most studies included in the review tested terlipressin as vasoconstrictor; 2 papers addressed noradrenalin. Clinicians have been so far reluctant to choose noradrenalin because of the fear of aggravating renal hypoperfusion, and noradrenalin stimulates afferent arteriolar vasoconstriction through α-1 adrenergic receptor stimulation.

Some small-sized RCTs have recently reported that noradrenalin may be a good alternative to terlipressin in improving renal function. According to a recent systematic review of the medical literature with a meta-analysis, 4 studies ($n = 154$ subjects)[71–74] were included to compare efficacy and safety of terlipressin versus noradrenalin in the management of HRS (**Fig. 3**). There was no difference in the reversal of HRS (RR 0.97, 95% CI 0.76–1.23), mortality at 30 days (RR 0.89, 95% CI 0.68–1.17), and recurrence of HRS (RR 0.72, 95% CI 0.36–1.45) between norepinephrine and terlipressin.[37] Also, most studies calculated that noradrenalin was less expensive than terlipressin.

THERAPY FOR HEPATORENAL SYNDROME: TRANSJUGULAR INTRAHEPATIC PORTOSYSTEMIC SHUNT

In addition to vasoconstrictor therapy, an alternative approach includes transjugular intrahepatic portosystemic shunt (TIPS). TIPS is a nonsurgical procedure of portal decompression used as an alternative therapy for cirrhotic patients bleeding from esophageal or gastric varices who do not respond to medical or endoscopic treatment. An interventional radiologist will place a side-to-side portocaval shunt that links

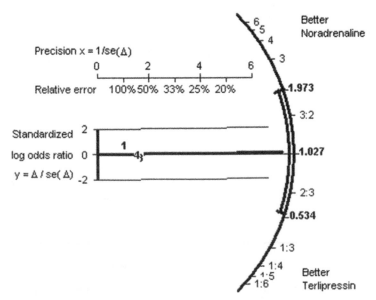

Fig. 3. Terlipressin versus noradrenalin for HRS: Galbraith plot.

the portal and hepatic veins within the hepatic parenchyma. TIPS reduces portal pressure and the filtration in the peritoneal space to a level that can be drained by the lymphatic system. TIPS returns some of the volume of blood pooled in the splanchnic circulation to the systemic circulation.

Within 4 weeks after TIPS, urinary sodium excretion and serum creatinine improve and, in combination with diuretics, can normalize within 6 to 12 months. This occurs in association with increases in urinary volume, glomerular filtration rate, and serum sodium concentration. The activity of vasoconstrictor and antinatriuretic systems such as RAAS, SNS, and arginine vasopressin is reduced, and an improvement of renal circulation occurs. The effect of TIPS on renal function and hemodynamics has been addressed by various investigators among patients with cirrhosis and refractory ascites.[75] TIPS have been proved to be effective even in patients with cirrhosis and parenchymal renal disease.[76] The activity of TIPS in the treatment of HRS has been explored in a few papers. Guevara and colleagues[77] were the first investigators to treat HRS patients by TIPS; renal function strongly improved in 6 out of 7 patients with type 1 HRS. Brensing and colleagues[78] treated 31 HRS patients (14 type 1 and 17 type 2), 77% (24 out of 31) exhibited sustained improvement in glomerular filtration rate. Cox regression analysis showed that bilirubin ($P<.001$) and HRS type ($P<.05$) were independent predictors of survival after TIPS. In a recent series of type 1 HRS subjects, Testino and colleagues[79,80] treated by TIPS 9 consecutive subjects who had severe acute alcoholic hepatitis; 30 days after TIPS insertion serum creatinine was 1.6 plus or minus 0.6 compared with 5.2 plus or minus 0.9 at baseline ($P<.04$).

However, there are some drawbacks associated with TIPS, including transcapsular puncture and shunt stenosis. Patients with advanced cirrhosis are not good candidates for TIPS procedure because they are at risk for worsening liver failure and/or hepatic encephalopathy. TIPS activity seems slow and beneficial in some patients only. Many clinical, biochemical, and neurohumoral parameters improve but do not fully reverse after TIPS insertion.

THERAPY FOR HEPATORENAL SYNDROME: RENAL REPLACEMENT THERAPY

Initiation of RRT is controversial in patients with type 1 HRS who are not candidates for LT due to poor life expectancy, high morbidity, and the mortality rates associated with RRT. Early studies demonstrated that initiation of RRT in cirrhotic patients is associated with greater mortality due in part to the increased risk of hypotension and hemorrhage.[81] Keller and colleagues[82] found that HRS patients who underwent RRT had greater survival than those who did not receive RT but 33% of the days gained were spent in hospital.

RRT should be considered a good choice for HRS patients who are nonresponders to vasoconstrictor agents or TIPS, and are on the waiting list for LT.[81] The choice between intermittent hemodialysis or continuous RRT (CRRT) should be individualized because evidence currently shows that neither has been demonstrated to be superior to the other; however, CRRT is probably better in unstable patients.[83–85]

Novel approaches are currently under evaluation for HRS patients, including the extracorporeal albumin dialysis molecular adsorbent recirculation system (MARS) or the Prometheus system. MARS is designed to cause clearance of albumin-bound toxins (ie, bile acids) and water-soluble cytokines (ie, interleukin-6), which have been implicated in the pathogenesis of HRS. A prospective, clinical, RCT has demonstrated that MARS is better than CRRT in type 1 HRS population because it offers greater survival and improved clinical and biochemical parameters.[86] Another study showed that MARS is ineffective in the management of type 1 HRS in subjects with cirrhosis and ascites who did not respond to medical treatment with vasoconstrictors. A transient reduction in serum creatinine was found but MARS was ineffective in improving systemic hemodynamics in 6 subjects with type 1 HRS.[87] A more recent study on 32 type 1 HRS subjects reported a rate of complete renal response of 28% (9 out of 32).[88] Extremely limited information is now available for the Prometheus system, which is a plasma filtration treatment coupling adsorption (FPSA) and hemodialysis to perform blood purification in liver failure. The Prometheus system was used in 12 patients with acute or acute-on-chronic liver insufficiency: 8 cirrhosis, 1 post-transplant dysfunction, and 3 secondary liver insult (2 cardiogenic shock and 1 rhabdomyolysis). All patients were severely hyperbilirubinemic, hyperchloremic, and hyperammonemic. The mean total bilirubin decreased from 33.6 plus or minus 20 to 22.2 plus or minus 13.6 mg/dL ($P<.001$); the reduction ratios for cholic acid and ammonia were 48.6% and 51.6%, respectively. The before and after session urea reduction was 57.6% plus or minus 9.5% and creatinine 42.7% plus or minus 10%. The hemodynamics were stable during treatments. Two patients received LT. The overall survival at 30 days was 41.6% (5 out of 12 patients). Prometheus, based on FPSA, produced high clearance for protein-bound and water soluble markers, which resulted in high treatment efficacy.[89] The Prometheus system has not yet been studied among HRS patients, and has been studied in hepatic failure only. MARS and Prometheus can work as a bridge to LT but controlled trials are needed.

SUMMARY

Various causes of renal failure among cirrhotics exist and outcomes after LT are worse for patients with ATN than those with HRS. HRS is still a frequent complication of cirrhosis and plays a detrimental role in survival before and after LT, compared with non-HRS patients. The diagnostic criteria of AKI for the diagnosis of HRS have been recently revised to allow prompt recognition of kidney disease and earlier treatment; studies are in progress to demonstrate the benefits of the revised classification. Treatment of HRS now includes surgery (TIPS), medical management (vasoconstrictors), and support therapy (RRT or extracorporeal artificial liver). However, LT remains the treatment of choice because it allows both the liver disease and the associated renal failure to be cured.

REFERENCES

1. Fagundes C, Gines P. Hepatorenal syndrome: a severe, but treatable, cause of kidney failure in cirrhosis. Am J Kidney Dis 2012;59:874–85.
2. Garcia-Tsao G, Parikh C, Viola A. Acute kidney injury in cirrhosis. Hepatology 2008;48:2064–77.
3. Moreau R, Lebrec D. Acute renal failure in patients with cirrhosis: perspectives in the age of MELD. Hepatology 2003;37:233–43.
4. Angeli A, Merkel C. Pathogenesis and management of hepatorenal syndrome in patients with cirrhosis. J Hepatol 2008;48:S93–103.
5. Gines A, Escorsell A, Gines P, et al. Incidence, predictive factors, and prognosis of the hepatorenal syndrome in cirrhosis and ascites. Gastroenterology 1993;105: 229–36.
6. Martin-Llahi M, Guevara M, Torre A, et al. Prognostic importance of the cause of renal failure in patients with cirrhosis. Gastroenterology 2011;140:488–96.
7. Nadim M, Genyk Y, Tokin C, et al. Impact of the aetiology of acute kidney injury on outcomes following liver transplantation: acute tubular necrosis versus hepatorenal syndrome. Liver Transpl 2012;18:539–45.

8. Frerichs F. Tratado practico de las Enfermedades del Higado, de los Vasos Hepaticos y de las Vias Biliares. Madrid: Libreria Extranjera y Nacional, Scientifica y Literaria; 1877.
9. Flint A. Clinical report on hydro-peritoneum, based on analysis of forty-six cases. Am J Med Sci 1863;45:306–39.
10. Wilenski A. Occurrence, distribution, and pathogenesis of so called liver death and/or hepatorenal syndrome. Arch Surg 1939;38:625–31.
11. Orr T, Helwig F. Liver trauma and the hepatorenal syndrome. Ann Surg 1939;110: 683–92.
12. Hecker R, Sherlock S. Electrolyte and circulatory changes in terminal liver failure. Lancet 1956;271:1121–5.
13. Koppel M, Coburn J, Mims M, et al. Transplantation of cadaveric kidneys from patients with hepatorenal syndrome. Evidence for the functional nature of renal failure in advanced liver disease. N Engl J Med 1969;280:1367–71.
14. Epstein M, Berk D, Hollenberg N, et al. Renal failure in the patient with cirrhosis. The role of active vasoconstriction. Am J Med 1970;49:175–85.
15. Anonimous. Hepatorenal syndrome or hepatic nephropathy? Lancet 1980;315: 801–2.
16. Arroyo V, Gines P, Gerbes A, et al. Definition and diagnostic criteria of refractory ascites and hepatorenal syndrome in cirrhosis. Hepatology 1996;23:164–76.
17. Salerno F, Gerbes A, Gines P, et al. Diagnosis, prevention, and treatment of hepatorenal syndrome in cirrhosis. Gut 2007;56:1310–8.
18. Wadei H, Mai M, Ahsan N, et al. Hepatorenal syndrome: pathophysiology and management. Clin J Am Soc Nephrol 2006;1:1066–79.
19. Schrier R, Arroyo V, Bernardi M, et al. Peripheral arterial vasodilatation hypothesis: a proposal for the initiation of renal sodium and water retention in cirrhosis. Hepatology 1988;8:1151–7.
20. Wong F. Cirrhotic cardiomyopathy. Hepatol Int 2009;3:294–304.
21. Angeli P, Gines P, Wong F, et al. Diagnosis and management of acute kidney injury in patients with cirrhosis: revised consensus recommendations of the International Club of Ascites. J Hepatol 2015;62:968–74.
22. Boyer T, Sanyal A, Garcia-Tsao G, et al. Predictors of response to terlipressin plus albumin in hepatorenal syndrome type 1: relationship of serum creatinine to hemodynamics. J Hepatol 2011;55:315–21.
23. Fagundes C, Pepin M, Guevara M, et al. Urinary neutrophil gelatinase –associated lipocalin as biomarkers in the differential diagnosis of impairment of kidney function in cirrhosis. J Hepatol 2012;57:267–73.
24. Fabrizi F, Aghemo A, Messa P. Hepatorenal syndrome and novel advances in its management. Kidney Blood Press Res 2013;37:588–601.
25. Gonwa T, Morris C, Goldstein R, et al. Long-term survival and renal function following liver transplantation in patients with and without hepatorenal syndrome-experience in 300 cases. Transplantation 1991;51:428–30.
26. Distant D, Gonwa T. The kidney in liver transplantation. J Am Soc Nephrol 1993;4: 129–36.
27. Ruiz R, Barri Y, Jennings L, et al. Hepatorenal syndrome: a proposal for kidney after liver transplantation. Liver Transpl 2007;13:838–43.
28. Kiser T, Fish D, Obritsch M, et al. Vasopressin, not octreotide, may be beneficial in the treatment of hepatorenal syndrome: a retrospective study. Nephrol Dial Transplant 2005;20:1813–20.

29. Guevara M, Gines P, Fernandez-Esparrach G, et al. Reversibility of hepatorenal syndrome by prolonged administration of ornipressin and plasma volume expansion. Hepatology 1998;27:35–41.

30. Gulberg V, Bilzer M, Gerbes A. Long-term therapy and retreatment of hepatorenal syndrome type 1 with ornipressin and dopamine. Hepatology 1999;30:870–5.

31. Kaffy F, Borderie C, Chagneau C, et al. Octreotide in the treatment of hepatorenal syndrome in cirrhotic patients. J Hepatol 1999;30:174.

32. Pomier-Layrargues G, Pasquin S, Hassoun Z, et al. Octreotide in hepatorenal syndrome: a novel randomized, double-blind, placebo-controlled, crossover study. Hepatology 2003;38:238–43.

33. Angeli P, Volpin R, Gerunda G, et al. Reversal of type-1 hepatorenal syndrome with the administration of midodrine and octreotide. Hepatology 1999;30:174.

34. Esrailian E, Pantangco E, Kyulo N, et al. Octreotide/midrodine therapy significantly improve renal function and 30-day survival in patients with type 1 hepatorenal syndrome. Dig Dis Sci 2007;52:742–8.

35. Durkin R, Winter S. Reversal of hepatorenal syndrome with the combination of norephrine and dopamine. Crit Care Med 1995;23:202–4.

36. Duvoux C, Zanditenas DF, Hezode C, et al. Effects of noradrenalin and albumin in patients with type 1 hepatorenal syndrome. A pilot study. Hepatology 2002;36: 374–80.

37. Nasar A, Farias A, d'Albuquerque L, et al. Terlipressin versus norepinephrine in the treatment of hepatorenal syndrome: a systematic review and meta-analysis. PLoS One 2014;9:e107466.

38. Restuccia T, Ortega R, Guevara M, et al. Effects of treatment of hepatorenal syndrome before transplantation on post-transplantation outcome. A case-control study. J Hepatol 2004;40:140–6.

39. Fabrizi F, Dixit V, Martin P. Meta-analysis: terlipressin therapy for the hepatorenal syndrome. Aliment Pharmacol Ther 2006;24:935–44.

40. Ganne-Carie N, Hadengue A, Mathurin P, et al. Hepatorenal syndrome. Long-term treatment with terlipressin as a bridge to liver transplantation. Dig Dis Sci 1996;41:1054–6.

41. Hadengue A, Gadano A, Moreau R, et al. Beneficial effects of the 2-day administration of terlipressin in patients with cirrhosis and hepatorenal syndrome. J Hepatol 1998;29:565–70.

42. Le Moine O, el Nawar A, Jagodzinski R, et al. Treatment with terlipressin as a bridge to liver transplantation in a patient with hepatorenal syndrome. Acta Gastroenterol Belg 1998;61:268–70.

43. Duhamel C, Mauillon J, Berkelmans I, et al. Hepatorenal syndrome in cirrhotic patients: terlipressin is a safe and efficient treatment; propanolol and digital treatment: precipitating and preventing factors? Am J Gastroenterol 2000;95:2984–5.

44. Uriz J, Gines P, Cardenas A, et al. Terlipressin plus albumin infusion: an effective and safe therapy of hepatorenal syndrome. J Hepatol 2000;33:43–8.

45. Mulkay J, Louis H, Donckier V, et al. Long-term terlipressin administration improves renal function in cirrhotic patients with type 1 hepatorenal syndrome: a pilot study. Acta Gastroenterol Belg 2001;64(1):15–9.

46. Yang Y, Dan Z, Liu N, et al. Efficacy of terlipressin in the treatment of liver cirrhosis with hepatorenal syndrome. J Inter Intensive Med 2001;7:123–5.

47. Ortega R, Gines P, Uriz J, et al. Terlipressin therapy with and without albumin for patients with hepatorenal syndrome: results of a prospective, non randomised study. Hepatology 2002;36:941–8.

48. Halimi C, Bonnard P, Bernard B, et al. Effect of terlipressin (glypressin) on hepatorenal syndrome in cirrhotic patients: results of a multicentre pilot study. Eur J Gastroenterol Hepatol 2002;14:153–8.
49. Colle I, Durand F, Pessione F, et al. Clinical course, predictive factors, and prognosis in patients with cirrhosis and type 1 hepatorenal syndrome treated with terlipressin: a retrospective analysis. J Gastroenterol Hepatol 2002;17:882–8.
50. Moreau R, Durand F, Poynard T, et al. Terlipressin in patients with cirrhosis and type 1 hepatorenal syndrome: a retrospective multicenter study. Gastroenterology 2002;122:923–30.
51. Moreau R, Asselah T, Condat B, et al. Comparison of the effect of terlipressin and albumin on arterial blood volume in patients with cirrhosis and tense ascites treated by paracentesis: a randomised pilot study. Gut 2002;50:90–4.
52. Alessandria C, Debernardi Venon W, Marzano A, et al. Renal failure in cirrhotic patients: role of terlipressin in clinical approach to hepatorenal syndrome type 2. Eur J Gastroenterol Hepatol 2002;14:1363–8.
53. Saner F, Fruhaut N, Schafers R, et al. Terlipressin plus hydroxyethyl starch infusion: an effective treatment for hepatorenal syndrome. Eur J Gastroenterol Hepatol 2003;15:925–7.
54. Saner F, Kavuk I, Lang H, et al. Terlipressin and gelafundin: safe therapy of hepatorenal syndrome. Eur J Med Res 2004;9:78–82.
55. Kalambokis G, Economou M, Paraskevi K, et al. Effects of somatostatin, terlipressin and somatostatin plus terlipressin on portal and systemic hemodynamics and renal sodium excretion in patients with cirrhosis. J Gastroenterol Hepatol 2005;20:1075–81.
56. Piano S, Morando F, Fasolato S, et al. Continuous recurrence of type 1 hepatorenal syndrome and long-term treatment with terlipressin and albumin: a new exception to MELD score in the allocation system to liver transplantation? J Hepatol 2011;55:491–6.
57. Caraceni P, Santi L, Mirici F, et al. Long-term treatment of hepatorenal syndrome as a bridge to liver transplantation. Dig Liver Dis 2011;43:242–5.
58. Lee J, Lee H, Jung S, et al. A case of peripheral ischemic complication after terlipressin therapy. Korean J Gastroenterol 2006;47:454–7.
59. Cardenas A. Hepatorenal syndrome: a dreaded complication of end-stage liver disease. Am J Gastroenterol 2005;100:460–7.
60. Lata J. Hepatorenal syndrome. World J Gastroenterol 2012;28:4978–84.
61. Fabrizi F, Martin P, Messa P. Recent advances in the management of hepatorenal syndrome. Acta Clin Belg 2007;62:S393–6.
62. Solanki P, Chawla A, Garg R, et al. Beneficial effects of terlipressin in hepatorenal syndrome: a prospective, randomized placebo-controlled clinical trial. J Gastroenterol Hepatol 2003;18:152–6.
63. Neri S, Pulvirenti D, Malaguarnera M, et al. Terlipressin and albumin in patients with cirrhosis and type I hepatorenal syndrome. Dig Dis Sci 2008;53:830–5.
64. Martin-Llahi M, Pepin M, Guevara M, et al, for the TAHRS investigators. Terlipressin and albumin vs. albumin in patients with cirrhosis and hepatorenal syndrome: a randomized study. Gastroenterology 2008;134:1352–9.
65. Sanyal A, Boyer T, Garcia-Tsao G, et al, The Terlipressin Study Group. A randomized, prospective, double-blind, placebo-controlled trial of terlipressin for type 1 hepatorenal syndrome. Gastroenterology 2008;134:1360–8.
66. Boyer T, Sanyal A, Wong F, et al, The Reverse Study Investigators. Terlipressin plus albumin is more effective than albumin alone in improving renal function in

patients with cirrhosis and hepatorenal syndrome type 1. Gastroenterology 2016; 150:1579–89.

67. Fabrizi F, Dixit V, Messa PG, et al. Terlipressin for hepatorenal syndrome: a meta-analysis of randomized trials. Int J Artif Organs 2009;32:133–40.

68. Gluud L, Christensen K, Christensen E, et al. Systematic review of randomized trials on vasoconstrictor drugs for hepatorenal syndrome. Hepatology 2010;51: 576–84.

69. Cavallin M, Piano S, Romano A, et al. Terlipressin given by continuous intravenous infusion versus intravenous boluses in the treatment of hepatorenal syndrome: a randomized controlled study. Hepatology 2016;63:983–92.

70. Velez J, Nietert P. Therapeutic response to vasoconstrictors in hepatorenal syndrome parallels increase in mean arterial pressure: a pooled analysis of clinical trials. Am J Kidney Dis 2011;58:928–38.

71. Alessandria C, Ottobrelli A, Debernardi-Venon W, et al. Noradrenalin versus terlipressin in patients with hepatorenal syndrome: a prospective, randomized, unblinded, pilot study. J Hepatol 2007;47:499–505.

72. Sharma P, Kumar A, Sharma B, et al. An open label, pilot, randomized controlled trial of noradrenaline versus terlipressin in the treatment of type 1 hepatorenal syndrome and predictors of response. Am J Gastroenterol 2008;103:1–9.

73. Singh V, Ghosh S, Singh B, et al. Noradrenalin vs. terlipressin in the treatment of hepatorenal syndrome: a randomized study. J Hepatol 2012;56:1293–8.

74. Ghosh S, Choudhary N, Sharma K, et al. Noradrenaline versus terlipressin in the treatment of type 2 hepatorenal syndrome: a randomized pilot study. Liver Int 2013;33:1187–93.

75. Rossle M, Gerbes A. TIPS for the treatment of refractory ascites, hepatorenal syndrome and hepatic hydrothorax: a critical update. Gut 2010;59:988–1000.

76. Hollò S, Pacitti A, Ottobrelli A, et al. Acute renal failure treatment in liver cirrhosis: the role of transjugular intrahepatic portosystemic shunts. G Ital Nefrol 2001;18: 666–72.

77. Guevara M, Ginès P, Bandi J, et al. Transjugular intrahepatic portosystemic shunt in hepatorenal syndrome: effects on renal function and vasoactive systems. Hepatology 1998;28:416–22.

78. Brensing K, Textor J, Perz J, et al. Long term outcome after transjugular intrahepatic portosystemic stent-shunt in non-transplant cirrhotics with hepatorenal syndrome: a phase 2 study. Gut 2000;47:288–95.

79. Testino G, Ferro C, Sumberaz A, et al. Type-2 hepatorenal syndrome and refractory ascites: role of of transjugular intra-hepatic portosystemic stent-shunt in eighteen patients with advanced cirrhosis awaiting orthotopic liver transplantation. Hepatogastroenterology 2000;50:1753–6.

80. Testino G, Leone S, Ferro C, et al. Severe acute alcoholic hepatitis and hepatorenal syndrome: role of transjugular portosystemic stent shunt. J Med Life 2012;5: 203–5.

81. Gonwa T, Wadei H. The challenges of providing renal replacement therapy in decompensated liver cirrhosis. Blood Purif 2012;33:144–8.

82. Keller F, Heinze H, Jochimsen F, et al. Risk factors and outcome of 107 patients with decompensated liver disease and acute renal failure: the role of haemodialysis. Ren Fail 1995;17:135–46.

83. Davenport A, Will E, Davison A. Effect of renal replacement therapy on patients with combined acute renal and fulminant hepatic failure. Kidney Int 1993;41: S245–51.

84. Gonwa T, Mai M, Melton L, et al. Renal replacement therapy and orthotopic liver transplantation: the role of continuous veno-venous haemodialysis. Transplantation 2001;71:1424–8.
85. Witzke O, Baumann M, Patschan D, et al. Which patients benefit from haemodialysis therapy in hepatorenal syndrome? J Gastroenterol Hepatol 2004;19: 1369–73.
86. Mitzner S, Stange J, Klammt S, et al. Improvement of hepatorenal syndrome with extracorporeal albumin dialysis MARS: results of a prospective, randomized, controlled clinical trial. Liver Transpl 2002;6:277–86.
87. Wong F, Raina N, Richardson R. Molecular adsorbent recirculating system is ineffective in the management of type 1 hepatorenal syndrome in patients with cirrhosis and ascites who have failed vasoconstrictor treatment. Gut 2010;59: 381–6.
88. Lavayssiere L, Kallab S, Cardeau-Desangles I, et al. Impact of molecular adsorbent recirculating system on renal recovery in type-1 hepatorenal syndrome patients with chronic liver failure. J Gastroenterol Hepatol 2013;28:1019–24.
89. Santoro A, Faenza S, Mancini E, et al. Prometheus system: a technological support in liver failure. Transplant Proc 2006;38:1078–82.

De Novo and Recurrence of Nonalcoholic Steatohepatitis After Liver Transplantation

 CrossMark

Matthew Kappus, MD, Manal Abdelmalek, MD, MPH*

KEYWORDS

- Nonalcoholic fatty liver disease • Insulin resistance • Hyperlipidemia • Hypertension
- Obesity • Metabolic syndrome • Cryptogenic cirrhosis

KEY POINTS

- Metabolic risk factors for recurrent nonalcoholic steatohepatitis (NASH) and de novo nonalcoholic fatty liver disease (NAFLD) are similar to the risk factors associated with NASH acquisition and progression in nontransplant cohorts.
- All liver transplant recipients have modifiable and nonmodifiable risk factors for the development of recurrent or de novo NAFLD or NASH.
- Therapeutic targets are multiple and require a multidisciplinary approach to treatment.

INTRODUCTION

Nonalcoholic fatty liver disease (NAFLD) is a heterogeneous disease for which most patients have no associated liver-related morbidity or mortality. Isolated hepatic steatosis (intrahepatic fat accumulation) is unlikely to progress to more advanced stages of hepatic fibrosis or cirrhosis. However, when hepatic steatosis is accompanied by hepatic necroinflammation and hepatic fibrosis (nonalcoholic steatohepatitis [NASH]), progression is variable with approximately 11% of patients with NASH progressing to cirrhosis within 15 years.[1] Progression to cirrhosis carries an associated risk decompensation from portal hypertension, diminished liver synthetic function, or increased risk for hepatocellular carcinoma.[2–4] The probability of developing hepatic decompensation or hepatocellular carcinoma is 2% to 3% in patients without cirrhosis with NASH, and up to 13% in patients with NASH and cirrhosis.[5–7] The increase in liver-related morbidity and mortality in patients with NASH is dictated by the severity of hepatic fibrosis; patients with advanced hepatic fibrosis (Brunt stage ≥3) have the

Conflict of Interest: The authors have nothing to disclose.
Division of Gastroenterology, Duke University Medical Center, 40 Duke Medicine Circle, PO Box 3913, Durham, NC 27710, USA
* Corresponding author.
E-mail address: manal.abdelmalek@duke.edu

highest rate of mortality compared with patients with lower fibrosis stages.[8,9] Metabolic syndrome is strongly associated with NASH with the risk of hepatic fibrosis significantly increasing with age, three or more clinical features of metabolic syndrome, and in particular the presence of diabetes mellitus.[10,11]

Although liver transplantation resolves the complications of NASH-related cirrhosis, the metabolic risk factors for NASH persist and potentially worsen in the setting of posttransplant immunosuppression thereby increasing the risk for de novo or recurrent NASH.[12–14] The inherent metabolic risk factors of the transplant recipient, coupled with the diabetogenic risks of immunosuppression, contribute to high (40%–60%) recurrence rate of hepatic steatosis in the allograft within the first year posttransplant.[12–14] The development of recurrent NAFLD posttransplant is a risk factor for NASH and recurrent hepatic fibrosis. In a single-center study of patients who underwent transplantation for NASH cirrhosis (n = 98), recurrent NAFLD, NASH, and at least stage 2 hepatic fibrosis developed respectively at a mean of 18 months in 70%, 25%, and 18% of those recipients.[15] Issues pertaining to the risk for de novo and/or recurrence of NASH post liver transplantation pose a unique set of challenges to the transplant community.

This article reviews the donor-, recipient-, and transplant-specific factors that contribute to de novo and recurrent NAFLD and NASH following liver transplantation (**Fig. 1**) and discusses potential approaches to management and treatment of recurrent NAFLD and NASH.

DONOR FACTORS: RISK FOR DE NOVO NONALCOHOLIC FATTY LIVER DISEASE POST LIVER TRANSPLANT

There is no known association between donor clinical risk factors for NAFLD or NASH and the risk for de novo or recurrent hepatic steatosis in the transplant recipients. However, use of donor livers with increased (>30%) hepatic steatosis increase the risk for primary nonfunction.[16] With NAFLD estimated to affect nearly 25% to 30% of the general US population, many potential donor livers will be steatotic. Severely (>60%) steatotic grafts are associated with increased risk of poor graft function,

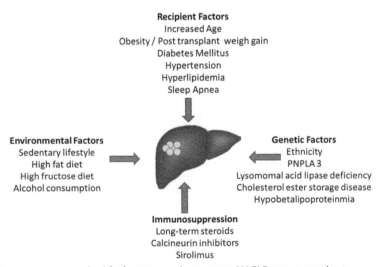

Recipient Factors
Increased Age
Obesity / Post transplant weigh gain
Diabetes Mellitus
Hypertension
Hyperlipidemia
Sleep Apnea

Environmental Factors
Sedentary lifestyle
High fat diet
High fructose diet
Alcohol consumption

Genetic Factors
Ethnicity
PNPLA 3
Lysomomal acid lipase deficiency
Cholesterol ester storage disease
Hypobetalipoproteinmia

Immunosuppression
Long-term steroids
Calcineurin inhibitors
Sirolimus

Fig. 1. Factors associated with de novo and recurrent NAFLD posttransplant.

whereas moderate-severe (>30%) steatotic grafts are associated with decreased graft survival. The prevalence of steatosis in the donor liver increases with age (>30 years old), obesity, diabetes mellitus, and serum triglyceride levels.[17] Approximately 70% of patients with diabetes mellitus have fatty liver disease as assessed by abdominal ultrasound.[18] Although steatotic grafts have historically been considered unsuitable for deceased donor liver transplantation because of unacceptably high risk for primary nonfunction and graft loss, recent data suggest that severely steatotic liver grafts from low-risk donors could be safely transplanted with excellent outcomes, if caution was exercised, particularly in high Model for End-State Liver Disease score recipients.[19]

The limited use of donor allografts known to have hepatic steatosis and lack of surveillance or protocol posttransplant liver biopsies leaves a challenge in defining the prevalence, incidence, and/or natural history of donor hepatic steatosis on de novo or recurrent NAFLD and the associated transplant outcomes. The inherent selection bias to use (or not use) steatotic grafts for transplantation may confound outcomes.[20] The assessment of the quality of liver grafts relies heavily on the procurement surgeon's intraoperative judgment because imaging studies and/or liver biopsy may not be available. Surgeons may have a higher tendency not to accept livers from patients with risk factors for severe hepatic steatosis to avoid the potential risk of primary graft nonfunction. However, instead of discarding all severely steatotic liver grafts, the transplant community should aim at alternative strategies to minimize hepatic fat and/or modify the approach by which to facilitate such organs being used successfully for liver transplantation. Although donor steatosis status influences graft survival, there is no evidence to suggest that it is a predictor for de novo or recurrent NAFLD posttransplant.

RECIPIENT-SPECIFIC FACTORS FOR DE NOVO AND RECURRENT NONALCOHOLIC FATTY LIVER DISEASE AGE

Advancements in surgical technique and immunosuppressant management and improved clinical outcomes have provided increased opportunity for use of allografts from older donors.[21] Age is a strong independent predictor for hepatic fibrosis in patients with NASH.[10,22]

The rising prevalence of NASH, coupled with the slower rate of fibrosis progression with NASH as compared with hepatitis C virus or alcohol-related liver disease has resulted in a steady increase in liver transplantation rates especially in those more than 65 years old.[23] Although it remains controversial whether age alone confers poorer outcomes with liver transplantation,[24,25] increased age and metabolic syndrome does confer increased risk for comorbidities (ie, obesity, diabetes, cardiovascular disease),[26–29] and therefore the associated risk for recurrent NAFLD.

Ethnic Risk Factors

The pathogenesis of NASH cirrhosis demonstrates significant ethnic and genetic variability.[23,30–32] In an urban population-based study of 2287 patients, Latinos had the highest prevalence of hepatic steatosis, followed by white persons, and then African-Americans.[33] The ethnic differences in NAFLD were not attributable to differences in body mass index (BMI), insulin sensitivity, or ethanol ingestion. The variability of NAFLD across different ethnic groups has been reported in other studies[31,34,35] with suggestions that African-Americans may not develop progressive liver disease even when fatty liver disease is present. Both Asian and Hispanic ethnicity confer increased risk for NASH at lower BMI threshold (average BMI, 26 kg/m^2),[31] keeping in mind that the World Health Organization definition of obesity varies by racial-ethnic groups.[36]

The ethnic differences in the prevalence of NAFLD and NASH pretransplant (white persons > Latinos > African Americans)[37,38] may account for the reported variance in incidence across ethnicities of de novo and recurrent NAFLD posttransplant.[23]

Gender

Whether gender plays a role in the risk prevalence of de novo or recurrent NAFLD after liver transplantation is unknown. Early epidemiologic studies in NAFLD using the National Health and Nutrition Examination Survey data suggested NAFLD to be more prevalent in men than in women.[33,39] However, earlier data ascertained from the National Health and Nutrition Examination Survey were subject to ascertainment bias because this was not initially designed as data acquire from random sampling of the general population. Younossi and colleagues,[40] however, demonstrated that among a lean cohort of patients with NASH, there was a female predominance. Likewise, the prevalence of biopsy-proven NAFLD, as defined by the NASH Clinical Research Network, reported a 2:1 female predominance of NAFLD.[41] Whether the reported gender differences are true pathophysiologic variances for disease, or referral bias (more women pursing health care) is unclear. Although noteworthy that most patients wait-listed for the indication of NAFLD are women,[42] it is unclear whether women are at higher risk for de novo or recurrent NASH post liver transplantation. If such differences exist, variances fat depots and/or sex-hormone metabolism may contribute.[43–45]

Genetic Factors

Familial and twin studies suggest genetic predisposition NAFLD, and NASH-related cirrhosis.[46,47] In recent years, genome-wide association studies have helped to determine genetic determinants of steatosis. Gene variants, such as the patatin-like phospholipase domain—containing 3 (PNPLA3) and transmembrane 6 superfamily member 2 (TM6SF2) E167K, have been shown to be involved in hepatocellular lipid droplet remodeling and interference of very-low-density lipoprotein secretion, and may be stimulated in early NALFD.[48–50] Additional studies demonstrate the importance other genetic variants play in inflammation,[51] insulin sensitivity,[52] oxidative stress, iron metabolism,[53] and fibrotic remodeling, all of which play key roles in the spectrum of fatty liver disease toward NASH-related cirrhosis. In the setting of posttransplant NAFLD, the role of PNPLA3 has been evaluated specifically. Finkenstedt and colleagues[54] assessed in 237 transplant recipients and 255 organ donors the risk of macrovesicular steatosis as assessed by computed tomography 5 years after liver transplantation. Donor genotypes were not associated with the development of graft steatosis. The PNPLA3 variant was significantly more frequent in transplant recipients than in donors (42% vs 28%; $P<.001$). A prevalence of graft steatosis of greater than or equal to 30% significantly increased from 11.6% at 1 year after liver transplantation to 32.6% at 5 years after transplantation. Five years after liver transplantation, steatosis was present in 63.2% of patients homozygous for the rs738409-G allele, in 31.4% of heterozygous recipients, and in 12.0% of rs738409-CC recipients ($P = .002$).[54] In multivariate regression analysis, recipients who carried rs738409-GG had a 13.7-fold higher risk of graft steatosis than recipients who carried rs738409-CC ($P = .022$), independent of recipient age, weight gain after liver transplantation, or the underlying disease.[54]

In a study of long-term recipients (n = 65) with a survival exceeding 10 years, Liu and colleagues[55] demonstrated that de novo NAFLD was more frequent in PNPLA3 GG carriers (0.33 vs 0.10 for GG vs CC + CG carriers; $P = .018$), whereas the genetic impact on NAFLD susceptibility was insignificant when categorized by the TM6SF2 polymorphism. Multicovariate analysis revealed that *PNPLA3* exerted a significant genetic effect on de novo NAFLD following a recessive model (GG vs CC + CG; odds ratio, 14.2; 95% confidence interval, 1.78–113; $P = .012$). Hepatic steatosis was highly prevalent (71.4%) in *PNPLA3* GG carriers with obesity conferring substantial increased risk for recurrent NAFLD and NASH following liver transplantation in obese recipients with *PNPLA3* gene variants.

Another potential genetic cause for liver transplantation for the indication of NAFLD or cryptogenic cirrhosis is early or late onset lysosomal acid lipase deficiency (LALD), previously referred to as cholesteryl ester storage disorder. LALD is a rare lysosomal storage disorder characterized by accumulation of cholesteryl esters. LALD has a heterogeneous clinical phenotype including abdominal pain, poor growth, hyperlipidemia with vascular complications, hepatosplenomegaly, and rapid progression to end-stage liver disease. A few reports of successful liver transplantation for known cases of LALD exist. However, given the lack of routine testing for LALD, liver transplantation may be performed in the absence of a known diagnosis and for what otherwise seems to be cryptogenic- or NAFLD-related cirrhosis. Patients with LALD may present with complications of portal hypertension, splenomegaly, NASH-related cirrhosis, cryptogenic cirrhosis, or hepatopulmonary or portopulmonary syndrome.[56] It is conceivable that historic cases of rapid recurrent of NASH posttransplant may have been associated with undiagnosed cases of LALD.[57,58] Evaluation for LALD by enzyme assay should be considered for patients with recurrent NASH because enzyme-replacement therapy could potentially salvage patient and graft survival.[59,60]

Rapid Weight Gain After Transplantation

Posttransplant weight gain is common after orthotopic liver transplantation, irrespective of the cause of their chronic liver disease. Most weight gain has been reported to occur within the first 16 months following transplant with pretransplant overweight status being a strong predictor of posttransplant overweight or obese status. To complicate this matter, the percentage of liver transplant candidates obese at the time of transplant has increased from 15% to 25% as of 2003, and 35.4% by 2012.[61,62] Mean rate of weight gain for overweight compared with nonoverweight patients during the first 16 months after transplant was 1.5 ± 0.9 kg/month versus 0.4 ± 0.4 kg/month for those not overweight.[63] Another study reported the median weight gain at 1 and 3 years was 5.1 kg and 9.5 kg above dry weight pretransplant.[64] By 1 and 3 years, 24% and 31% had become obese. The weight gain was not associated with gender, pretransplant obesity, or those who received corticosteroids for greater than 3 months. A pretransplant BMI greater than 30 was a strong indicator that the patient would still have a BMI greater than 30 at 3 years. There was no effect of the type of immunosuppression on weight gain.[64] Posttransplant overweight status was associated with more hypertension, hypercholesterolemia, hypertriglyceridemia, and abnormal liver aminotransferases,[63] potentially reflecting associated NASH. In one single-center, observational study the percentage of overweight status at 6 months after transplantation increased from 16% to 30.7% and obese status increased from 17.3% to 40%.[65] Excess weight gain after transplantation (up to 10 kg) 1 year after transplant has been well described in not only liver transplant recipients, but also in the renal and cardiac transplant population.[64,66,67] There is conflicting evidence to implicate immunosuppressive regimens or low-dose prednisone therapy in posttransplant weight gain.[68–70] In several studies involving liver patients, there has been no significant difference in weight gain between patients taking steroids and those on steroid-free regimens or between patients on longer versus shorter regimens of steroids.[64,65] Some authors have found cyclosporine use to be a predictor of obesity after transplantation,[66] whereas others have not confirmed this.[64,65] Unfortunately, a large systematic review of the United Network for Organ Sharing database to assess the risk and clinical consequences of posttransplant weight gain has not been published.[71] Although there are limited data about the association of posttransplant weight with de novo and/or recurrent NAFLD, the increased incidence of metabolic syndrome with posttransplant weight gain likely confers an associated risk for de novo or recurrent NAFLD.

Comorbid Metabolic Syndrome

NAFLD is the hepatic manifestation of metabolic syndrome. The presence of obesity and diabetes confers increased risk for NAFLD. NAFLD occurs in 80% to 100% of patients with obesity and diabetes.[72,73] Patients receiving a liver transplant for the indication of NASH-related cirrhosis are more likely to be white, have diabetes, and have higher BMI.[74] All patients who undergo liver transplant, irrespective of indication, are at risk metabolically for hyperlipidemia, diabetes mellitus, hypertension, and cardiovascular disease and therefore are at increased risk for de novo or recurrent NAFLD. A third of patients who are transplanted for non-NASH-related causes develop insulin resistance in less than 3 years from the time of transplant.[75,76] The incidence of diabetes mellitus after transplantation increased from 15% before transplant to 30% to 40% after transplant.[77,78] Hyperlipidemia is present in 45% to 69% of liver transplant recipients.[79,80] Hyperlipidemia is an independent risk factor for cardiovascular disease. Overall, the metabolic syndrome is found in 45% to 58% of patients transplanted within 6 months.[81] Posttransplant weight gain and metabolic syndrome need to be managed with dietary and lifestyle modification to minimize the risk for de novo and/or recurrent NAFLD acquisition and progression.

Pretransplant Alcoholic Liver Disease

NAFLD mimics alcohol-related fatty liver disease histologically. Patients with a pretransplant diagnosis of alcoholic cirrhosis have an increased risk of de novo NAFLD.[82] One potential explanation is the potential that pretransplant social alcohol use could serve as a cofactor for NAFLD progression in patients who otherwise have risk factors for NAFLD. Alternatively, patients with alcohol use disorder could have been misdiagnosed as NAFLD pretransplant because of denial of their overuse or abuse and/or fear that openness about alcohol addiction could deprive them of life-saving therapy. Therefore, in the absence of treatment of alcohol use disorder, de novo hepatic steatosis or recurrent "NAFLD" may in fact be a reflection of recurrent or surreptitious alcohol-related fatty liver disease.

TRANSPLANT-SPECIFIC FACTORS

Aside from the multitude of metabolic risk factors that place patients at risk for the development of de novo or recurrent NAFLD, immunosuppression can lead to or exacerbate metabolic risk factors for NAFLD. Commonly used maintenance immunosuppressant agents are steroids, calcineurin inhibitors (CNIs), mammalian targets of rapamycin (mTOR) inhibitors, and mycophenolate mofetil. Here we examine the contribution of immunosuppressive agents on the worsening of the metabolic profile, therefore contributing to the development of de novo NAFLD.

Corticosteroids

Glucocorticoids are effective prophylaxis against allograft rejection in the immediate and short-term posttransplant period. They decrease interleukin-1, -2, and -6 activities and nonspecifically inhibit T-cell activation. Steroid-related side effects include hypertension, hyperglycemia, hypercholesterolemia, and obesity. Glucocorticoids contribute to obesity and insulin insensitivity, thereby also implicating them as potential risk factors in the pathogenesis of de novo NAFLD. Patients with glucocorticoid excess (Cushing syndrome) develop obesity, insulin resistance, and hepatic steatosis in a significant proportion of cases.[83] Glucocorticoids affect lipid metabolism and storage in a tissue-specific manner. Glucocorticoids promote gluconeogenesis and glycogenolysis thereby increasing the availability of glucose as a substrate for de novo lipogenesis in the liver.[84] Glucocorticoids promote insulin-induced lipogenesis in rodent hepatocytes, and are potent regulators of genes that drive lipogenesis including fatty acid synthase and acetyl-CoA carboxylase 1 and 2.[85,86] Whether glucocorticoids alone, or in concert with insulin, contribute to lipid accumulation in the hepatocytes is unclear.

Aside from affecting fat metabolism and storage, glucocorticoids also contribute to hypertension, dyslipidemia, and insulin resistance. Although corticosteroids are a necessary component of the posttransplant immunosuppression strategy, they are associated with a risk profile that should be recognized as a risk for developing de novo fatty liver disease. To minimize such steroid-related effects, most immunosuppressant strategies include a progressive steroid taper to steroid-free regimens in the long term.

Calcineurin Inhibitors

CNIs (ie, cyclosporine and tacrolimus) inhibit the action of the phosphatase calcineurin. CNIs have been a staple of immunosuppression since the discovery of cyclosporine in 1971 and its approval in 1983 in the prevention of transplant rejection. CNIs have increased 1-year survival to greater than 80%,[87] and they are associated with improved patient survival and decreased rates of acute cellular rejection in sold-organ transplant recipients.[88] Tacrolimus, similar in mechanism to cyclosporine, was discovered in 1987, and was approved by the Food and Drug Administration (FDA) for transplantation in 1994. Although highly effective in minimizing risk for cellular rejection, CNIs are associated with hypertension, hyperlipidemia, new-onset diabetes, and chronic renal disease after liver transplantation.

The impact of tacrolimus on lipid profiles has been debated for several years. Tarantino and colleagues[89] reported significant changes in plasma lipid concentrations and glycemic imbalance among kidney transplant recipients (n = 29) on tacrolimus treatment for 6 years. The liver enzyme activity showed a modest derangement during the tacrolimus treatment, suggesting the presence of lipid accumulation in the liver.[89] Cyclosporine A causes a dose–dependent inhibition of mitochondrial 27-hydroxylase (CYP27A1) and therefore increases the expression of 3-hydroxy-3-methyl-glutaryl-CoA reductase, a key regulatory enzyme in cholesterol synthesis.[90] Cyclosporine A impairs the clearance of very-low-density lipoprotein and low-density lipoprotein (LDL) cholesterol by binding to the LDL receptor, and increases the activity of hepatic lipase. Hepatic lipase converts intermediate-density lipoprotein to LDL.[91] This effect on lipid metabolism is compounded by the concomitant use of steroids. The prevalence of calcineurin-related dyslipidemia is worse in recipients with as opposed to without metabolic syndrome pretransplant (70% vs 40%, respectively).[78] CNI withdrawal and replacement with mycophenolate mofetil has been shown to improve posttransplant dyslipidemia.[92] In 41 patients where this strategy was used, blood cholesterol decreased in 76% and blood triglyceride decreased in 89% of those patients who underwent CNI withdrawal.[92] Different strategies to reduce the metabolic risk profile of the CNI, including combination with other agents, such as mycophenolate mofitil, have been used. Although tacrolimus and cyclosporine share a similar mechanism, tacrolimus has a lower rate of acute rejection, and produces a more favorable cardiovascular profile,[93,94] causing many transplant centers to favor tacrolimus as the favored CNI for long-term immunosuppression management.

Sirolimus

Sirolimus is part of the mTOR inhibitor family. Sirolimus increases triglyceride production, with 55% of patients developing dyslipidemia,[95] and alters insulin signaling pathways. Of 92 patients having undergone transplantation, patients treated with mTORs were at higher risk for hyperlipidemia and insulin insensitivity when compared with patients on CNIs.[96] Although immunosuppression is a necessity of transplantation, tailoring of immunosuppressive medication requires knowledge of the recipient's overall health and potential for specific immunosuppressive drug to worsen underlying comorbidities. In animal models, sirolimus caused glucose intolerance, increased storage of lipids in the liver and skeletal muscle, decreased the insulin-stimulated glucose uptake in isolated adipocytes, and increased genes and/or proteins involved in hepatic lipogenesis and gluconeogenesis. Moreover, there was an increase in interleukin-6 gene expression in adipose tissue in the sirolimus-treated rats, suggesting stimulation of lipolysis.[97] Sirolimus led to metabolic alterations in liver, muscle, and adipose tissue, which may contribute to the development of dyslipidemia and insulin resistance and therefore confer increased risk for de novo or recurrent NAFLD. Because of its antiproliferative effect, there was enthusiasm early that it may prolong survival and attenuate nephrotoxicity and carcinoma risk; however, sirolimus has been associated with increased risk for acute cellular rejection thereby leaving CNIs as the preference backbone for long-term immunosuppression.

MANAGEMENT OF DE NOVO NONALCOHOLIC FATTY LIVER DISEASE

There are no pharmacologic therapies for de novo or recurrent NAFLD following liver transplantation. Transplant programs can deploy approaches to manage individual patients with NASH by identifying and treating underlying risk factors for NAFLD acquisition and modifying risk factors associated with fibrosis progression. Lifestyle modification with routine physical activity is a mandatory change in current norms of being a sedentary society. Patients, particularly those with obesity and diabetes, should be clearly informed that in addition to cardiovascular, metabolic, and kidney complications of metabolic syndrome, their obese status poses risk for liver-related morbidity and mortality. With knowledge comes the opportunity to help patients help themselves. Community-based lifestyle modification programs and the use of cognitive behavioral therapy is effective in reducing and normalizing liver fat in patients with NAFLD[98,99] and are worthy of consideration in posttransplant management of recurrent NAFLD. In nontransplant cohorts of patients with NAFLD, sustained lifestyle changes associated with a greater extent of weight loss ($\geq$10%) can resolve or reduce steatohepatitis and regress hepatic fibrosis (25%, 47%, and 19%, respectively).[100] Although such interventions have not been systematically studied in transplanted cohorts, modification of risk factors (ie, increased dietary fructose consumption,[101] alcohol consumption,[102] cigarette smoking,[103] obstructive sleep apnea[104]) associated with fibrosis progression is cost-effective and may improve total and liver-related outcomes.

Optimal treatment targets include improving obesity before or after transplantation, rapid weight gain after transplant, insulin resistance, dyslipidemia, hypertension, and/or the improvement of pathogenic mechanisms for transition to steatohepatitis and hepatic fibrosis (ie, oxidative stress cytokine production, stellate cell activation).[105]

Immunosuppression management poses additional clinical challenges but provides the opportunity for further investigation.

Bariatric surgery is the most effective treatment of morbid obesity and its associated metabolic comorbidities. Although data suggest that patients with indications for bariatric surgery also have improvement in the histologic and biochemical parameters of NAFLD,[106,107] no studies have evaluated liver-related mortality or the role of bariatric surgery as a treatment of de novo or recurrent NAFLD following liver transplantation.

Despite the lack of FDA-approved therapy for NASH, encouraging results from recent studies lend the opportunity for clinicians to effectively treat comorbidities for NAFLD in a manner that may also improve recurrent NAFLD or NASH. Specifically, vitamin E may be a consideration for patients without diabetes with NASH,[108] whereas insulin-sensitizing agents (ie, pioglitazone or liraglutide) may be beneficial for patients with diabetes with NASH,[108,109] thereby allowing for such therapies to also be used within the scope of their FDA-approved indications. Enhanced use of statins, when indicated in patients with NAFLD and dyslipidemia, not only decreases cardiovascular morbidity and mortality, but may also resolve NASH.[110] No studies evaluating such interventions following transplantation currently exist. The ultimate goal is to harmonize a myriad of different approaches to mitigate risk for de novo or recurrent NAFLD and risk for chronic liver injury in the allograft. Unfortunately, practice guidelines to guide the clinical care and immunosuppression management of liver transplant recipients with de novo and recurrent NAFLD are currently lacking.

SUMMARY

With the rise of obesity and diabetes mellitus, NAFLD will likely become the leading indication for liver transplantation in the United States in the near future. Although transplantation cures the complications of end-stage liver disease for those patients transplanted for the indication of NAFLD-related cirrhosis, the metabolic risk factors associated with de novo and recurrent NAFLD persist and may worsen in the setting of chronic immunosuppression. Thoughtful evaluation of modifiable risk factors for NAFLD and lifestyle modification, before and after transplantation, is important to decreasing recurrent hepatitis steatosis and steatosis-related liver injury. Although emerging therapies for NAFLD are currently under investigation, FDA approval for such therapies is years away. The role of pharmacologic approaches and bariatric surgery for treatment of NAFLD following liver transplant requires further investigation. NAFLD-specific liver transplant practice guidelines are needed to guide posttransplant care and immunosuppression management of patients with de novo or recurrent NAFLD.

REFERENCES

1. Torres DM, Williams CD, Harrison SA. Features, diagnosis, and treatment of nonalcoholic fatty liver disease. Clin Gastroenterol Hepatol 2012;10(8):837–58.
2. Ong JP, Younossi ZM. Epidemiology and natural history of NAFLD and NASH. Clin Liver Dis 2007;11(1):1–16, vii.
3. Ratziu V, Goodman Z, Sanyal A. Current efforts and trends in the treatment of NASH. J Hepatol 2015;62(1 Suppl):S65–75.
4. Vernon G, Baranova A, Younossi ZM. Systematic review: the epidemiology and natural history of non-alcoholic fatty liver disease and non-alcoholic steatohepatitis in adults. Aliment Pharmacol Ther 2011;34(3):274–85.
5. Mittal S, El-Serag HB, Sada YH, et al. Hepatocellular carcinoma in the absence of cirrhosis in United States veterans is associated with nonalcoholic fatty liver disease. Clin Gastroenterol Hepatol 2016;14(1):124–31.e1.

6. Schuppan D, Schattenberg JM. Non-alcoholic steatohepatitis: pathogenesis and novel therapeutic approaches. J Gastroenterol Hepatol 2013;28(Suppl 1): 68–76.

7. White DL, Kanwal F, El-Serag HB. Association between nonalcoholic fatty liver disease and risk for hepatocellular cancer, based on systematic review. Clin Gastroenterol Hepatol 2012;10(12):1342–59.e2.

8. Younossi ZM, Stepanova M, Rafiq N, et al. Pathologic criteria for nonalcoholic steatohepatitis: interprotocol agreement and ability to predict liver-related mortality. Hepatology 2011;53(6):1874–82.

9. Angulo P, Kleiner DE, Dam-Larsen S, et al. Liver fibrosis, but No other histologic features, is associated with long-term outcomes of patients with nonalcoholic fatty liver disease. Gastroenterology 2015;149(2):389–97.e10.

10. Angulo P, Keach JC, Batts KP, et al. Independent predictors of liver fibrosis in patients with nonalcoholic steatohepatitis. Hepatology 1999;30(6):1356–62.

11. Ong JP, Elariny H, Collantes R, et al. Predictors of nonalcoholic steatohepatitis and advanced fibrosis in morbidly obese patients. Obes Surg 2005;15(3): 310–5.

12. Charlton M. Evolving aspects of liver transplantation for nonalcoholic steatohepatitis. Curr Opin Organ Transplant 2013;18(3):251–8.

13. Friman S. Recurrence of disease after liver transplantation. Transplant Proc 2013;45(3):1178–81.

14. Ong J, Younossi ZM, Reddy V, et al. Cryptogenic cirrhosis and posttransplantation nonalcoholic fatty liver disease. Liver Transpl 2001;7(9):797–801.

15. Malik SM, Devera ME, Fontes P, et al. Recurrent disease following liver transplantation for nonalcoholic steatohepatitis cirrhosis. Liver Transpl 2009;15(12): 1843–51.

16. Marsman WA, Wiesner RH, Rodriguez L, et al. Use of fatty donor liver is associated with diminished early patient and graft survival. Transplantation 1996; 62(9):1246–51.

17. Hines CD, Frydrychowicz A, Hamilton G, et al. T(1) independent, T(2) (*) corrected chemical shift based fat-water separation with multi-peak fat spectral modeling is an accurate and precise measure of hepatic steatosis. J Magn Reson Imaging 2011;33(4):873–81.

18. Kosmalski M, Kasznicki J, Drzewoski J. Relationship between ultrasound features of nonalcoholic fatty liver disease and cardiometabolic risk factors in patients with newly diagnosed type 2 diabetes. Pol Arch Med Wewn 2013; 123(9):436–42.

19. Wong TC, Fung JY, Chok KS, et al. Excellent outcomes of liver transplantation using severely steatotic grafts from brain-dead donors. Liver Transpl 2016; 22(2):226–36.

20. Tanaka T, Sugawara Y, Tamura S, et al. Living donor liver transplantation for nonalcoholic steatohepatitis: a single center experience. Hepatol Res 2014;44(10): E3–10.

21. Aduen JF, Sujay B, Dickson RC, et al. Outcomes after liver transplant in patients aged 70 years or older compared with those younger than 60 years. Mayo Clin Proc 2009;84(11):973–8.

22. Shimada M, Hashimoto E, Kaneda H, et al. Nonalcoholic steatohepatitis: risk factors for liver fibrosis. Hepatol Res 2002;24(4):429–38.

23. Kemmer N, Neff GW, Franco E, et al. Nonalcoholic fatty liver disease epidemic and its implications for liver transplantation. Transplantation 2013;96(10):860–2.

24. Collins BH, Pirsch JD, Becker YT, et al. Long-term results of liver transplantation in older patients 60 years of age and older. Transplantation 2000;70(5):780–3.
25. Emre S, Mor E, Schwartz ME, et al. Liver transplantation in patients beyond age 60. Transplant Proc 1993;25(1 Pt 2):1075–6.
26. Ford ES, Giles WH, Dietz WH. Prevalence of the metabolic syndrome among US adults: findings from the third National Health and Nutrition Examination Survey. JAMA 2002;287(3):356–9.
27. Hildrum B, Mykletun A, Hole T, et al. Age-specific prevalence of the metabolic syndrome defined by the International Diabetes Federation and the National Cholesterol Education program: the Norwegian HUNT 2 study. BMC Public Health 2007;7:220.
28. Ravaglia G, Forti P, Maioli F, et al. Metabolic syndrome: prevalence and prediction of mortality in elderly individuals. Diabetes Care 2006;29(11):2471–6.
29. Saad MA, Cardoso GP, Martins Wde A, et al. Prevalence of metabolic syndrome in elderly and agreement among four diagnostic criteria. Arq Bras Cardiol 2014; 102(3):263–9.
30. Chatterjee A, Basu A, Chowdhury A, et al. Comparative analyses of genetic risk prediction methods reveal extreme diversity of genetic predisposition to nonalcoholic fatty liver disease (NAFLD) among ethnic populations of India. J Genet 2015;94(1):105–13.
31. Weston SR, Leyden W, Murphy R, et al. Racial and ethnic distribution of nonalcoholic fatty liver in persons with newly diagnosed chronic liver disease. Hepatology 2005;41(2):372–9.
32. Graham RC, Burke A, Stettler N. Ethnic and sex differences in the association between metabolic syndrome and suspected nonalcoholic fatty liver disease in a nationally representative sample of US adolescents. J Pediatr Gastroenterol Nutr 2009;49(4):442–9.
33. Browning JD, Szczepaniak LS, Dobbins R, et al. Prevalence of hepatic steatosis in an urban population in the United States: impact of ethnicity. Hepatology 2004;40(6):1387–95.
34. Giday SA, Ashiny Z, Naab T, et al. Frequency of nonalcoholic fatty liver disease and degree of hepatic steatosis in African-American patients. J Natl Med Assoc 2006;98(10):1613–5.
35. Solga SF, Clark JM, Alkhuraishi AR, et al. Race and comorbid factors predict nonalcoholic fatty liver disease histopathology in severely obese patients. Surg Obes Relat Dis 2005;1(1):6–11.
36. WHO Expert Consultation. Appropriate body-mass index for Asian populations and its implications for policy and intervention strategies. Lancet 2004; 363(9403):157–63.
37. Deurenberg P, Yap M, van Staveren WA. Body mass index and percent body fat: a meta-analysis among different ethnic groups. Int J Obes Relat Metab Disord 1998;22(12):1164–71.
38. Okosun IS, Dever GE. Abdominal obesity and ethnic differences in diabetes awareness, treatment, and glycemic control. Obes Res 2002;10(12):1241–50.
39. Ruhl CE, Everhart JE. Determinants of the association of overweight with elevated serum alanine aminotransferase activity in the United States. Gastroenterology 2003;124(1):71–9.
40. Younossi ZM, Stepanova M, Negro F, et al. Nonalcoholic fatty liver disease in lean individuals in the United States. Medicine (Baltimore) 2012;91(6):319–27.

41. Neuschwander-Tetri BA, Clark JM, Bass NM, et al. Clinical, laboratory and histological associations in adults with nonalcoholic fatty liver disease. Hepatology 2010;52(3):913–24.
42. Rodriguez-Castro KI, De Martin E, Gambato M, et al. Female gender in the setting of liver transplantation. World J Transplant 2014;4(4):229–42.
43. Suzuki A, Abdelmalek MF, Unalp-Arida A, et al. Regional anthropometric measures and hepatic fibrosis in patients with nonalcoholic Fatty liver disease. Clin Gastroenterol Hepatol 2010;8(12):1062–9.
44. Yang JD, Abdelmalek MF, Pang H, et al. Gender and menopause impact severity of fibrosis among patients with nonalcoholic steatohepatitis. Hepatology 2014;59(4):1406–14.
45. Yang JD, Abdelmalek MF, Guy CD, et al. Patient sex, reproductive status, and synthetic hormone use associate with histologic severity of nonalcoholic steatohepatitis. Clin Gastroenterol Hepatol 2016;15(1):127–31.e2.
46. Guerrero R, Vega GL, Grundy SM, et al. Ethnic differences in hepatic steatosis: an insulin resistance paradox? Hepatology 2009;49(3):791–801.
47. Schwimmer JB, Celedon MA, Lavine JE, et al. Heritability of nonalcoholic fatty liver disease. Gastroenterology 2009;136(5):1585–92.
48. Dongiovanni P, Donati B, Fares R, et al. PNPLA3 I148M polymorphism and progressive liver disease. World J Gastroenterol 2013;19(41):6969–78.
49. Romeo S, Kozlitina J, Xing C, et al. Genetic variation in PNPLA3 confers susceptibility to nonalcoholic fatty liver disease. Nat Genet 2008;40(12):1461–5.
50. Zelber-Sagi S, Salomone F, Yeshua H, et al. Non-high-density lipoprotein cholesterol independently predicts new onset of non-alcoholic fatty liver disease. Liver Int 2014;34(6):e128–35.
51. Mohamed J, Nazratun Nafizah AH, Zariyantey AH, et al. Mechanisms of diabetes-induced liver damage: the role of oxidative stress and inflammation. Sultan Qaboos Univ Med J 2016;16(2):e132–41.
52. Dongiovanni P, Valenti L, Rametta R, et al. Genetic variants regulating insulin receptor signalling are associated with the severity of liver damage in patients with non-alcoholic fatty liver disease. Gut 2010;59(2):267–73.
53. Valenti L, Rametta R, Dongiovanni P, et al. The A736V TMPRSS6 polymorphism influences hepatic iron overload in nonalcoholic fatty liver disease. PLoS One 2012;7(11):e48804.
54. Finkenstedt A, Auer C, Glodny B, et al. Patatin-like phospholipase domain-containing protein 3 rs738409-G in recipients of liver transplants is a risk factor for graft steatosis. Clin Gastroenterol Hepatol 2013;11(12):1667–72.
55. Liu ZT, Chen TC, Lu XX, et al. PNPLA3 I148M variant affects non-alcoholic fatty liver disease in liver transplant recipients. World J Gastroenterol 2015;21(34):10054–6.
56. Leone L, Ippoliti PF, Antonicelli R, et al. Treatment and liver transplantation for cholesterol ester storage disease. J Pediatr 1995;127(3):509–10.
57. Jankowska I, Socha P, Pawlowska J, et al. Recurrence of non-alcoholic steatohepatitis after liver transplantation in a 13-yr-old boy. Pediatr Transplant 2007;11(7):796–8.
58. Molloy RM, Komorowski R, Varma RR. Recurrent nonalcoholic steatohepatitis and cirrhosis after liver transplantation. Liver Transpl Surg 1997;3(2):177–8.
59. Hamilton J, Jones I, Srivastava R, et al. A new method for the measurement of lysosomal acid lipase in dried blood spots using the inhibitor Lalistat 2. Clin Chim Acta 2012;413(15–16):1207–10.

60. Valayannopoulos V, Malinova V, Honzik T, et al. Sebelipase alfa over 52 weeks reduces serum transaminases, liver volume and improves serum lipids in patients with lysosomal acid lipase deficiency. J Hepatol 2014;61(5):1135–42.
61. Kim WR, Smith JM, Skeans MA, et al. OPTN/SRTR 2012 annual data report: liver. Am J Transplant 2014;14(Suppl 1):69–96.
62. Leonard J, Heimbach JK, Malinchoc M, et al. The impact of obesity on long-term outcomes in liver transplant recipients-results of the NIDDK liver transplant database. Am J Transplant 2008;8(3):667–72.
63. Palmer M, Schaffner F, Thung SN. Excessive weight gain after liver transplantation. Transplantation 1991;51(4):797–800.
64. Richards J, Gunson B, Johnson J, et al. Weight gain and obesity after liver transplantation. Transpl Int 2005;18(4):461–6.
65. Wawrzynowicz-Syczewska M, Karpinska E, Jurczyk K, et al. Risk factors and dynamics of weight gain in patients after liver transplantation. Ann Transplant 2009;14(3):45–50.
66. Everhart JE, Lombardero M, Lake JR, et al. Weight change and obesity after liver transplantation: incidence and risk factors. Liver Transpl Surg 1998;4(4):285–96.
67. Rezende Anastacio L, Garcia Ferreira L, Costa Liboredo J, et al. Overweight, obesity and weight gain up to three years after liver transplantation. Nutr Hosp 2012;27(4):1351–6.
68. Aberg F, Jula A, Hockerstedt K, et al. Cardiovascular risk profile of patients with acute liver failure after liver transplantation when compared with the general population. Transplantation 2010;89(1):61–8.
69. Dolgos S, Hartmann A, Jenssen T, et al. Determinants of short-term changes in body composition following renal transplantation. Scand J Urol Nephrol 2009;43(1):76–83.
70. van den Ham EC, Kooman JP, Christiaans MH, et al. Weight changes after renal transplantation: a comparison between patients on 5-mg maintenance steroid therapy and those on steroid-free immunosuppressive therapy. Transpl Int 2003;16(5):300–6.
71. Beckmann S, Ivanovic N, Drent G, et al. Weight gain, overweight and obesity in solid organ transplantation-a study protocol for a systematic literature review. Syst Rev 2015;4:2.
72. Subichin M, Clanton J, Makuszewski M, et al. Liver disease in the morbidly obese: a review of 1000 consecutive patients undergoing weight loss surgery. Surg Obes Relat Dis 2015;11(1):137–41.
73. Prashanth M, Ganesh HK, Vima MV, et al. Prevalence of nonalcoholic fatty liver disease in patients with type 2 diabetes mellitus. J Assoc Physicians India 2009;57:205–10.
74. Wong RJ, Aguilar M, Cheung R, et al. Nonalcoholic steatohepatitis is the second leading etiology of liver disease among adults awaiting liver transplantation in the United States. Gastroenterology 2015;148(3):547–55.
75. Pagadala M, Dasarathy S, Eghtesad B, et al. Posttransplant metabolic syndrome: an epidemic waiting to happen. Liver Transpl 2009;15(12):1662–70.
76. Sprinzl MF, Weinmann A, Lohse N, et al. Metabolic syndrome and its association with fatty liver disease after orthotopic liver transplantation. Transpl Int 2013;26(1):67–74.
77. Laryea M, Watt KD, Molinari M, et al. Metabolic syndrome in liver transplant recipients: prevalence and association with major vascular events. Liver Transpl 2007;13(8):1109–14.

78. Pfitzmann R, Nussler NC, Hippler-Benscheidt M, et al. Long-term results after liver transplantation. Transpl Int 2008;21(3):234–46.
79. Gisbert C, Prieto M, Berenguer M, et al. Hyperlipidemia in liver transplant recipients: prevalence and risk factors. Liver Transpl Surg 1997;3(4):416–22.
80. Neal DA, Tom BD, Luan J, et al. Is there disparity between risk and incidence of cardiovascular disease after liver transplant? Transplantation 2004;77(1):93–9.
81. Watt KD, Charlton MR. Metabolic syndrome and liver transplantation: a review and guide to management. J Hepatol 2010;53(1):199–206.
82. Dumortier J, Giostra E, Belbouab S, et al. Non-alcoholic fatty liver disease in liver transplant recipients: another story of "seed and soil." Am J Gastroenterol 2010; 105(3):613–20.
83. Rockall AG, Sohaib SA, Evans D, et al. Hepatic steatosis in Cushing's syndrome: a radiological assessment using computed tomography. Eur J Endocrinol 2003; 149(6):543–8.
84. Mueller KM, Kornfeld JW, Friedbichler K, et al. Impairment of hepatic growth hormone and glucocorticoid receptor signaling causes steatosis and hepatocellular carcinoma in mice. Hepatology 2011;54(4):1398–409.
85. Dolinsky VW, Douglas DN, Lehner R, et al. Regulation of the enzymes of hepatic microsomal triacylglycerol lipolysis and re-esterification by the glucocorticoid dexamethasone. Biochem J 2004;378(Pt 3):967–74.
86. Wang JC, Gray NE, Kuo T, et al. Regulation of triglyceride metabolism by glucocorticoid receptor. Cell Biosci 2012;2(1):19.
87. Waki K. UNOS Liver Registry: ten year survivals. Clin Transplant 2006;29–39.
88. Hong JC, Kahan BD. Immunosuppressive agents in organ transplantation: past, present, and future. Semin Nephrol 2000;20(2):108–25.
89. Tarantino G, Palmiero G, Polichetti G, et al. Long-term assessment of plasma lipids in transplant recipients treated with tacrolimus in relation to fatty liver. Int J Immunopathol Pharmacol 2010;23(4):1303–8.
90. Gueguen Y, Ferrari L, Souidi M, et al. Compared effect of immunosuppressive drugs cyclosporine A and rapamycin on cholesterol homeostasis key enzymes CYP27A1 and HMG-CoA reductase. Basic Clin Pharmacol Toxicol 2007;100(6): 392–7.
91. Derfler K, Hayde M, Heinz G, et al. Decreased postheparin lipolytic activity in renal transplant recipients with cyclosporin A. Kidney Int 1991;40(4):720–7.
92. Orlando G, Baiocchi L, Cardillo A, et al. Switch to 1.5 grams MMF monotherapy for CNI-related toxicity in liver transplantation is safe and improves renal function, dyslipidemia, and hypertension. Liver Transpl 2007;13(1):46–54.
93. Bakar F, Keven K, Dogru B, et al. Low-density lipoprotein oxidizability and the alteration of its fatty acid content in renal transplant recipients treated with cyclosporine/tacrolimus. Transplant Proc 2009;41(5):1630–3.
94. Sandrini S, Aslam N, Tardanico R, et al. Tacrolimus versus cyclosporine for early steroid withdrawal after renal transplantation. J Nephrol 2012;25(1):43–9.
95. Neff GW, Montalbano M, Tzakis AG. Ten years of sirolimus therapy in orthotopic liver transplant recipients. Transplant Proc 2003;35(3 Suppl):209S–16S.
96. Zimmermann A, Zobeley C, Weber MM, et al. Changes in lipid and carbohydrate metabolism under mTOR- and calcineurin-based immunosuppressive regimen in adult patients after liver transplantation. Eur J Intern Med 2016;29: 104–9.
97. Fuhrmann A, Lopes P, Sereno J, et al. Molecular mechanisms underlying the effects of cyclosporin A and sirolimus on glucose and lipid metabolism in liver,

skeletal muscle and adipose tissue in an in vivo rat model. Biochem Pharmacol 2014;88(2):216–28.

98. Wong VW, Chan RS, Wong GL, et al. Community-based lifestyle modification programme for non-alcoholic fatty liver disease: a randomized controlled trial. J Hepatol 2013;59(3):536–42.

99. Marchesini G, Petta S, Dalle Grave R. Diet, weight loss, and liver health in nonalcoholic fatty liver disease: pathophysiology, evidence, and practice. Hepatology 2016;63(6):2032–43.

100. Vilar-Gomez E, Martinez-Perez Y, Calzadilla-Bertot L, et al. Weight loss through lifestyle modification significantly reduces features of nonalcoholic steatohepatitis. Gastroenterology 2015;149(2):367–78.e5 [quiz: e14–5].

101. Abdelmalek MF, Suzuki A, Guy C, et al. Increased fructose consumption is associated with fibrosis severity in patients with nonalcoholic fatty liver disease. Hepatology 2010;51(6):1961–71.

102. Hejlova I, Honsova E, Sticova E, et al. Prevalence and risk factors of steatosis after liver transplantation and patient outcomes. Liver Transpl 2016;22(5): 644–55.

103. Liu Y, Dai M, Bi Y, et al. Active smoking, passive smoking, and risk of nonalcoholic fatty liver disease (NAFLD): a population-based study in China. J Epidemiol 2013;23(2):115–21.

104. Pulixi EA, Tobaldini E, Battezzati PM, et al. Risk of obstructive sleep apnea with daytime sleepiness is associated with liver damage in non-morbidly obese patients with nonalcoholic fatty liver disease. PLoS One 2014;9(4):e96349.

105. Gitto S, Vitale G, Villa E, et al. Treatment of nonalcoholic steatohepatitis in adults: present and future. Gastroenterol Res Pract 2015;2015:732870.

106. Aguilar-Olivos NE, Almeda-Valdes P, Aguilar-Salinas CA, et al. The role of bariatric surgery in the management of nonalcoholic fatty liver disease and metabolic syndrome. Metabolism 2016;65(8):1196–207.

107. Bower G, Toma T, Harling L, et al. Bariatric surgery and non-alcoholic fatty liver disease: a systematic review of liver biochemistry and histology. Obes Surg 2015;25(12):2280–9.

108. Sanyal AJ, Chalasani N, Kowdley KV, et al. Pioglitazone, vitamin E, or placebo for nonalcoholic steatohepatitis. N Engl J Med 2010;362(18):1675–85.

109. Armstrong MJ, Gaunt P, Aithal GP, et al. Liraglutide safety and efficacy in patients with non-alcoholic steatohepatitis (LEAN): a multicentre, double-blind, randomised, placebo-controlled phase 2 study. Lancet 2016;387(10019): 679–90.

110. Kargiotis K, Athyros VG, Giouleme O, et al. Resolution of non-alcoholic steatohepatitis by rosuvastatin monotherapy in patients with metabolic syndrome. World J Gastroenterol 2015;21(25):7860–8.

Management of Immunosuppression in Liver Transplantation

Renumathy Dhanasekaran, MD

KEYWORDS

- Transplantation • Rejection • Calcineurin • Immunosuppression • Hepatitis C

KEY POINTS

- The liver has a unique tolerogenic immune environment; thus, liver transplantation is usually well tolerated and rejection is easily managed.
- Newer steroid-free regimens with T-cell–depleting antibodies and IL-2R antibodies are effective and safe for induction of posttransplant immunosuppression.
- Antibody-mediated rejection is increasingly recognized as a contributor to graft dysfunction.

INTRODUCTION

Liver transplantation (LT) is a life-saving surgery for patients with liver failure, cirrhosis, and early-stage hepatocellular carcinoma (HCC). The first LT was performed as early as 1963 by Dr Thomas Starzl,[1] but throughout the 1960s and 1970s, the procedure was not very popular because it was fraught with complications, and 1-year survival was less than 25%.[2] However, the introduction of cyclosporine in the 1980s, as the immunosuppressant of choice, rapidly changed the scenario because it led to significantly decreased rates of rejection and improved survival.[3] Subsequently, multiple other challenges have been overcome, and the 1-year survival rate after LT is now 85% to 95%. For the past 20 years, around 4000 to 6000 LTs are performed annually in the United States alone,[4] and worldwide, more than 20,000 LTs have been performed since 2008.[5] Several advances related to LT in the control of infection, treatment of rejection, and improvisation of surgical techniques have also contributed to improved graft and patient survival. However, it is true that the tremendous progress made in the field of LT is mainly due to the advent of safe and effective immunosuppression agents. Various features of these agents are discussed in this review.

The author has nothing to disclose.
Division of Gastroenterology and Hepatology, Stanford University, 750 Welch Road, Suite 210, Palo Alto, CA 94304, USA
E-mail address: dhanaser@stanford.edu

The liver, as an organ, is unique in several aspects relevant to this discussion on immunosuppression. The liver is supplied by dual blood supply—the portal venous system and the hepatic arterial system. The portal venous system, which is the predominant source of blood supply, drains the intestinal system. The liver is thus exposed to multiple gut microbial products, metabolic products, and toxins constantly, and hence, has developed mechanisms to circumvent overreaction to this antigen load. Some of the major mechanisms include effective scavenging of antigens by Kupffer cells and dendritic cells; abundance of tolerogenic antigen-presenting cells (APCs) in the liver; expression of interleukin-10 (IL-10) and transforming growth factor-β, which induce regulatory T cells, and a low level of expression of major histocompatibility (MHC) class of proteins.[6–8] It overall has a distinctive immune environment, which has been coined as being "tolerogenic." Compared with other organ transplants like the kidney or the heart, patients who undergo LT usually need lower doses of immunosuppression, and LT is associated with less frequent episodes of rejection. Also, interestingly, when dual organ transplants are performed along with the liver, like liver and kidney or liver and heart, the LT reduces the chance of rejection of the second organ.[9,10]

Despite the relatively tolerogenic environment in the liver, rejection remains a dreaded complication and approximately 25% of the patients suffer at least one episode of rejection after transplantation.[11,12] Hence, adequate immunosuppression that can prevent rejection and prevent graft loss while being accompanied by minimal adverse effects is essential. Broadly speaking, there are 3 periods in the utilization of posttransplant immunosuppression: (1) induction phase (early posttransplant); (2) maintenance phase (long term); and (3) treatment of rejection. In this review, the author broadly discusses the immune environment of the liver, management of posttransplant immunosuppression, treatment of rejection, immunosuppression in special populations, and future directions.

PATHOPHYSIOLOGY OF IMMUNE RESPONSE AFTER LIVER TRANSPLANTATION

In general, the immune response elicited after LT is predominantly driven by T cells. Antibody-mediated rejection (AMR) is relatively uncommon in ABO-compatible LTs compared with other organs (like kidney), although it is being increasingly recognized as an important phenomenon influencing graft survival.[13,14] The immunologic response elicited by the donor liver is immediate, swift, and complicated.[15–18] **Fig. 1** provides an outline of the immune response after LT and also demonstrates the mechanism of action of the different classes of immunosuppressants. The basic steps can be broken down into the following:

1. *Antigen presentation:* The alloantigens in the donor liver are complexed with MHC proteins existing on donor and recipient APCs (like Kupffer cells and dendritic cells) and are presented to recipient's T-cell receptors. Simultaneously, ligands on APCs engage costimulatory receptors on T cells like CD28 and CD154.
   Drugs affecting this step: Antithymocyte globulin (ATG)[19] and antilymphocyte globulin (ALG) can prevent antigen presentation because they can deplete the recipient's T cells.
2. *T-cell activation and expansion:* Once the alloantigen is presented to the TCR in the presence of the appropriate costimulation, the receptor complex is internalized. Internalization of T cell receptor complex activates a downstream activation mechanism that involves immunophilin and calcineurin, ultimately resulting in activation of nuclear factor of T-cell activation (NFAT). NFAT translocates to the nucleus and enhances transcription of IL-2. IL-2 plays the crucial role of driving clonal expansion of T cells.

Drugs affecting this step: Calcineurin inhibitors (CNIs), cyclosporine[20] and tacro-limus,[21] block targets of calcineurin (cyclophilin and FK binding protein, respectively), thus preventing activation of NFAT and IL-2 transcription. Basi-liximab[22] and daclizumab[23] are monoclonal antibodies against the IL-2 recep-tor, and they block T-cell expansion. Sirolimus[24] and everolimus,[25] which inhibit mammalian target of rapamycin (mTOR) pathway, also act at this step. Azathioprine and mycophenolate mofetil (MMF)[26] are antimetabolites, which inhibit DNA synthesis and hence block T-cell clonal expansion.

3. Inflammation—final common pathway: The clonal expansion of T cells leads to cell-mediated cytotoxicity facilitated by release of cytokines and chemokines, which recruit inflammatory cells like neutrophils and result in tissue inflammation and destruction, which if untreated can lead to graft loss.

Drugs affecting this step: Steroids are master inhibitors of inflammation, and they execute this by several mechanisms, including downregulation of IL-2, IL-6, and interferon gamma synthesis by T cells.

MAJOR CLASSES OF IMMUNOSUPPRESSIVE DRUGS

The pharmacokinetics, pharmacodynamics, and adverse effect profile of the different classes of immunosuppressants are briefly described.

Corticosteroids

Despite several advances in the field of immunosuppression, corticosteroids remain the most commonly used drug for induction and also for treatment of rejection.

Mechanism of action
Steroids inhibit inflammation by multiple mechanisms, including decreased migration of neutrophils, decreased tissue accumulation and activation of macrophages, decreased production of interleukins (IL-1, IL-2, IL-6), and decreased transcription of proinflammatory genes.[27,28]

Dose and protocol
Steroids are used for induction of immunosuppression and for treatment of acute rejection. The dose and protocol vary widely between centers and are also modified based on patient risk factors. In general, the first 2 to 3 doses are the highest and range from 250 to 1000 mg of intravenous (IV) methylprednisolone. Subsequently, they are tapered over the first couple of weeks to 10 to 20 mg per day and maintained on lower doses for the first 3 to 6 months after transplant. For treatment of acute cellular rejection (ACR), a similar starting dose is used, but the taper down is much faster over 10 to 14 days.

Adverse effects
Glucocorticoids are associated with several side effects, especially with chronic use. In patients receiving high doses, delirium can be a common early problem. The other common adverse effects include hyperglycemia, hypertension, hyperlipidemia, and weight gain.[29–31] There are specific side effects that are relevant from a transplant standpoint. Risk of opportunistic infections is high in immunosuppressed patients; wound healing can be delayed, and also, there is concern for early and aggressive post-transplant hepatitis C recurrence, which is discussed in detail later in this review.[32,33]

Calcineurin Inhibitors

CNIs form the cornerstone of long-term immunosuppression after LT. There are 2 main drugs in this class: cyclosporine and tacrolimus.

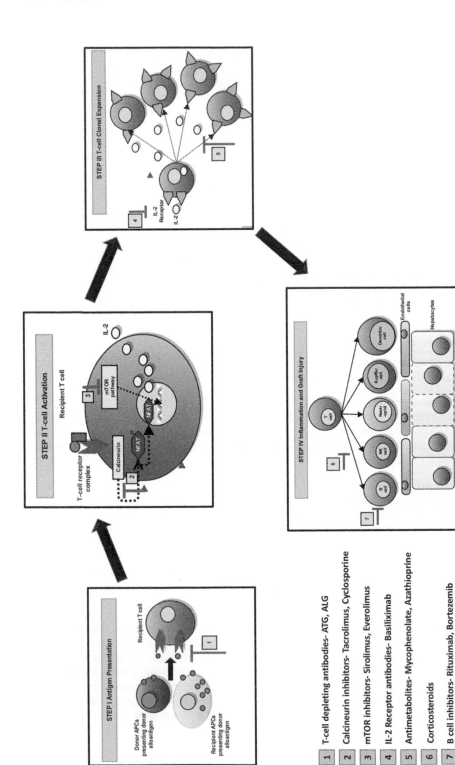

Fig. 1. Schematic representation of the immune response elicited after LT. Step I antigen presentation: the alloantigens in the donor liver are com-plexed with MHC proteins and presented to recipient's T-cell receptors. Step II T-cell activation: the T-cell receptor complex is internalized, and it

Mechanism of action
As mentioned above, the CNIs block T-cell activation by binding to specific receptors and inhibiting activation of NFAT and thus reducing IL-2 transcription.

Dose and protocol
Tacrolimus is the preferred CNI in LT. Tacrolimus is started within 1 to 3 days after transplant, allowing time for renal recovery. The dosage protocol again differs between centers. The author usually started with a low dose (0.1–0.15 mg/kg per day) orally and modified based on trough levels. The IV formulation of tacrolimus is associated with seizures and hence is used very sparingly. The target 12-hour trough levels also vary based on renal function, patient tolerance, and center preference. The author generally targets trough levels of 10 to 12 ng/mL for the first 1 to 2 months, levels of 7 to 9 ng/mL for 3 to 6 months, and 5 to 8 ng/mL subsequently. Cyclosporine is rarely used following liver transplant; it is reserved for patients who have significant adverse effects with tacrolimus. The usual starting dose is 5 to 15 mg/kg and titrated based on trough levels. Again, the target 12-hour trough levels vary. The author usually aims for 200 to 250 mg/dL in the first 3 months and a level of 100 to 150 mg/dL subsequently.

Adverse effects
The major side effect of CNIs is their nephrotoxicity, which can lead to acute kidney injury, and also cumulative use over several years can result in chronic renal insufficiency.[34,35] Other major side effects for tacrolimus include hypertension, hyperkalemia, headaches, tremors, seizures, hyperglycemia, hyperlipidemia, and opportunistic infections. Side effects more specific to cyclosporine include hypertrichosis, gingival hyperplasia, and edema.[20]

Antimetabolites—Mycophenolic Acid and Azathioprine

These drugs are usually used as second line of therapy for maintenance immunosuppression in combination with CNIs. Mycophenolate is the more commonly used antimetabolites, and azathioprine is only used occasionally.[36,37]

Mechanism of action
Mycophenolic acid (MPA) inhibits the formation of guanosine monophosphate by blocking inosine monophosphate dehydrogenase.[26] Azathioprine is a prodrug of 6-Merceptopurine. Both drugs ultimately lead to inhibition of purine synthesis and depletion of both B and T lymphocytes.

Dose and protocol
MMF is used as a second-line immunosuppressant in conjunction with CNI either to reduce CNI dose to prevent nephrotoxicity or as a part of a steroid-sparing regimen. MMF is much better tolerated if it started at a lower dose and titrated upwards. The author usually starts at 500 mg twice daily and increases it to 1000 mg oral twice daily.[38] Azathioprine is rarely used in the posttransplant setting. However, when

---

activates calcineurin and leads to nuclear translocation of NFAT and enhanced transcription of IL-2. Step III T-cell clonal expansion: IL-2 plays the crucial role of driving clonal expansion and maturation of T cells. Step IV inflammation and graft injury: the clonal expansion of T cells leads to cell-mediated cytotoxicity facilitated by release of cytokines and chemokines, which recruit inflammatory cells like neutrophils, NK cells, and macrophages and result in tissue inflammation and destruction. The numbered boxes show the different sites at which various classes of immunosuppressants act.

used, it is dosed at 1.5 to 2.0 mg/kg per day. Thiopurine methyltransferase or thiopurine S-methyltransferase levels or genotype need to be checked before dosing.

Adverse effects
MPA does not have nephrologic or neurologic side effects like CNI. One of the main side effects is dose-dependent leukopenia, which usually improves with dose reduction. Gastrointestinal side effects like nausea, vomiting, and diarrhea are also common.[39] Dose reduction and switching to a different formulation like mycophenolate sodium (Myfortic) also helps at times. The main side effects of azathioprine are cytopenias, pancreatitis, hepatotoxicity, and risk for neoplasia with long-term use.

Mammalian Target of Rapamycin Inhibitors—Sirolimus and Everolimus

Mechanism of action
Both sirolimus and everolimus inhibit activation of T cells by binding to a different site on the same protein that binds tacrolimus, FKBP-12, and inhibiting the regulatory kinase, mTOR. Inhibition of mTOR pathway leads to blunting of cytokine-mediated T-cell activation and proliferation.[40]

Dose and protocol
Sirolimus is not routinely used as first-line immunosuppressant after LT. It is usually used in patients who cannot tolerate CNI, those who have renal dysfunction, or those with high-risk HCCs.[41,42] The usual loading dose for sirolimus is 4 to 6 mg daily followed by a maintenance dose of 2 mg daily. The target trough level is 6 to 10 ng/mL. Everolimus is preferably used on an empty stomach. A starting dose of 0.75 mg twice daily with a target trough level of 3 to 8 ng/dL is standard.

Adverse effects
The main adverse effect of both sirolimus and everolimus is hyperlipidemia.[43] Sirolimus has also been reported to be associated with hepatic artery thrombosis and hence should be avoided in the early posttransplant period.[44,45] Both drugs also cause delayed wound healing. Other adverse effects include oral ulcers, hypertension, hyperlipidemia, peripheral edema, and cytopenias.[43,46]

Antibodies

Specific antibodies that inhibit or deplete T cells can be used for steroid-free induction of immunosuppression and for treatment of steroid-resistant ACR.[47] The major drugs in this category are ATG (thymoglobulin), ALG, anti-CD3 antibody (muromonab-CD3 [OKT3]), monoclonal antibodies to IL-2 receptor (basiliximab and daclizumab), and monoclonal anti-CD52 antibody (alemtuzumab).

Mechanism of action
ATG and ALG are polyclonal antibodies to multiple T-cell antigens, CD2, CD3, CD4, and CD8. Treatment with them induces opsonization of lymphocytes and subsequent complement-medicated cell lysis, thus eventually leading to lymphocyte depletion.[48] OKT3 is a monoclonal antibody that targets CD3 on mature T cells and leads to inactivation and apoptosis of T cells.[49] Basiliximab and daclizumab are humanized monoclonal antibodies to IL-2 receptor, which prevent T-cell proliferation.[50] Alemtuzumab (campath-1H) is a monoclonal antibody against CD52 receptors on peripheral mononuclear cells; it leads to depletion of lymphocytes and profound immunosuppression.[51]

Dosage and protocol

Thymoglobulin is used for steroid-free induction regimens and for steroid refractory rejection. The author uses thymoglobulin induction at her center, and the protocol followed is to administer a single dose of methylprednisolone intraoperatively and subsequently induce with ATG 1 to 1.5 mg/kg per dose for 3 doses (after premedication with diphenhydramine/hydrocortisone/Tylenol). Basiliximab induction is carried out with 2 doses: 20 mg IV on day 0 and day 4. Alemtuzumab is used as a single dose of 30 mg IV given intraoperatively.

Adverse effects

The polyclonal antibodies can induce allergic reaction and also serum sickness–like illness with arthralgias, nephritis, rash, and fever. With the monoclonal antibodies, there is higher concern for cytomegalovirus (CMV) infection and posttransplant lymphoproliferative disorder (PTLD). OKT-3 was reported to be associated with a 3.6-fold higher risk of PTLD,[52] and the manufacturer has currently discontinued this drug. Basiliximab was not found to be associated with higher risk for CMV or PTLD in one study,[53] and another study actually suggests that risk of CMV infection may be lower when daclizumab is used in combination with tacrolimus compared with tacrolimus combined to steroids.[54] Alemtuzumab is associated with severe immunosuppression, and case reports of hepatitis C reactivation, zoster infection, and cryptococcus after LT has raised cautions about using this drug.[55–57]

EVIDENCE-BASED APPROACH TO IMMUNOSUPPRESSION REGIMENS FOR LIVER TRANSPLANTATION

There are 2 main stages in application of immunosuppression after LT: (1) induction and (2) maintenance. **Fig. 2** shows the evolution of immunosuppressive regimens between 1998 and 2012 based on data from the Organ Procurement and Transplantation Network (OPTN).[58] In this section, the author discusses some of the major trials on the various immunosuppressive regimens for each phase.

Induction Phase

The induction phase is the early posttransplant phase when the recipient immune system is inundated with alloantigens from the donor liver, and more intense immunosuppression is needed in the first few days to prevent acute rejection and preserve graft

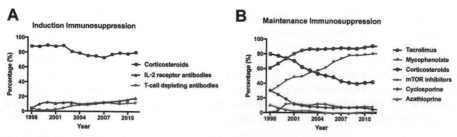

Fig. 2. The evolution of immunosuppressive regimens between 1998 and 2012 based on data from OPTN. (*A*) Induction immunosuppression. The graph shows that glucocorticoids remain the most commonly used medications for induction but the use of T-cell depleting antibodies and IL-2 receptor antibodies like basiliximab is increasing. (*B*) The trend in the use of maintenance immunosuppression. CNI tacrolimus is the most commonly used medication for this phase, but the use of mycophenolate has been slowly increasing. The use of steroids as maintenance therapy has been steadily dropping.

function. As mentioned above, corticosteroids have been the main component of induction regimens for a long time, but recognition of severe steroid-related adverse effects has led to the emergence of antibody-based steroid-free regimens for induction. Glucocorticoid induction has been shown to associate with higher incidence of post-transplant diabetes, hypertension, and CMV infection when compared with steroid-sparing regimens.[59,60] One of the biggest concerns for steroid induction has been acceleration of HCC recurrence in patients with hepatitis C virus (HCV)-related cirrhosis (discussed later), but avoiding repeated pulses and slowing down the taper of steroids[61,62] have been shown to be associated with less risk for recurrence of HCV. The alternative is to consider switching to a steroid-free induction regimen in patients with hepatitis C. Although this should theoretically ameliorate the risk of HCV recurrence and the rapid progression to graft cirrhosis, the results from randomized controlled trials (RCT) have been conflicting. After a multicenter RCT, Klintmalm and colleagues[63] reported that the severity of HCV recurrence was not different between the cohorts that received steroids versus those who received the steroid-free induction regimen using daclizumab. Also, Kato and colleagues[64] reported that there was no difference in HCV-induced fibrosis among patients receiving steroids and steroid-free induction. Interestingly, in a recent meta-analysis of 16 completed randomized clinical trials including 1347 patients, steroid-free induction regimens were actually found to be associated with higher incidence of acute rejection.[59] Therefore, overall, despite occurrence of adverse events, steroid induction still has a role after LT, especially in non-HCV patients.

An attractive option for steroid-free induction is use of polyclonal antibodies like thymoglobulin (ATG) or monoclonal antibodies like basiliximab. Eason and colleagues[65] reported a prospective RCT in which they found that ATG induction was associated with a trend toward lower rejection rate, decreased incidence of post-OLT diabetes, decreased recurrent hepatitis C, and decreased CMV infection when compared with steroid induction. Also, low-dose induction was shown to be associated with lower rates of rejection and better graft survival than induction with basiliximab.[66] Also, a single-center retrospective study of long-term follow-up of 1000 patients who received ATG for induction reports that it is associated with low rejection rates and excellent survival.[67] Finally, evidence that basiliximab or daclizumab induction is safe and effective for induction is accumulating. In a multicenter RCT, daclizumab induction was compared with steroid induction, and daclizumab was associated with lower incidence of diabetes, viral infection, and a lower incidence of steroid-resistant acute rejection (SRAR).[54] Another significant factor impacting the decision to switch to steroid-free induction regimens is the high cost of antibody induction. However, given the improved adverse effect profile, data from other organ transplants point out that ATG or basiliximab induction is likely cost-effective.[68]

Overall, steroids remain the most commonly used induction agent, and there is no strong objective evidence that steroid-free antibody–based induction regimens are associated with improved graft or patient survival. However, given the improved side-effect profile of antibody therapies, more and more transplant centers are embracing steroid-free induction regimens.

Maintenance Immunosuppression

CNIs remain the cornerstone of long-term maintenance immunosuppression after LT. Cyclosporine was the first CNI to be used after LT, and it showed significant improvement in graft survival compared with conventional immunosuppression with azathioprine and steroids.[69,70] Tacrolimus was subsequently introduced in the early 1990s, and it was shown to have better graft survival and lower rates of rejection than cyclosporine[71,72]; thus, it quickly replaced cyclosporine as the drug of choice for LT. A meta-analysis of 16 RCTs confirmed the findings from individual trials and established the safety and efficacy of tacrolimus over cyclosporine.[73] The main concern of long-term tacrolimus monotherapy is renal insufficiency. Multiple strategies are used to avoid this complication and prevent progression to end-stage renal disease. These strategies included targeting lower trough of tacrolimus, adding an auxiliary agent like mycophenolate[74] or switching to an mTOR inhibitor like sirolimus[75] or everolimus.[76] Modest improvement in renal function has been noted with the above approaches, but this has to be balanced with the fact that tacrolimus appears to provide the strongest defense against ACR. The CNIs are both metabolized by the cytochrome P450 system and hence necessitate close monitoring for drug-drug interactions.

Mycophenolate is commonly used as second-line therapy in combination with tacrolimus to preserve renal function. Leukopenias and gastrointestinal side effects are the chief concerns with this medication. Rarely, it can be used as monotherapy in a subset of patients who are several years out of transplantation.[77,78] Sirolimus monotherapy is rarely used as the first line for maintenance immunosuppression given concerns for hepatic artery thrombosis, especially within the first 30 days. However, it is usually used in patients who do not tolerate CNIs due to adverse events or those who develop early renal insufficiency.[79] Patients who have chronic renal insufficiency or those who have pre-existing renal disease do not appear to benefit from switching to sirolimus.[80] Everolimus is another mTOR inhibitor that has been approved for LT. Monotherapy with everolimus was associated with higher rates of rejection; hence, it should only be used in combination with a CNI. However, it does facilitate use of a lower dose of tacrolimus and thus potentially can preserve renal function.[81] More prospective data on everolimus are needed before it is used more widely.

Overall, tacrolimus monotherapy remains the maintenance immunosuppression regimen of choice. In patients with renal dysfunction, an approach of dual immunosuppression with tacrolimus (targeting lower trough) and mycophenolate is probably desirable. However, switching such patients to sirolimus or everolimus might not definitively lead to improvement in renal function while being associated with several adverse events.

REJECTION AFTER LIVER TRANSPLANTATION

LT in general only requires ABO compatibility, and HLA matching is not performed because the liver is not considered to be susceptible to alloantibody-induced humoral rejection, unlike the kidney or the heart. The main mechanism of rejection is T-cell–mediated cellular rejection. The major types of rejection after LT include ACR, steroid-resistant rejection, and AMR. Chronic ductopenic rejection is not common after LT and occurs in less than 5% of patients. In this section, the role of immunosuppression drugs in the management of acute rejection is briefly discussed.

Acute Cellular Rejection

Early rejection is defined as those episodes occurring within 90 days of transplantation; this is relatively common, occurring in 25% to 65% of patients.[12,82–84] The patients may present with fever, abdominal pain, hepatomegaly, or other nonspecific symptoms like fatigue. Early rejection is accompanied by elevation of transaminases, bilirubin, and gamma glutamate transferase. The diagnosis is made on liver biopsy, and the classical features are endothelitis, portal mixed inflammatory infiltrate, and cholangitis/biliary damage.[85] Banff score can be used to grade the severity of rejection, and this grade has been shown to predict clinical outcome. The differential diagnosis for acute rejection is broad and includes HCV recurrence, drug toxicity, preservation injury, CMV hepatitis, and large duct obstruction. Hence, close collaboration with an experienced liver pathologist is essential. Once the diagnosis is established, then prompt treatment should be initiated. Steroid therapy is the treatment of choice and methylprednisolone 500- to 1000-mg bolus followed by a slow taper over 10 to 14 days usually results in resolution of ACR in 70% to 80% of the cases.[86] A small percentage of patients does not respond to the initial treatment with steroids and are re-treated with another course of steroid bolus. Clinically, this is confirmed by normalization of the liver enzymes and bilirubin, although some centers perform a posttreatment biopsy to confirm resolution of rejection. During treatment with high-dose steroids, vigilance needs to be maintained for complications like CMV reactivation, psychosis, hyperglycemia, and other steroid-related adverse effects mentioned above.

Steroid-Resistant Acute Rejection

Around 10% of the patients do not respond even after 2 courses of steroids and thus need further therapy. Thymoglobulin is used as first line of treatment of steroid-resistant rejection in most centers.[87,88] A dose of 1.5 mg/kg per day is used for 5 doses, with standard premedication. Because ATG can cause severe cytopenias, HCV, or CMV reactivation, these patients need to be closely monitored for adverse events. Basiliximab has also been successfully reported to treat ACR in small cohorts of patients,[89,90] but more evidence regarding its efficacy is needed before it can used as first-line agent for SRAR. Once there is resolution of SRAR, the maintenance immunosuppression will usually need to be modified to either increase the target trough levels of CNI or to add another class of immunosuppressant like mycophenolate or sirolimus.

Antibody-Mediated Rejection

As mentioned above, the liver is generally considered to be resistant to allo-AMR. However, recent evidence suggests that AMR does occur in concurrence with ACR or independently and is likely an underrecognized phenomenon.[91–93] Diagnosis of AMR can be made on biopsy specimen, which shows biliary injury with bile ductular reaction, canalicular cholestasis, feathery degeneration, and portal edema. A high index of suspicion needs to be maintained because these changes can be seen with other causes of biliary obstruction. Diffuse immunohistochemical staining for C4d, a complement product, can be used as a tissue biomarker to confirm the diagnosis.[94] When AMR is suspected based on the biopsy specimen, donor-specific antibodies need to be measured because they provide further evidence for the occurrence of AMR. Treatment of AMR is with anti-B-cell agents like rituximab, IV immunoglobulin, and bortozemib (antiproteasome antibody that depletes plasma cells).[13,95,96]

IMMUNOSUPPRESSION IN SPECIAL POPULATIONS
Liver Transplant for Hepatitis C

Hepatitis C is one of the most common indications for LT in the United States. Recurrence of HCV after LT is almost universal, if the patient is viremic at the time of transplantation.[97] The diagnosis and treatment of posttransplant HCV recurrence still remain important issues. The main issue surrounding use of immunosuppression in HCV patients is regarding the use of high-dose steroids. Numerous studies have clearly documented that steroid use in this setting can result in rapid and severe recurrence of HCV.[98–100] Hence, several centers have attempted to use steroid-free regimens for induction of immunosuppression with either thymoglobulin or IL-2R antibodies like basiliximab. Also, for maintenance immunosuppression regimens, cyclosporine has been theoretically proposed to be safer than tacrolimus for HCV patients.[101] However, overall, there is no strong objective evidence to suggest that any particular induction regimen or any particular CNI is associated with better outcomes in HCV patients. The arrival of direct-acting antivirals has completely changed the landscape of posttransplant hepatitis C management. Sustained virologic response of more than 90% can now be achieved even in this challenging population without significant drug-drug interactions or adverse events.[102] Given this, the concern for steroid use in this population might not be very relevant in the near future.

Immunosuppression in Pregnant Patients

There are several fertility-related questions that female patients of reproductive age face after LT, including questions regarding contraception, timing, and safety of pregnancy, infertility management, and fetal risks. Many women with end-stage liver disease suffer from infertility, and LT restores fertility in such patients, thus allowing them to get pregnant and bear children. These pregnancies are considered high risk and should be handled by specialists who have experience in their management.[103] In general, a planned pregnancy is associated with better outcomes, and patients should discuss this in advance with their transplant hepatologists. Pregnancy is considered to be safer after at least 1 year of transplantation because most patients by then are likely to be on CNI monotherapy for immunosuppression. Steroids may still be needed for management if ACR occurs during pregnancy. If this happens, then the patient should be monitored for hyperglycemia, hypertension, and infections. CNIs are considered to be relatively safe during pregnancy, and no fetal adverse events have been reported.[104] However, metabolic complications like hyperglycemia, hypertension, and renal insufficiency still remain concerning, and close monitoring of trough levels will be needed during pregnancy. MMF has been reported to be associated with teratogenic effects, and it should be stopped at least 6 to 8 weeks before planned pregnancy.[105] There are insufficient data on sirolimus in pregnant women and it is generally avoided in favor of CNI.

Immunosuppression in Patients with Hepatocellular Carcinoma

Recurrence of HCC after transplantation can occur in 10% to 15% of patients and is associated with significant morbidity and mortality. Studies have shown that patients with HCC are at increased risk for tumor recurrence with higher levels of immunosuppression[106]; hence, they need to be maintained on minimum required immunosuppression that will prevent rejection while also lowering the risk of HCC recurrence. Among the CNIs, there are no good data to suggest that one is better than the other, but it is rather the trough levels of CNIs that appear to matter. Sirolimus has been reported to have a beneficial effect in patients with HCC because it has been shown to block angiogenesis by inhibiting the vascular endothelial growth factor pathway. A few small studies showed that sirolimus immunosuppression was associated with lower recurrence rates, and a meta-analysis confirmed this association.[107] However, given the side-effect profile of sirolimus (described above) and lack of large, prospective studies, current guidelines do not recommend switching from CNI to sirolimus based on the pretransplant diagnosis of HCC alone. However, a recent RCT has shown that sirolimus provides improved recurrence-free survival and overall survival benefit in the first 3 to 5 years after LT in patients with HCC.[108] Further good quality data supporting the use of sirolimus will possibly lead to a change in the guidelines for immunosuppression in recipients with a history of HCC.

SUMMARY AND FUTURE DIRECTIONS

Liver has a tolerogenic immune environment, making allograft rejection less frequent than other solid organ transplants. However, acute rejection still does occur after LT and can lead to graft loss and poor survival. The introduction of CNIs for immunosuppression several decades ago significantly improved outcomes after LT. Over the past few years, the understanding of the immune response that follows LT has expanded significantly, and several new targeted therapies have been introduced. Improvement in the safety and efficacy profile of immunosuppressant drugs has significantly prolonged post-LT graft and patient survival. However, many challenges nevertheless exist, including developing newer molecular targeted therapies, improving the safety profile of the drugs, developing noninvasive drug monitoring technologies, and identifying noninvasive biomarkers for rejection. It is hoped that further research in these areas will lead to personalized design of immunosuppressive regimens that are tailored to each individual patient and are associated with minimal side effects while still effectively prolonging graft and patient survival.

REFERENCES

1. Starzl TE, Marchioro TL, Vonkaulla KN, et al. Homotransplantation of the liver in humans. Surg Gynecol Obstet 1963;117:659–76.
2. Meirelles RF, Salvalaggio P, de Rezende MB, et al. Liver transplantation: history, outcomes and perspectives. Einstein (Sao Paulo) 2015;13(1):149–52.
3. Calne RY, Rolles K, White DJ, et al. Cyclosporin A initially as the only immunosuppressant in 34 recipients of cadaveric organs: 32 kidneys, 2 pancreases, and 2 livers. Lancet 1979;2(8151):1033–6.
4. Based on OPTN data as of September 19, 2016.
5. Available at: http://www.who.int/transplantation/gkt/statistics/en/. Accessed September 15, 2016.
6. Thomson AW, Knolle PA. Antigen-presenting cell function in the tolerogenic liver environment. Nat Rev Immunol 2010;10(11):753–66.
7. Invernizzi P. Liver auto-immunology: the paradox of autoimmunity in a tolerogenic organ. J Autoimmun 2013;46:1–6.
8. Cheng EY. Tolerogenic mechanisms in liver transplantation. SOJ Immunol 2015; 3(4):1–13.
9. Abu-Elmagd KM, Costa G, Bond GJ, et al. Five hundred intestinal and multivisceral transplantations at a single center: major advances with new challenges. Ann Surg 2009;250(4):567–81.
10. Taner T, Heimbach JK, Rosen CB, et al. Decreased chronic cellular and antibody-mediated injury in the kidney following simultaneous liver-kidney transplantation. Kidney Int 2016;89(4):909–17.
11. Seiler CA, Renner EL, Czerniak A, et al. Early acute cellular rejection: no effect on late hepatic allograft function in man. Transpl Int 1999;12(3):195–201.
12. Fisher LR, Henley KS, Lucey MR. Acute cellular rejection after liver transplantation: variability, morbidity, and mortality. Liver Transpl Surg 1995;1(1):10–5.
13. Hubscher SG. Antibody-mediated rejection in the liver allograft. Curr Opin Organ Transplant 2012;17(3):280–6.
14. O'Leary JG, Michelle Shiller S, Bellamy C, et al. Acute liver allograft antibody-mediated rejection: an inter-institutional study of significant histopathological features. Liver Transpl 2014;20(10):1244–55.
15. Sood S, Testro AG. Immune monitoring post liver transplant. World J Transplant 2014;4(1):30–9.

16. Takaki A, Yagi T, Yamamoto K. Contradictory immune response in post liver transplantation hepatitis B and C. Int J Inflamm 2014;2014:15.
17. Heymann F, Tacke F. Immunology in the liver—from homeostasis to disease. Nat Rev Gastroenterol Hepatol 2016;13(2):88–110.
18. Pons JA, Revilla-Nuin B, Ramirez P, et al. Development of immune tolerance in liver transplantation. Gastroenterol Hepatol 2011;34(3):155–69 [in Spanish].
19. Gaber AO, Monaco AP, Russell JA, et al. Rabbit antithymocyte globulin (thymoglobulin): 25 years and new frontiers in solid organ transplantation and haematology. Drugs 2010;70(6):691–732.
20. Matsuda S, Koyasu S. Mechanisms of action of cyclosporine. Immunopharmacology 2000;47(2–3):119–25.
21. Vicari-Christensen M, Repper S, Basile S, et al. Tacrolimus: review of pharmacokinetics, pharmacodynamics, and pharmacogenetics to facilitate practitioners' understanding and offer strategies for educating patients and promoting adherence. Prog Transplant 2009;19(3):277–84.
22. Ramirez CB, Marino IR. The role of basiliximab induction therapy in organ transplantation. Expert Opin Biol Ther 2007;7(1):137–48.
23. Mottershead M, Neuberger J. Daclizumab. Expert Opin Biol Ther 2007;7(10):1583–96.
24. Kawahara T, Asthana S, Kneteman NM. m-TOR inhibitors: what role in liver transplantation? J Hepatol 2011;55(6):1441–51.
25. Trotter JF, Lizardo-Sanchez L. Everolimus in liver transplantation. Curr Opin Organ Transplant 2014;19(6):578–82.
26. Kaltenborn A, Schrem H. Mycophenolate mofetil in liver transplantation: a review. Ann Transplant 2013;18:685–96.
27. Vacca A, Martinotti S, Screpanti I, et al. Transcriptional regulation of the interleukin 2 gene by glucocorticoid hormones. Role of steroid receptor and antigen-responsive 5'-flanking sequences. J Biol Chem 1990;265(14):8075–80.
28. Vacca A, Felli MP, Farina AR, et al. Glucocorticoid receptor-mediated suppression of the interleukin 2 gene expression through impairment of the cooperativity between nuclear factor of activated T cells and AP-1 enhancer elements. J Exp Med 1992;175(3):637–46.
29. Neal DA, Brown MJ, Wilkinson IB, et al. Mechanisms of hypertension after liver transplantation. Transplantation 2005;79(8):935–40.
30. Fernandez-Miranda C, Guijarro C, de la Calle A, et al. Lipid abnormalities in stable liver transplant recipients—effects of cyclosporin, tacrolimus, and steroids. Transpl Int 1998;11(2):137–42.
31. Zaydfudim V, Feurer ID, Landman MP, et al. Reduction in corticosteroids is associated with better health-related quality of life after liver transplantation. J Am Coll Surg 2012;214(2):164–73.
32. Oberholzer J, Al-Saghier M, Kneteman NM. Steroid avoidance in liver transplantation. Can J Gastroenterol 2004;18(Suppl C):5c–11c.
33. Lake JR. Immunosuppression and outcomes of patients transplanted for hepatitis C. J Hepatol 2006;44(4):627–9.
34. Campo A. Chronic renal failure after transplantation of a nonrenal organ. N Engl J Med 2003;349(26):2563–5 [author reply: 2565].
35. Magee C, Pascual M. The growing problem of chronic renal failure after transplantation of a nonrenal organ. N Engl J Med 2003;349(10):994–6.
36. Klupp J, Bechstein WO, Platz KP, et al. Mycophenolate mofetil added to immunosuppression after liver transplantation—first results. Transpl Int 1997;10(3):223–8.

37. Mele TS, Halloran PF. The use of mycophenolate mofetil in transplant recipients. Immunopharmacology 2000;47(2–3):215–45.
38. Staatz CE, Tett SE. Clinical pharmacokinetics and pharmacodynamics of mycophenolate in solid organ transplant recipients. Clin Pharmacokinet 2007;46(1): 13–58.
39. Staatz CE, Tett SE. Pharmacology and toxicology of mycophenolate in organ transplant recipients: an update. Arch Toxicol 2014;88(7):1351–89.
40. Halloran PF. Molecular mechanisms of new immunosuppressants. Clin Transplant 1996;10(1 Pt 2):118–23.
41. Neff GW, Montalbano M, Tzakis AG. Ten years of sirolimus therapy in orthotopic liver transplant recipients. Transplant Proc 2003;35(3 Suppl):209s–16s.
42. Trotter JF. Sirolimus in liver transplantation. Transplant Proc 2003;35(3 Suppl): 193s–200s.
43. Morard I, Dumortier J, Spahr L, et al. Conversion to sirolimus-based immunosuppression in maintenance liver transplantation patients. Liver Transpl 2007; 13(5):658–64.
44. Ventura-Aguiar P, Campistol JM, Diekmann F. Safety of mTOR inhibitors in adult solid organ transplantation. Expert Opin Drug Saf 2016;15(3):303–19.
45. Massoud O, Wiesner RH. The use of sirolimus should be restricted in liver transplantation. J Hepatol 2012;56(1):288–90.
46. Montalbano M, Neff GW, Yamashiki N, et al. A retrospective review of liver transplant patients treated with sirolimus from a single center: an analysis of sirolimus-related complications. Transplantation 2004;78(2):264–8.
47. Wall WJ. Use of antilymphocyte induction therapy in liver transplantation. Liver Transpl Surg 1999;5(4 Suppl 1):S64–70.
48. Yu LZ, Fang Y, Zhu L, et al. Immunomodulation of human CD8(+) T cells by thymoglobulin in vitro. Transplant Proc 2012;44(4):1052–4.
49. Janssen O, Wesselborg S, Kabelitz D. Immunosuppression by OKT3–induction of programmed cell death (apoptosis) as a possible mechanism of action. Transplantation 1992;53(1):233–4.
50. Kapic E, Becic F, Kusturica J. Basiliximab, mechanism of action and pharmacological properties. Med Arh 2004;58(6):373–6.
51. Levitsky J, Thudi K, Ison MG, et al. Alemtuzumab induction in non-hepatitis C positive liver transplant recipients. Liver Transpl 2011;17(1):32–7.
52. Kremers WK, Devarbhavi HC, Wiesner RH, et al. Post-transplant lymphoproliferative disorders following liver transplantation: incidence, risk factors and survival. Am J Transplant 2006;6(5 Pt 1):1017–24.
53. Ramirez CB, Doria C, di Francesco F, et al. Basiliximab induction in adult liver transplant recipients with 93% rejection-free patient and graft survival at 24 months. Transplant Proc 2006;38(10):3633–5.
54. Boillot O, Mayer DA, Boudjema K, et al. Corticosteroid-free immunosuppression with tacrolimus following induction with daclizumab: a large randomized clinical study. Liver Transpl 2005;11(1):61–7.
55. Alcaide ML, Abbo L, Pano JR, et al. Herpes zoster infection after liver transplantation in patients receiving induction therapy with alemtuzumab. Clin Transplant 2008;22(4):502–7.
56. Peleg AY, Husain S, Kwak EJ, et al. Opportunistic infections in 547 organ transplant recipients receiving alemtuzumab, a humanized monoclonal CD-52 antibody. Clin Infect Dis 2007;44(2):204–12.

57. Safdar N, Smith J, Knasinski V, et al. Infections after the use of alemtuzumab in solid organ transplant recipients: a comparative study. Diagn Microbiol Infect Dis 2010;66(1):7–15.

58. 2014 Annual Report of the U.S. Organ Procurement and Transplantation Network and the Scientific Registry of Transplant Recipients: transplant data 1998-2012. Department of Health and Human Services. Available at: https://optn.transplant.hrsa.gov/data/. Accessed September 15, 2016.

59. Fairfield C, Penninga L, Powell J, et al. Glucocorticosteroid-free versus glucocorticosteroid-containing immunosuppression for liver transplanted patients. Cochrane Database Syst Rev 2015;(12):CD007606.

60. Penninga L, Wettergren A, Wilson CH, et al. Antibody induction versus corticosteroid induction for liver transplant recipients. Cochrane Database Syst Rev 2014;(5):CD010252.

61. Vivarelli M, Burra P, La Barba G, et al. Influence of steroids on HCV recurrence after liver transplantation: a prospective study. J Hepatol 2007;47(6):793–8.

62. Berenguer M, Aguilera V, Prieto M, et al. Significant improvement in the outcome of HCV-infected transplant recipients by avoiding rapid steroid tapering and potent induction immunosuppression. J Hepatol 2006;44(4):717–22.

63. Klintmalm GB, Davis GL, Teperman L, et al. A randomized, multicenter study comparing steroid-free immunosuppression and standard immunosuppression for liver transplant recipients with chronic hepatitis C. Liver Transpl 2011;17(12):1394–403.

64. Kato T, Gaynor JJ, Yoshida H, et al. Randomized trial of steroid-free induction versus corticosteroid maintenance among orthotopic liver transplant recipients with hepatitis C virus: impact on hepatic fibrosis progression at one year. Transplantation 2007;84(7):829–35.

65. Eason JD, Loss GE, Blazek J, et al. Steroid-free liver transplantation using rabbit antithymocyte globulin induction: results of a prospective randomized trial. Liver Transpl 2001;7(8):693–7.

66. Laftavi MR, Alnimri M, Weber-Shrikant E, et al. Low-dose rabbit antithymocyte globulin versus basiliximab induction therapy in low-risk renal transplant recipients: 8-year follow-up. Transplant Proc 2011;43(2):458–61.

67. Mangus RS, Fridell JA, Vianna RM, et al. Immunosuppression induction with rabbit anti-thymocyte globulin with or without rituximab in 1000 liver transplant patients with long-term follow-up. Liver Transpl 2012;18(7):786–95.

68. Woodroffe R, Yao GL, Meads C, et al. Clinical and cost-effectiveness of newer immunosuppressive regimens in renal transplantation: a systematic review and modelling study. Health Technol Assess 2005;9(21):1–179, iii-iv.

69. Gordon RD, Shaw BW Jr, Iwatsuki S, et al. Indications for liver transplantation in the cyclosporine era. Surg Clin North Am 1986;66(3):541–56.

70. Iwatsuki S, Starzl TE, Todo S, et al. Experience in 1,000 liver transplants under cyclosporine-steroid therapy: a survival report. Transplant Proc 1988;20(1 Suppl 1):498–504.

71. O'Grady JG, Burroughs A, Hardy P, et al. Tacrolimus versus microemulsified ciclosporin in liver transplantation: the TMC randomised controlled trial. Lancet 2002;360(9340):1119–25.

72. Kelly D, Jara P, Rodeck B, et al. Tacrolimus and steroids versus ciclosporin microemulsion, steroids, and azathioprine in children undergoing liver transplantation: randomised European multicentre trial. Lancet 2004;364(9439):1054–61.

73. McAlister VC, Haddad E, Renouf E, et al. Cyclosporin versus tacrolimus as primary immunosuppressant after liver transplantation: a meta-analysis. Am J Transplant 2006;6(7):1578–85.

74. Lake J, Patel D, David K, et al. The association between MMF and risk of progressive renal dysfunction and death in adult liver transplant recipients with HCV. Clin Transplant 2009;23(1):108–15.

75. Watson CJ, Gimson AE, Alexander GJ, et al. A randomized controlled trial of late conversion from calcineurin inhibitor (CNI)-based to sirolimus-based immunosuppression in liver transplant recipients with impaired renal function. Liver Transpl 2007;13(12):1694–702.

76. Castroagudin JF, Molina E, Romero R, et al. Improvement of renal function after the switch from a calcineurin inhibitor to everolimus in liver transplant recipients with chronic renal dysfunction. Liver Transpl 2009;15(12):1792–7.

77. Schmeding M, Kiessling A, Neuhaus R, et al. Mycophenolate mofetil monotherapy in liver transplantation: 5-year follow-up of a prospective randomized trial. Transplantation 2011;92(8):923–9.

78. Creput C, Blandin F, Deroure B, et al. Long-term effects of calcineurin inhibitor conversion to mycophenolate mofetil on renal function after liver transplantation. Liver Transpl 2007;13(7):1004–10.

79. Fairbanks KD, Eustace JA, Fine D, et al. Renal function improves in liver transplant recipients when switched from a calcineurin inhibitor to sirolimus. Liver Transpl 2003;9(10):1079–85.

80. Lam P, Yoshida A, Brown K, et al. The efficacy and limitations of sirolimus conversion in liver transplant patients who develop renal dysfunction on calcineurin inhibitors. Dig Dis Sci 2004;49(6):1029–35.

81. De Simone P, Nevens F, De Carlis L, et al. Everolimus with reduced tacrolimus improves renal function in de novo liver transplant recipients: a randomized controlled trial. Am J Transplant 2012;12(11):3008–20.

82. Levitsky J, Goldberg D, Smith AR, et al. Acute rejection increases risk of graft failure and death in recent liver transplant recipients. Clin Gastroenterol Hepatol 2016. [Epub ahead of print].

83. Klintmalm GB, Nery JR, Husberg BS, et al. Rejection in liver transplantation. Hepatology 1989;10(6):978–85.

84. Farges O, Saliba F, Farhamant H, et al. Incidence of rejection and infection after liver transplantation as a function of the primary disease: possible influence of alcohol and polyclonal immunoglobulins. Hepatology 1996;23(2):240–8.

85. Neil DA, Hubscher SG. Current views on rejection pathology in liver transplantation. Transpl Int 2010;23(10):971–83.

86. Goddard S, Adams DH. Methylprednisolone therapy for acute rejection: too much of a good thing? Liver Transpl 2002;8(6):535–6.

87. Aydogan C, Sevmis S, Aktas S, et al. Steroid-resistant acute rejections after liver transplant. Exp Clin Transplant 2010;8(2):172–7.

88. Lee JG, Lee J, Lee JJ, et al. Efficacy of rabbit anti-thymocyte globulin for steroid-resistant acute rejection after liver transplantation. Medicine 2016; 95(23):e3711.

89. Fernandes ML, Lee YM, Sutedja D, et al. Treatment of steroid-resistant acute liver transplant rejection with basiliximab. Transplant Proc 2005;37(5):2179–80.

90. Shigeta T, Sakamoto S, Uchida H, et al. Basiliximab treatment for steroid-resistant rejection in pediatric patients following liver transplantation for acute liver failure. Pediatr Transplant 2014;18(8):860–7.

91. O'Grady J. Antibody-mediated injury to the transplanted liver: receiving the sages' wisdom. Am J Transplant 2016;16:2773–4.
92. Demetris AJ, Bellamy C, Hubscher SG, et al. 2016 comprehensive update of the Banff Working Group on liver allograft pathology: introduction of antibody-mediated rejection. Am J Transplant 2016;16:2816–35.
93. Trotter JF. Current issues in liver transplantation. Gastroenterol Hepatol 2016; 12(4):214–9.
94. Muro M, Moya-Quiles MR, Mrowiec A. Humoral response in liver allograft transplantation: a review of the role of anti-human leukocyte antigen (HLA) antibodies. Curr Protein Pept Sci 2016;17(8):776–84.
95. Honda M, Sakamoto S, Sakamoto R, et al. Antibody-mediated rejection after ABO-incompatible pediatric living donor liver transplantation for propionic acidemia: a case report. Pediatr Transplant 2016;20(6):840–5.
96. Galian JA, Mrowiec A, Muro M. Molecular targets on B-cells to prevent and treat antibody-mediated rejection in organ transplantation. Present and future. Expert Opin Ther Targets 2016;20(7):859–67.
97. Dhanasekaran R, Firpi RJ. Challenges of recurrent hepatitis C in the liver transplant patient. World J Gastroenterol 2014;20(13):3391–400.
98. Berenguer M, Ferrell L, Watson J, et al. HCV-related fibrosis progression following liver transplantation: increase in recent years. J Hepatol 2000;32(4): 673–84.
99. Neumann UP, Berg T, Bahra M, et al. Long-term outcome of liver transplants for chronic hepatitis C: a 10-year follow-up. Transplantation 2004;77(2):226–31.
100. Bahra M, Neumann UP, Jacob D, et al. Repeated steroid pulse therapies in HCV-positive liver recipients: significant risk factor for HCV-related graft loss. Transplant Proc 2005;37(4):1700–2.
101. Nakagawa M, Sakamoto N, Enomoto N, et al. Specific inhibition of hepatitis C virus replication by cyclosporin A. Biochem Biophys Res Commun 2004; 313(1):42–7.
102. Coilly A, Roche B, Duclos-Vallée J-C, et al. News and challenges in the treatment of hepatitis C in liver transplantation. Liver Int 2016;36:34–42.
103. Deshpande NA, James NT, Kucirka LM, et al. Pregnancy outcomes of liver transplant recipients: a systematic review and meta-analysis. Liver Transpl 2012;18(6):621–9.
104. Christopher V, Al-Chalabi T, Richardson PD, et al. Pregnancy outcome after liver transplantation: a single-center experience of 71 pregnancies in 45 recipients. Liver Transpl 2006;12(7):1138–43.
105. Sifontis NM, Coscia LA, Constantinescu S, et al. Pregnancy outcomes in solid organ transplant recipients with exposure to mycophenolate mofetil or sirolimus. Transplantation 2006;82(12):1698–702.
106. Rodriguez-Peralvarez M, Tsochatzis E, Naveas MC, et al. Reduced exposure to calcineurin inhibitors early after liver transplantation prevents recurrence of hepatocellular carcinoma. J Hepatol 2013;59(6):1193–9.
107. Finn RS. Current and future treatment strategies for patients with advanced hepatocellular carcinoma: role of mTOR inhibition. Liver Cancer 2012;1(3–4): 247–56.
108. Schnitzbauer AA, Zuelke C, Graeb C, et al. A prospective randomised, open-labeled, trial comparing sirolimus-containing versus mTOR-inhibitor-free immunosuppression in patients undergoing liver transplantation for hepatocellular carcinoma. BMC Cancer 2010;10:190.

Liver Transplantation in Alpha-1 Antitrypsin Deficiency

Virginia C. Clark, MD, MS

KEYWORDS

- Alpha-1 antitrypsin • Liver transplantation • Chronic obstructive pulmonary disease

KEY POINTS

- Liver transplantation for Alpha-1 antitrypsin deficiency accounts for a small portion of total liver transplants in the United States.
- The recipient assumes the phenotype of the donor; thus, liver transplantation is considered a cure for the underlying metabolic deficiency.
- Long-term outcomes and preservation of lung function after transplant are not well studied.
- Increased risk of hepatocellular carcinoma requiring liver transplantation is controversial.

INTRODUCTION

Alpha-1 antitrypsin (AAT) deficiency is a genetic condition that increases the risk for liver disease and chronic obstructive pulmonary disease (COPD). The protein deficiency was first described in 1963, and it was recognized that 3 of 5 patients had emphysema at a young age.[1] Several years later, the connection to liver cirrhosis in children was recognized.[2] Research over the last 50 years has led to a better understanding of the pathophysiology and the clinical consequences of both lung and liver disease.[3] However, highly effective therapies remain elusive. Liver transplantation (LT) is considered a "cure" for the condition because the donor liver is able to produce adequate serum levels of AAT. However, transplant is not a practical treatment for everyone affected with AAT, and consideration of LT is limited to those with complications of cirrhosis.

EPIDEMIOLOGY AND GENETICS

AAT deficiency is defined as the inheritance of 2 severe deficiency alleles in the *SERPINA1* gene (**Table 1**). It is an autosomal-recessive disorder with codominant

The author has nothing to disclose.
Division of Gastroenterology, Hepatology, and Nutrition, University of Florida, 1600 Southwest Archer Road, Room M440, Gainesville, FL 32601, USA
E-mail address: Virginia.Clark@medicine.ufl.edu

Table 1
Phenotype, genotype, and disease risk in alpha-1 antitrypsin deficiency

Inherited Alleles	Phenotype	Serum Protein Levels[a]	Risk of Liver Disease
MM	M	Normal (100%)	None
ZZ	Z	Very low (<15%)	High
MZ	MZ	Intermediate (60%)	Possibly increased
SZ	SZ	Low (35%)	Possibly increased
MS	MS	Intermediate (80%)	None

[a] Serum protein levels are approximations of what is expected in an MM; heterozygotes can have levels that overlap with normal ranges.

expression, with each allele contributing equally to the total circulating level of protein. More than 100 genetic variants of AAT have been described, but most are not associated with liver disease. The most common allele for the AAT gene is designated "M," and the predominant phenotype in the US population is PI*MM. Under these conditions, AAT is present in normal serum concentrations of 120 to 200 mg/dL. The deficiency allele classically associated with clinical disease states is designated as "Z." Individuals who are homozygous (PI*ZZ) have the lowest serum concentration of AAT, usually less than 50 mg/dL, and are at risk for both liver and lung disease. Population screening studies estimate the prevalence for PI*ZZ to range from 1 in 2000 to 1 in 5000.[4–6] The risk of liver disease in carriers (PI*MZ) has also been reported because they are typically overrepresented among individuals with chronic liver disease.[7] The S variant is another common deficiency allele, but it is not associated with liver disease unless a Z is also present. Rare alleles, M_{Malton} and M_{Duarte}, deserve mention because they are also associated with liver disease.[8] Null variants are also rare, but they are highly informative about mechanisms of disease because no liver disease occurs in this phenotype. Null mutations generally occur due to the presence of a premature stop codon, which results in essentially zero production of AAT. No abnormal AAT protein accumulates in the liver.[9]

PATHOGENESIS

The signature feature of AAT deficiency on a liver biopsy specimen is the presence of periodic acid-Schiff-positive (PAS+), diastase-resistant globules. The globules represent the polymerization of the abnormally folded Z protein retained within the hepatocyte. It is the retention of the AAT within the endoplasmic reticulum of the hepatocyte that is the inciting event in the pathogenesis of liver disease. Normal cellular mechanisms such as endoplasmic reticulum–associated degradation and macroautophagy dispose of the AAT, but when the capacity of these processes is overwhelmed, AAT polymerization and accumulation occur. It is hypothesized that the cells with differing burdens of AAT accumulation (high vs low) may have different fates, but ultimately, cell death, liver fibrosis, and cirrhosis can occur.[10] Detailed discussion is beyond the scope of this review, but several excellent reviews of the pathogenesis have been recently published.[11,12]

ALPHA-1 ANTITRYPSIN DEFICIENCY AND LIVER DISEASE IN CHILDREN

Most AAT-deficient infants are clinically healthy and remain so throughout childhood. Evidence for this comes from a Swedish neonatal screening study of 200,000 infants, which detected 127 PI*ZZ individuals and followed them prospectively into adulthood.[4,13] Prolonged cholestasis was present in 11% of the infants, and another 6% had clinical symptoms of liver disease without jaundice. Clinical signs of liver disease in infants were present in 11% who had prolonged cholestasis and 6% with clinical symptoms of liver disease without jaundice. Four deaths occurred in the cholestasis group: 2 from cirrhosis, 1 from aplastic anemia who was found to have cirrhosis, and 1 from an motor vehicle accident. Most children had abnormal liver enzymes at least once during follow-up. By age 18, no additional children had developed any clinical signs of liver disease.

Descriptions of the clinical presentation of pediatric PI*ZZ liver emphasize how variable the disease can be. Most commonly, neonatal hepatitis and cholestasis are present, but severe liver failure can occur in infants. Children and adolescents can present with signs of portal hypertension without ever having cholestasis as infants.[14] The variability suggests that other genetic and environmental modifiers are required for the development of childhood liver disease. Furthermore, it appears that LT only becomes necessary for a small proportion of affected children.

LIVER DISEASE IN ADULTS
Risk of Cirrhosis in PI*ZZ Adults

The link between classic AAT deficiency and cirrhosis in adults was recognized in the 1970s.[15,16] No population-based studies in adults have been completed to date. The strength of the association between PI*ZZ and chronic liver disease has been estimated by comparing the prevalence in combined cohorts with liver disease (0.8%) to the expected population frequency (0.04%). The prevalence of PI*ZZ in chronic liver disease is 20 times higher, suggesting increased risk in homozygous individuals.[14] The true prevalence of advanced liver disease in adults with AAT is not known. The best estimate comes from a population-based, case-control study from Sweden. The prevalence of cirrhosis was 43%, and the relative risk of cirrhosis was 8.3 (95% confidence interval [CI], 3.8–18.3).[17]

Several important risk factors for cirrhosis have been established. Foremost, older age has a higher risk, especially in men.[18] In a relatively large cohort of 246 PI*ZZ adults evaluated by age groups, cirrhosis was present in 2% of those ages 20 to 50. However, it was present in 19% of those older than 50.[19] The risk of cirrhosis is particularly high in the nonsmoking A1ATD population, who survive longer.[20]

Risk of Cirrhosis in PI*MZ Adults

The question regarding heterozygosity as risk for LT is often asked, but a conclusive answer has not been reached. It is thought that a "second hit" may be necessary for liver disease to develop, but no prospective population-based study to evaluate this question has been performed. Evaluation of cirrhotic patients referred for LT provides some evidence of a small risk (<3%) of liver disease in heterozygotes.[14]

EARLY EXPERIENCE IN LIVER TRANSPLANTATION AND ALPHA-1 ANTITRYPSIN DEFICIENCY

The first case reports of LT for AAT deficiency shed light on the crucial role of the liver in the disease state. The first lesson learned was that AAT deficiency is similar to other inborn errors of metabolism, such as Wilson disease, in that replacement of the liver corrects the underlying metabolic problem. Although the first 2 children transplanted for AAT deficiency died within a month, normal levels of AAT were detected in their blood soon after transplant.[21,22] The corresponding phenotype change was demonstrated in a subsequent case report of a 16-year-old girl transplanted for AAT deficiency. Not only did the serum AAT level return to normal but also the patient's phenotype changed from ZZ to MM. This patient eventually underwent a second transplant, and by chance, the donor was MZ, so a second phenotypic conversion occurred.[23] These first observations of sustained normal levels of AAT and recipient phenotype change were confirmed in the first small case series of AAT-deficient individuals transplanted.[24] The first successful LT occurred before even a basic understanding of the mechanisms that cause liver disease, so investigators were not sure if disease would recur. Repeat liver biopsies performed 1 year after LT demonstrated the noticeable lack of AAT accumulation as measured by PAS-D$^+$ globules.[25]

Early graft and patient outcomes in LT for AATD are reflective of the LT outcomes for other causes of end-stage liver disease (ESLD) in that era. A large case series of LTs from 1980 to 1986 in Pittsburgh reported the experience in adults separately from children.[26] The 10 adults ranged in age from 18 to 48 years (mean 34), and all presented with complications of advanced liver disease at the time of diagnosis of AAT deficiency. Average time between symptom onset and LT was 3 years (range 1–9), and only 1 individual reported COPD. The 29 ZZ children were transplanted at an average age of 5 years (range, 8 months to 13 years). Reported 5-year survival was 60% and 83% for adult and pediatric recipients, respectively.[26] The diagnosis of AATD accounted for 2.94% (10/339) of the total adult LTs and 13% (29/223) children performed at this center during this time. An additional study from the United Kingdom reported similar findings as the US experience. Reported survival at 1 year for adults was 73% and 87.5% for children.[25] With advances in immunosuppression, surgical techniques, and use of split grafts for children, outcomes for LT have improved over time.

The landmark paper describing success in children with LT for any indication included 29 individuals with AAT deficiency. It was the second most common diagnosis in the cohort and represented 11% of the children transplanted.[27] As LT eventually became a more realistic option for severely liver affected AAT children at multiple centers, questions remained around optimal timing and if surgical shunting was a viable alternative.[28,29] The clinical heterogeneity and unpredictable progression of liver disease created the clinical challenge of determining the most appropriate time to list for transplant. Initially, abnormal results of anticoagulation test and persistently elevated bilirubin were recommended as criteria for placement on LT list based on a single center's experience.[30] However, it came with the caveat that each patient should be considered individually. In addition to these indications, other groups used hypoalbuminemia, ascites, and variceal bleeding to prompt listing.[31] In a large referral center in the United Kingdom, 97 children were evaluated for AAT liver disease over a period of 10 years: 24.7% required LT, and 73.3% were alive without transplant.[32] The median time from presentation to liver failure was 2.5 years (range, 1.2 months to 13 years) in those who presented with neonatal hepatitis. In the group that presented with chronic liver disease, the time to transplant was 4.5 years (range, presentation to 13 years). Complication rates were similar to those in other reported LT series. Survival rates were 96% and 92% at 1 and 5 years, respectively.[32] The authors concluded that in the era of successful LT, an overall survival of 98% for liver affected children was exceptional.

LIVER TRANSPLANTATION FOR ALPHA-1 ANTITRYPSIN DEFICIENCY IN CHILDREN

Over the last 20 years, what has emerged is a picture of slowly progressive liver disease in some children, even in the presence of portal hypertension and cirrhosis.[33] Liver disease presents as mild in many children, and even those with significant cholestasis at presentation can go on to improve without requiring LT.[34] At this time, the prognosis regarding eventual LT in children cannot be reliably based on the clinical features of liver disease. A large overlap exists between those with mild and severe liver disease, including age at initial presentation.[35] In a baseline analysis of a longitudinal cohort of children with AAT deficiency, portal hypertension was found to be a common complication (29%) of AAT deficiency in children. Growth patterns and quality of life are normal in most.[35]

Unfortunately, a small percentage of children with AAT deficiency will eventually require LT. A review of the United Network for Organ Sharing (UNOS) database provides insight on the scope of LT in the United States.[36] From 1995 to 2004, a total of 161 LT were performed in the pediatric age group for AAT deficiency. The diagnosis accounted for 3.51% of all pediatric LT with a trend toward fewer transplants performed in more recent years.[36] Median age at time of transplant was 3 years (range, 0.5–17), and 60.9% were male patients. Graft survival was excellent at 1, 3, and 5 years with rates of 84%, 81%, and 78%. Patient survival at 1, 3, and 5 years was 92%, 90%, and 90%. Long-term outcomes after LT in 35 AAT children have been reported as a single-center experience to show the influence of immunosuppression regimen on survival.[37] Children transplanted in the tacrolimus era (n = 12) had 100% survival compared with 76.5% survival during the CSA era (n = 17) and 33.3% survival pre-CSA.[37]

LIVER TRANSPLANTATION FOR ALPHA-1 ANTITRYPSIN DEFICIENCY IN ADULTS

As detailed above, the original descriptions of population of AAT individuals requiring LT were children and young adults, and most of the literature available has focused on pediatric disease. Understandably, the impression that most clinicians have regarding AAT liver disease is that children are primarily affected and that adults are stricken with lung disease. Recently, this question has been revisited to evaluate where the burden of liver disease from AAT deficiency truly lies. Answering this question directly is difficult because many people with AAT deficiency escape diagnosis. From survey data of individuals (n = 1953) diagnosed with AAT deficiency, only 2.4% (n = 47) report a history of LT.[38] Meanwhile, it is known that cirrhosis is a significant cause of morbidity and mortality in adults with AAT deficiency. In the National Heart, Lung, and Blood Institute (NHLBI) registry, cirrhosis accounted for 10% of deaths in the NHLBI Registry and has been reported as the primary cause of death in 28% of PI*ZZ nonsmokers.[39,40]

The extent and success of LT performed in adults with AAT deficiency have been evaluated retrospectively by reviewing large national transplant databases as well as in single transplant center series. The UNOS transplant database from 1995 to 2004 included 406 adults with AAT deficiency.[36] Overall, it was the indication for 1.06% of all adults transplanted during this time period. The demographics of the adults transplanted reflect the reported risk factors of age and sex for advanced liver disease. Seventy-two percent were men, and the median age at transplant was 52 years (range, 18–70). Graft survival was excellent with 1-, 3-, and 5-year survival of 83%, 79%, and 77%. Patient survival was also excellent with 1-, 3-, and 5-year survival of 89%, 85%, and 83%. Three patients had a prior lung transplant. The limitations of the UNOS database must be considered when interpreting these results. No phenotype was available, so the adult population could reflect both ZZ and MZ individuals. It also does not have information on contributing factors such as hepatitis C virus (HCV), obesity, and alcohol.

A recent re-analysis of the Organ Procurement and Transplantation Network (OPTN) database as well as 2 other large US transplant databases was performed to determine the age distribution of LT for AAT deficiency.[41] Interestingly, the peak age range for LT was between 50 and 64, and men had greater risk for LT than women. In the early time period studied from 1991 to 1997, a significantly higher proportion of LT for AAT deficiency went to children, but the trends have changed with time. In the model for end stage-liver disease (MELD)/pediatric end-stage liver disease era from 2002 to 2012, less than 20 children each year had an LT for AAT deficiency. Adults represented 87% of the total population of AAT-deficient individuals transplanted. As noted before, the OPTN dataset does not have AAT deficiency phenotype data, so the phenotype distribution (ZZ, SZ, MZ) in this dataset this remains uncertain. In 2 large LT databases where phenotype data are available, ZZ and SZ phenotypes accounted for 31.6% of AAT LT. Applying this phenotype distribution to the OPTN dataset, it was estimated that 2.5 times as many adults as children require LT secondary to AAT deficiency.[41]

The best characterized adult AAT LT population comes from a large retrospective study that combines the experience of 3 large transplant centers in a single health system from 1987 to 2012.[42] Only confirmed PI*ZZ (n = 50) and PI*SZ (n = 23) individuals were included, and a group of PI*MZ heterozygotes was used for comparison. What emerged was a similar picture to the UNOS/OPTN database: middle-aged men represented most of the individuals transplanted for AAT deficiency. Again, AAT deficiency represented a low percentage (1.4%) of the total number of LT, but most (97%) of those transplanted for AAT deficiency were adults. Survival at 1 and 5 years was 86% and 82%. Only 1 person died of a pulmonary complication 9.3 years after LT.

What should be emphasized from this series is that a diagnosis of hepatitis C, primary biliary cirrhosis, primary sclerosing cholangitis, alcoholic liver disease, or hemochromatosis was found in 8% of PI*ZZ and 43.5% of PI*SZ groups. The description of AAT deficiency as a co-morbid condition with other liver diseases highlights the importance of testing every person with cirrhosis for alpha-1. Furthermore, it is notable that in the PI*MZ group, 90% had a coexisting liver disease, which is consistent with the idea that heterozygosity requires an additional injury to cause cirrhosis. Other investigators have since confirmed these observations with reports of HCV, ETOH abuse, and obesity as comorbid diseases in liver disease from AAT deficiency.[17]

The literature for LT for individuals affected with AAT deficiency has several limitations. The natural history of liver disease is not well described, and there is wide clinical variability in presentation. Studying a rare condition makes achieving adequate numbers of patients to draw conclusions difficult. As a result, the literature on LT in AAT deficiency is from single-center experiences across multiple countries, generally is retrospective, has small numbers of AAT individuals, and spans different eras of LT. Therefore, liver allocation systems and immunosuppression regimens were different even within an individual study, and the impact this had on outcomes is not accounted for. Second, how investigators defined AAT deficiency liver disease varies from study to study, which makes direct comparisons difficult. Ideally, only well-characterized and clearly phenotyped PI*ZZ or PI*SZ individuals would be included because these are the individuals at risk for liver disease. Given the retrospective nature of the studies performed, phenotype was not always available. To circumvent this, investigators defined liver disease from AAT deficiency broadly and occasionally included individuals who are PI*MZ. For example, in 1 study, the presence of PAS-D⁺ globules on biopsy specimen, which are not specific for the diagnosis of AAT deficiency, was sufficient for inclusion. In another study, diagnosis codes without a confirmed phenotype were used to define the cohort. Both of these strategies led to the inclusion of heterozygotes, that have a different risk profile for liver disease. Clinically significant liver problems in PI*MZ do not appear to develop during childhood, so this is a limitation in the literature most relevant to the adult population.

HEPATOCELLULAR CARCINOMA AND ALPHA-1 ANTITRYPSIN DEFICIENCY

The reported risk and prevalence of hepatocellular carcinoma (HCC) in AAT deficiency are highly variable and dependent on the population studied. In a well-defined case control autopsy study from Sweden, the prevalence of HCC was reported at 28%, and the relative risk for developing HCC was 5 (95% CI 1.6–15.8).[17] In contrast, no cases of HCC were reported in the UNOS database, including 567 LT for AAT deficiency.[36] However, it may have lacked the clinical granularity to report this diagnosis because subsequent analysis of other large transplant databases report HCC prevalence from 10% to 19%.[41,42] The higher reported prevalence of HCC in the AAT liver transplant population should be interpreted with caution because allocation policies changed to prioritize HCC during the years reported. By 2008, 21% of those transplanted for any indication had HCC.[43] When this change is considered, the high prevalence described may just be a reflection of the increased prioritization of HCC over time. Only one study to date has addressed the cumulative incidence and risk of HCC in individuals with liver cirrhosis from AAT deficiency.[40] The overall incidence rate of HCC was significantly lower in the AAT deficiency group when compared with other causes of cirrhosis (8.5% vs 31%, P<.001). Furthermore, patients with ESLD due to AAT deficiency had the lowest yearly cumulative rate of HCC at 0.88% per year compared with 2.7% for those with HCV cirrhosis, 1.5% in patients with nonalcoholic steatohepatitis, and 0.9% in alcohol-induced liver disease (P<.001).[44]

GENOTYPE/PHENOTYPE MISMATCH AND OTHER DONOR ISSUES

After LT, the result of genotype testing reflects the recipient, whereas the result of phenotype testing will reflect the donor.[45] The most likely scenario is the genotype remains ZZ, a normal serum level of AAT is present, and the phenotype is MM (the most common). The prevalence of the carrier state PI*MZ is approximately 2% to 3% in the United States. It is also possible that an individual with AAT deficiency or any other LT recipient could receive a donor that is PI*MZ. Even more unlikely, an LT recipient could receive a graft that is PI*ZZ or PI*SZ if there is no obvious disease in the graft.[46,47] The recipient of an affected liver may go unnoticed clinically because testing for AAT post post-LT is not routinely performed. Testing should be considered part of an evaluation for unexplained post-LT liver function test abnormalities or if PAS + D globules are found on graft biopsies.

CONSIDERATIONS OF LUNG FUNCTION PARTICULAR TO ALPHA-1 ANTITRYPSIN DEFICIENCY

Adults are at risk for panacinar basilar emphysema, which has the potential to influence LT candidacy if lung disease is severe. COPD associated with AAT deficiency rarely develops before the age of 30 years,[48] so it is not a concern for pediatric LT. In adults, no specific guidelines are available on how advanced COPD would preclude safe LT.[49] Pulmonary function in ZZ and SZ individuals can range from normal to severe expiratory airflow obstruction depending on smoking and other exposure history. Lung disease progresses independent of the course of liver disease. Adults with AAT deficiency being considered for LT should undergo a thorough pulmonary evaluation, including a full set of pulmonary function tests (PFTs) as part of the LT evaluation. Studies of lung function in pre-LT patients are difficult to interpret as concurrent ascites, hepatic hydrothorax, malnutrition, and functional status may limit effort and ability of patients to perform spirometry.

The course of pulmonary disease after LT in both adults and children has been poorly studied. The first report of post-LT lung function was limited to 10/22 patients with full PFTs at a median of 28 months.[25] Only 2 had less than 70% predicted forced expiratory volume in 1 second (FEV_1), and no pre-LT PFTs or phenotypes were reported. A small series (n = 7) with pre-LT and post-LT PFTs showed no significant change in FEV_1 after a median of 30 months of follow-up post-LT. Two patients had dramatic changes in FEV_1, whereas the other 5 were steady, suggesting pulmonary decline could be slowed.[50] Ideally, pre-LT and post-LT PFTs collected regularly could show if LT halts the expected accelerated progression of lung function decline associated with AAT deficiency (46–87 mL/y). The largest series of paired pre-LT and post-LT PFTs includes 17 patients.[42] FEV_1 before LT was 2.79 ± 1.1 (0.93–4.5), which is 74.6% predicted. After LT, FEV_1 was 2.73 ± 1.34 (0.87–4.72). Individual data show a continued decline in 65% and improvement in 35% with wide variations. More importantly, 53% of the ZZ patients had an annual reduction in FEV_1 greater than the expected 30 mL/y from aging despite normalization of AAT levels after LT. Accelerated lung function decline could be an indication for earlier LT transplantation, but the available data do not justify MELD exception points.[49] Further study is needed to clarify the impact of LT on pulmonary function. Long-term pulmonary outcomes after pediatric LT are unknown.

The question of lung and LT occasionally arises when discussing ESLD in AAT-deficient adults if both organs are severely affected. It does not happen frequently. In the UNOS data, 3 liver-after-lung transplants were included.[36] Simultaneous lung and LTs could be an option for a select few. Data are limited to case reports of combined lung/liver transplants, which include 3 patients with AAT deficiency.[51,52] All are alive with 4, 7, and 13 years of follow-up. Identification of suitable candidates for multiorgan transplantation is complex and requires consideration of factors beyond what would be considered in a single organ.

SUMMARY

In conclusion, AAT deficiency is a genetic condition that in its most severe clinical presentation will require LT. Both children and adults are affected by liver disease, and transplantation is the only curative option for AAT deficiency. After LT, the phenotype of the recipient becomes that of the donor, and normal levels of AAT are detected in the blood after transplant. Overall survival after LT is excellent. The impact of LT on lung function is not well studied.

REFERENCES

1. Laurell CB, Eriksson S. The electrophoretic alpha-1 globulin pattern serum in alpha-1 antitrypsin deficiency. Scand J Clin Lab Invest 1963;15:132–40.
2. Sharp HL, Mathis R, Krivit W, et al. The liver in non-cirrhotic alpha-1-antitrypsin deficiency. J Lab Clin Med 1971;78:1012–3.
3. Silverman EK, Sandhaus RA. Alpha$_1$-antitrypsin deficiency. N Engl J Med 2009; 360:2749–57.
4. Sveger T. Liver disease in alpha 1-antitrypsin deficiency detected by screening of 200,000 infants. N Engl J Med 1976;294:1316–21.
5. O'Brien ML, Buist NR, Murphey WH. Neonatal screening for alpha-1 antitrypsin deficiency. J Pediatr 1978;92:1006–10.
6. Silverman EK, Miletich JP, Pierce JA, et al. Alpha-1 antitrypsin deficiency: high prevalence in the St. Louis area determined by direct population screening. Am Rev Respir Dis 1989;140:961–6.

7. Regev A, Guaqueta C, Molina EG, et al. Does the heterozygous state of alpha-1 antitrypsin deficiency have a role in chronic liver diseases? Interim results of a large case control study. J Pediatr Gastroenterol Nutr 2006;43: S30–5.

8. Reid CL, Wiener GJ, Cox DW, et al. Diffuse hepatocellular dysplasia and carcinoma associated with the M_{malton} variant of alpha$_1$-antitrypsin. Gastroenterology 1987;93:181–7.

9. Brantly M, Mukiwa T, Crystal RG. Molecular basis of alpha 1-antitrypsin deficiency. Am J Med 1988;84(Suppl 6A):13–31.

10. Greene CM, Marciniak SJ, Teckman J, et al. Alpha-1-antitrypsin deficiency. Nat Rev Dis Primers 2016;2:1–17.

11. Silverman GA, Pak SC, Perlmutter DH. Disorders of protein misfolding: alpha-1-antitrypsin deficiency as prototype. J Pediatr 2013;163:320–6.

12. Teckman JH, Mangalat N. Alpha-1 antitrypsin and liver disease: mechanisms of injury and novel interventions. Expert Rev Gastroenterol Hepatol 2015;9:261–8.

13. Sveger T, Eriksson S. The liver in adolescents with alpha$_1$-antitrypsin deficiency. Hepatology 1995;22:1316–21.

14. Stoller JK, Snider GL, Brantly ML, et al, American Thoracic Society, European Respiratory Society. American Thoracic Society/European Respiratory Society Statement: Standards for the diagnosis and management of individuals with alpha-1 antitrypsin deficiency. Am J Respir Crit Care Med 2003;168:818–900.

15. Berg NO, Eriksson S. Liver disease in adults with alpha-1 antitrypsin deficiency. N Engl J Med 1972;287:1264–7.

16. Triger DR, Millward-Sadler GH, Czaykowski AA, et al. Alpha-1 antitrypsin deficiency and liver in adults. Q J Med 1976;45:B51–72.

17. Elzouki AN, Eriksson S. Risk of hepatobiliary disease in adults with severe alpha1: an additional risk factor for cirrhosis and hepatocellular carcinoma? Eur J Gastroenterol Hepatol 1996;110:78–83.

18. Cox DW, Smth S. Risk for liver disease in adults with alpha-1-antitrypsin. Am J Med 1983;74:221–7.

19. Larsson C. Natural history and live expectancy in severe alpha-1 antitrypsin PiZ. Acta Med Scand 1978;294:345–51.

20. Eriksson S. Alpha-1-antitrypsin deficiency: natural course and therapeutic strategies. In: Boyer J, Blum HE, Maier KP, et al, editors. Cirrhosis and its development. Falk symposium 115. Dordrecht (The Netherlands): Kluwer Academic; 2000. p. 307–15.

21. Sharp HL. Alpha-1 antitrypsin deficiency. Hosp Prac 1971;6:83.

22. Sharp HL, Desnick RJ, Krivit W. The liver in inherited metabolic disease of childhood. In: Popper H, Schaffner F, editors. Progress in liver disease, vol. IV. New York: Grune and Stratton, Inc; 1972. p. 463–88.

23. Putnam CW, Porter KA, Peters RL, et al. Liver replacement for alpha-1 antitrypsin deficiency. Surgery 1977;81:258–61.

24. Hood JM, Koep LJ, Peters RL, et al. Liver transplantation for advanced liver disease with alpha-1 antitrypsin deficiency. N Engl J Med 1980;302(5):272–5.

25. Vennarecci G, Gunson BK, Ismail T, et al. Transplantation for end stage liver disease related to alpha-1 antitrypsin. Transplantation 1996;61(10):1488–95.

26. Esquivel CO, Vicente E, Van Thiel D, et al. Orthotopic liver transplantation for alpha-1 antitrypsin deficiency: an Experience in 29 children and ten adults. Transplant Proc 1987;19(5):3798–802.

27. Esquivel CO, Iwatsuki S, Gordon RD, et al. Indications for pediatric liver transplantation. J Pediatr 1987;111(6 Pt 2):1039–45.

28. Starzl TE, Porter KA, Francavilla A, et al. Reversal of hepatic alpha-1-antitrypsin deposition after portacaval shunt. Lancet 1983;2:424–6.
29. Starzl TE, Porter KA, Busuttil RW, et al. Portacaval shunt in three children with alpha-1 antitrypsin deficiency and cirrhosis: 9 to 12 1/3 years later. Hepatology 1990;11:152–4.
30. Ibarguen E, Gross CR, Savik SK, et al. Liver disease in alpha-1-antitrypsin deficiency: prognostic indicators. J Pediatr 1990;117:864–70.
31. Prachalias AA, Kalife M, Francavilla R, et al. Liver transplantation for alpha-1 antitrypsin deficiency in children. Transpl Int 2000;13:207–10.
32. Francavilla R, Castellaneta SP, Hadzic N, et al. Prognosis of alpha-1 antitrypsin deficiency-related liver disease in the era of paediatric liver transplantation. J Hepatol 2000;32:986–92.
33. Volpert D, Molleston JP, Perlmutter DH. α1-antitrypsin deficiency-associated liver disease progresses slowly in some children. J Pediatr Gastroenterol Nutr 2000; 31:258–63.
34. Bakula A, Socha J, Teisseyre M, et al. Good and bad prognosis of alpha-1 antitrypsin deficiency in children: when to list for liver transplantation. Transplant Proc 2007;39:3186–8.
35. Teckman JH, Rosenthal P, Abel R, et al. Baseline analysis of a young a-1-antitrypsin deficiency liver disease cohort reveals frequent portal hypertension. J Pediatr Gastroenterol Nutr 2015;61:94–101.
36. Kemmer N, Kaiser T, Zacharias V, et al. Alpha-1 antitrypsin deficiency: outcomes after liver transplantation. Transplant Proc 2008;40:1492–4.
37. Hughes MG, Khan KM, Gruessner AC, et al. Long-term outcome in 42 pediatric liver transplant patients with alpha 1-antitrypsin deficiency: a single-center experience. Clin Transplant 2011;25:731–6.
38. Strange C, Stoller JK, Sandhaus RA, et al. Results of a survey of patients with alpha-1 antitrypsin deficiency. Respiration 2006;73(2):185–90.
39. Stoller JK, Tomashefski J, Crystal R, et al. Mortality in individuals with severe deficiency of alpha-1 antitrypsin: findings from the National Heart, Lung, and Blood Institute registry. Chest 2005;127:1196–204.
40. Tanash HA, Nilsson PM, Nilsson JA, et al. Clinical course and prognosis of never smokers with severe alpha-1 antitrypsin deficiency (PiZZ). Thorax 2008;63: 1091–5.
41. Chu AS, Chopra KB, Perlmutter DH. Is severe progressive liver disease caused by alpha-1 antitrypsin deficiency more common in children or adults? Liver Transpl 2016;22:886–94.
42. Carey EJ, Iyer VN, Nelson DR, et al. Outcomes for recipients of liver transplantation for alpha-1-antitrypsin deficiency related cirrhosis. Liver Transplant 2013;19: 1370–6.
43. Ioannou GN, Perkins JD, Carithers RL Jr. Liver transplantation for hepatocellular carcinoma: impact of the MELD allocation system and predictors of survival. Gastroenterology 2008;134:1342–51.
44. Antoury C, Lopez R, Zein N, et al. Alpha-1 antitrypsin deficiency and the risk of hepatocellular carcinoma in end stage liver disease. World J Hepatol 2015; 7(10):1427–32.
45. Hackbarth JS, Tostrud LJ, Rumilla K, et al. Discordant alpha-1 antitrypsin phenotype and genotype results in a liver transplant patient. Clin Chim Acta 2010;411: 1146–8.
46. Arnal FM, Lorenzo MJ, Suarez F, et al. Acquired PiZZ alpha-1 antitrypsin deficiency in a liver transplant recipient. Transplantation 2004;77(12):1918–9.

47. Roelandt P, Dobbels P, Komuta M, et al. Herterozygous alpha-1 antitrypsin Z allele mutation in presumed healthy donors used for transplantation. Eur J Gastroenterol Hepatol 2013;25(11):1335–9.
48. Bernspang E, Sveger T, Piitulainen E. Respiratory symptoms and lung function in 30-year old individuals with alpha-1-antitrypsin deficiency. Respir Med 2007;101: 1971–6.
49. Krowka MJ, Wiesner RH, Heimbach JK. Pulmonary contraindications, indications and MELD exceptions for liver transplantation: a contemporary view and look forward. J Hepatol 2013;59:367–74.
50. Jain AB, Patil V, Sheikh B, et al. Effect of liver transplant on pulmonary functions in adults with alpha-1 antitrypsin deficiency: 7 cases. Exp Clin Transplant 2010;8(1): 4–8.
51. Grannas G, Neipp M, Hoeper MM, et al. Indications for and outcomes after combined lung and liver transplantation: a single center experience on 13 consecutive cases. Transplantation 2008;85:524–31.
52. Yi SG, Burroughs SG, Loebe M, et al. Combined lung and liver transplantation: analysis of a single center experience. Liver Transpl 2014;20:46–53.

Predictors of Cardiovascular Events After Liver Transplantation

Juan F. Gallegos-Orozco, MD[a], Michael R. Charlton, MD, FRCP[b],*

KEYWORDS

- Cardiovascular disease • Myocardial infarction • Atrial fibrillation • Ischemic stroke
- Heart failure • Cirrhotic cardiomyopathy • Liver transplant

KEY POINTS

- As a consequence of the success of liver transplants, we are now transplanting patients who are older and have more comorbid diseases, including cardiovascular (CV) disease.
- CV diseases (CVD), together with infectious and malignant diseases, account for the majority of posttransplant deaths.
- Patients with liver cirrhosis can develop heart disease through systemic diseases affecting the heart and the liver, cirrhosis-specific heart disease, or common CV conditions.
- To minimize negative outcomes and identify patients at risk for posttransplant CV events, the pretransplant evaluation must include a thorough cardiac evaluation.
- No single factor can predict posttransplant CV complications; however, a history of CVD and specific abnormalities on echocardiography, electrocardiography, or serum markers of heart disease imply complications, including cardiac-related death.

INTRODUCTION

Liver transplantation (LT) has become an integral part of the treatment of patients with end-stage liver disease (ESLD). With increasing medical and surgical expertise, we have liberalized the indications for LT and significantly expanded the number of patients that qualify for an LT. As a consequence, we are transplanting patients who are older and have more comorbid diseases, including cardiovascular (CV) disease (CVD), than ever before.[1,2] At the same time, high organ demand has resulted in rising acuity and severity of disease as reflected by higher Model for End-stage Liver

Disclosure: The authors have nothing to disclose pertaining to the subject matter of this review.
[a] Division of Gastroenterology, Hepatology and Nutrition, University of Utah School of Medicine, 30 North 1900 East SOM 4R118, Salt Lake City, UT 84132, USA; [b] Intermountain Transplant Center, Intermountain Medical Center, 5169 South Cottonwood Street, Suite 320, Murray, UT 84107, USA
* Corresponding author.
E-mail address: Michael.charlton@imail.org

Disease (MELD) scores at the time of transplant. Higher MELD scores also mean increased prevalence of acute and chronic renal dysfunction, which contributes to increased posttransplant morbidity and mortality.[3] In this setting, it is not unexpected that CVD, together with infectious and malignant diseases, account for the majority of the posttransplant deaths.[4–6]

The close physiologic interaction between the heart and the liver, which is more pronounced in cirrhosis, has been recognized for more than 60 years.[7,8] Patients with heart failure (HF) can develop congestive hepatopathy leading to cardiac cirrhosis[9]; similarly, patients with liver cirrhosis can develop heart disease through several mechanisms: (1) systemic diseases that affect both the heart and the liver, such as chronic alcohol use or hemochromatosis, (2) cirrhosis-specific heart disease, such as portopulmonary hypertension (POPH) and cirrhotic cardiomyopathy, or (3) common CV conditions that also affect the general population, such as ischemic heart disease.[10] All these situations are relevant in the LT setting because they affect short- and long-term outcomes.

Patients with ESLD commonly have hyperdynamic circulation, resulting in an increased cardiac output with decreased systemic vascular resistance and compromised ventricular response to stress, currently known as cirrhotic cardiomyopathy.[11,12] LT poses significant hemodynamic stress, especially early after liver reperfusion, when there is a sudden increase in cardiac preload. In the setting of cardiomyopathy, an increase in the pulmonary wedge pressure and/or reduction in the mean arterial pressure can result in severe hemodynamic instability and hepatic congestion.[1] In this setting, cardiac death may result from arrhythmia, acute HF, and myocardial infarction.[13,14] In an effort to minimize negative outcomes and identify patients at risk for post-LT CV events, the pretransplant evaluation incorporates a thorough cardiac evaluation.

CARDIOVASCULAR COMPLICATIONS AFTER LIVER TRANSPLANTATION

It is well-known that CVD is a leading cause of long-term complications and death after LT.[2,15] More recently, CVD has also been associated with early posttransplant morbidity and mortality.

In a retrospective review of 393 adult liver transplants from Mayo Clinic in Arizona, a total of 30 deaths occurred within the first 4 months after LT (7.6% overall early mortality); the majority were due to surgical or medical complications and only 3 were primary cardiac deaths (0.8% cardiac mortality rate for all LT). Of the 393 LT, 26 patients had an acute cardiac event (6.6%), including 13 arrhythmias, 7 cases of new-onset HF, and 6 myocardial infarctions. Twelve of the 13 significant intraoperative cardiac events were arrhythmias (92%), including 2 of the 3 cardiac deaths documented in this experience.[16]

In a study from the Ochsner Clinic, 389 consecutive adult LT patients were reviewed retrospectively to determine early (within 1 year of LT) or late (more than 1 year after LT) CV complications. Rates of 1-year CV morbidity and mortality were 15% and 2.8%, respectively. The most common CV events were acute coronary syndrome (5.5%), arrhythmia (3.3%) and severe HF with left ventricle ejection fraction of less than 40% (2.8%). Thirty-two of the 389 LT patients died within the first year (8.2% mortality rate): 11 patients died from CVD (2.8%), accounting for the main cause of death; followed by infection, malignancy, and graft failure. Of patients who survived more than 1 year, 4% developed CV morbidity and 2% died from CV complications, representing the third leading cause of death after graft failure and malignancy.[17]

According to the American Heart Association, CVD includes ischemic heart disease, HF, thromboembolism, and stroke.[18] To assess the prevalence and predictors of early

(30-day posttransplant) CVD as defined above, VanWagner and colleagues[3] performed an analysis of all adult recipients of primary LT in the Organ Procurement and Transplantation Network database from February 2002 to December 2012. Among close to 55,000 LT, there were 1576 deaths within 30 days after LT (3%). CVD was the leading cause of mortality (n = 633; 40%), followed by infection (n = 440; 28%) and graft failure (n = 193; 12%). The leading cause of CV mortality was cardiac arrest (48%), followed by stroke (12.5%), HF (12.3%), and pulmonary embolism (9.1%). Through multivariate analysis, the authors identified 9 significant predictors of early CVD mortality after LT: recipient age, preoperative hospitalization, intensive care unit status, ventilator status, calculated MELD score, portal vein thrombosis, national organ sharing, donor body mass index, and cold ischemia time.[19]

This same group recently reported on the prevalence and factors associated with major CV events (MACE) 30 and 90 days after LT. MACE were defined as myocardial infarction, HF, atrial fibrillation (AF), cardiac arrest, pulmonary embolism, and/or stroke. Of 32,810 recipients, MACE requiring hospitalization occurred in 8% and 11% of patients at 30 and 90 days, respectively. Recipients with MACE were older and more likely to have nonalcoholic steatohepatitis (NASH) and alcoholic cirrhosis, as well as history of myocardial infarction, HF, stroke, AF, chronic pulmonary disease and chronic kidney disease compared with recipients without MACE. In multivariable analysis, several factors were associated independently with MACE: recipient age greater than 65 years, NASH cirrhosis, alcoholic cirrhosis, pretransplant serum creatinine, baseline AF, and stroke. Importantly, the presences of MACE were associated with decreased 1-year post-LT survival (79% vs 88%; $P<.0001$).[20]

As we improve our ability to treat chronic hepatitis C, it is anticipated that alcoholic steatohepatitis and NASH cirrhosis will rapidly become the common indications for LT in the United States. By analyzing the Organ Procurement and Transplantation Network database, Charlton and colleagues[21] described a significant increase in NASH as the etiology for LT from 1.2% in 2001 to 9.7% in 2009, and on trajectory to become the most common indication. Although recipients with NASH as a primary indication for LT have comparable 1- and 3-year posttransplant patient and graft survivals, they tend on average to be older and have higher body mass indexes than recipients with other indications for LT.

One of the consequences of the increase of NASH as a cause for LT might be an increase in CV morbidity and mortality, because it has been associated with increased risk of MACE, as described previously. This was demonstrated in a retrospective analysis of 242 adult primary LT (115 NASH vs 127 alcoholic cirrhosis) from 2 transplant centers in Chicago. Recipients with NASH were older (58.4 years vs 53.3 years), more commonly female (45% vs 18%), morbidly obese (32% vs 9%), had dyslipidemia (25% vs 6%), or had hypertension (53% vs 38%). On multivariate analysis, compared with those with alcoholic cirrhosis, recipients with NASH were more likely to have a CV event within the first post-LT year (26% vs 8%; odds ratio, 4.12; 95% confidence interval, 1.9–8.9). The most common cardiac complications in both groups were acute pulmonary edema and new-onset AF. The majority of CV events occurred in the perioperative period (70%), and the occurrence of a CV event was associated with a 50% overall mortality. However, there were no differences in the 1-, 3-, and 5-year patient and graft survivals. Sepsis was the most common cause of death (11% vs 4% in the alcoholic cirrhosis group; $P = .11$), followed by CV causes in the NASH group (9% vs 1%; $P = .45$). These results demonstrate an increased risk of CV events among NASH recipients, even after controlling for preexisting comorbidities and despite extensive preoperative testing.[22]

In a follow-up study of the Organ Procurement and Transplantation Network database to examine the association between NASH and CV mortality after LT, among the more than 48,000 adult LT from 2002 to 2011, 5057 (10.5%) were performed for NASH. This population was found to be older, mostly female, obese, diabetic, and have a history of chronic kidney disease and CVD compared with other etiologies. NASH was associated with increased 30-day mortality compared with non-NASH recipients (3.8% vs 2.8%; P<.001). CVD was the most common cause of early mortality in both groups (accounting for more than 40% of all deaths), followed by infection (28%) and graft failure (12%). In the NASH group, cardiac arrest accounted for 53% of the deaths within 30 days, followed by thromboembolic disease (16%), HF (12%), and myocardial infarction (12%). Although there was no difference in all-cause mortality, both early (30-day) and long-term CVD-specific mortality was 30% to 40% higher among NASH patients. Interestingly, these associations were no longer significant after adjusting for pretransplant diabetes, renal dysfunction, or history of CVD. Using multivariate analysis, the authors identified risk factors associated with CV mortality and built a risk score that included recipient age 55 years or older, male sex, diabetes, and renal impairment (estimated glomerular filtration rate < 60 mL/min/1.73 m^2 or the need for renal replacement therapy) to categorize patients at different risk of CV mortality after LT. Compared with the low-risk recipients, patients with 3 or 4 of these risk factors were 2- to 3-fold more likely to die from CVD.[3]

Another contributor to increased CVD after LT is the frequent development of the metabolic syndrome or its individual components in many LT recipients. In a single-center retrospective study of 252 adult LT recipients from Israel, more than one-half (52%) developed the metabolic syndrome. Noticeably, these recipients had a 3-fold increase in major vascular events (defined as transient ischemic attack, stroke, acute coronary syndrome, or myocardial infarction) compared with recipients without metabolic syndrome (15% vs 5%, respectively; P<.007).[23] However, there was no difference in the mortality rate or cause of death between these 2 groups. Independent predictors of posttransplant metabolic syndrome included age, pre-LT NAFLD, body mass index, diabetes, and triglycerides.

PREOPERATIVE CARDIOVASCULAR EVALUATION IN LIVER TRANSPLANT CANDIDATES

The preoperative CV evaluation is a key component of the LT evaluation process. It aims not only to assess cardiac function, but also to identify patients with clinically significant coronary artery disease (CAD), as well as other relevant cardiopulmonary abnormalities, such as pulmonary hypertension, valvular heart disease, and cardiac arrhythmias, which might compromise the posttransplant outcomes (Fig. 1).

Although transplant programs differ in their approach to the CV evaluation, most rely heavily on stress echocardiography, nuclear medicine scans, and computed tomography coronary calcium scores. Some programs will also rely heavily on coronary angiography as the main tool to assess for CAD. Selected patients will need invasive testing with coronary angiography and possibly even revascularization before undergoing LT.[24]

There are some limited guidelines regarding the pretransplant cardiac evaluation. For example, in the section on cardiac disease, the American Association for the Study of Liver Diseases guidelines on pretransplant evaluation recommend the following[25]:

- Cardiac evaluation needs to an include assessment of cardiac risk factors with stress echocardiography as an initial screening test with cardiac catheterization as clinically indicated (1-B).

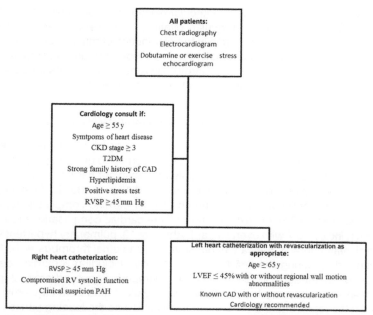

Fig. 1. Proposed cardiovascular assessment of patients undergoing pre-liver transplant evaluation. CAD, coronary artery disease; CKD, chronic kidney disease; LVEF, left ventricular ejection fraction; PAH, pulmonary artery hypertension; RV, right ventricle; RVSP, right ventricular systolic pressure; T2DM, type 2 diabetes mellitus.

- Cardiac revascularization should be considered in LT candidates with significant coronary artery stenosis before transplantation (2-C).

Similarly, the European Association for the Study of the Liver guideline recommends the following[26]:

- Electrocardiogram and transthoracic echocardiography should be performed in all liver transplant candidates (grade II-3).
- In patients with multiple CV risk factors, and in patients older than 50 years, a cardiopulmonary exercise test should be done. If the target heart rate is not achieved during a standard exercise test, a pharmacologic stress test is the test of choice (grade II-3).

Last, there are also recommendations from the American Heart Association and the American College of Cardiology Foundation on cardiac disease evaluation and management among liver transplant candidates[27]:

- Noninvasive stress testing may be considered in LT candidates with no active cardiac conditions based on the presence of multiple risk factors for CAD, regardless of functional status. Relevant risk factors among transplantation candidates include diabetes mellitus, prior CVD, left ventricular hypertrophy, age greater than 60 years, smoking, hypertension, and dyslipidemia. The specific number of risk factors that should be used to prompt testing remains to be determined, but the committee considers 3 or more to be reasonable (class IIb; level of evidence C).
- It may be reasonable for each program to identify a primary cardiology consultant for questions related to potential LT candidates (class IIb; level of evidence C).

- LT candidates who have a left ventricular ejection fraction of less than 50%, evidence of ischemic left ventricular dilation, exercise-induced hypotension, angina, or demonstrable ischemia in the distribution of multiple coronary arteries should be referred to a cardiologist for evaluation and long-term management according to American College of Cardiology/American Heart Association guidelines for the general population (class I; level of evidence B).

PREDICTORS OF POSTTRANSPLANT CARDIOVASCULAR COMPLICATIONS

Despite this extensive evaluation, CVD is prevalent among LT recipients and results in significant morbidity and mortality. As such, it is important to develop predictors of CV complications after LT, even after acceptable pretransplant cardiac evaluation.

Fouad and colleagues[28] reviewed the University of Alberta adult LT (age >40 years) experience to identify predictors of 6-month post-LT cardiac complications. In total, 82 of 197 recipients (42%) developed one or more cardiac complications (pulmonary edema = 61, including 7 with overt HF; arrhythmia = 13, pulmonary hypertension = 7, myocardial infarction = 3, pericardial effusion = 2, and atrial thrombus = 1). Twenty-one patients died during the first 6 months (10.6%), including 5 cardiac deaths (2 deaths occurred intraoperatively owing to postreperfusion syndrome, 2 patients died from severe pulmonary hypertension, and 1 patient died from cardiomyopathy). These 5 deaths represented 24% of all mortality and was the leading cause of death overall. By multivariate analysis, after adjusting for age and sex, independent predictors of 6-month cardiac complications in this cohort were intraoperative CV events, preoperative history of heart disease and integrated MELD score (incorporates MELD, sodium, and age).

Safadi and colleagues[29] reviewed the perioperative outcomes (nonfatal myocardial infarction and/or death within 30 days) in 400 LT recipients at the University of Indiana. There were 48 total events (12%)—25 myocardial infarction (7%) and 38 deaths (9%). On multivariate analysis, the main predictor of nonfatal myocardial infarction was a prior stroke (odd ratio [OR], 7.45; 95% confidence interval [CI], 1.7–32.7; P = .008); the predictors of death of any cause were postoperative sepsis (OR, 8.6; 95% CI, 3.5–21; P = .001) and increased interventricular septal thickness (OR, 2.8; 95% CI, 1.1–7.2; P = .03). The use of beta-blockers in the perioperative period was associated with a protective effect on death (OR, 0.07; 95% CI, 0.01–0.6; P = .01).

AF is the most common arrhythmia in the United States, with a prevalence of up to 2.3% in the general population.[30,31] However, it is more prevalent among men and older individuals.[32] AF is associated with increased CV morbidity and mortality. To assess the effects of AF on LT, Bargher and colleagues[33] performed a case-control study of LT recipients from Mayo Clinic Florida. They identified 32 of 717 recipients with pre-LT AF (4.5%) and matched them with 63 LT controls without AF. Recipients with pre-LT AF were more likely to have left ventricular hypertrophy, HF, and stroke or a transient ischemic attack. Intraoperative adverse cardiac events (28% vs 5%; P = .02) and AF-related postoperative events (28% vs 2%; P<.001) were more common in the AF group. However, overall patient and graft survival were comparable between cases and controls.[34]

Echocardiography is performed commonly as part of the pre-LT evaluation in most centers across the world. This has made it an attractive risk-stratifying tool and allowed us to identify pretransplant parameters that can predict posttransplant outcomes.[35] The presence of left ventricular hypertrophy has been associated with increased post-LT mortality,[36] whereas the presence of greater than mild tricuspid valve regurgitation was found to be associated with post-LT death in one study[37] but not in another one.[38] On multivariate analysis, Bushyhead and colleagues[39] described an increased risk of death after LT in patients with greater than mild tricuspid regurgitation (hazard ratio [HR], 1.68; 95% CI, 1.03–2.75; $P = .04$). Similarly, estimated pulmonary artery systolic pressure on echocardiography was associated independently with cardiac-related post-LT hospitalization (HF or myocardial infarction), with a subhazard ratio 1.79 per 5 mm Hg increase in pulmonary artery systolic pressure (95% CI, 1.48–2.17; $P<.001$).

Serum troponin levels have also been described as predictors of posttransplant CV events. It is well-known that troponin T is not only a marker of myocardial ischemia, but is also increased in multiple other cardiac pathologies. In the transplant realm, troponin T is known to be an excellent predictor of survival in patients with chronic kidney disease.[40–42] More recently, in a group of 1206 adult recipients, elevated troponin T levels before kidney transplantation were associated with an increased risk of death and cardiac events after transplantation. Persistently increased troponin T after kidney transplantation was also associated independently with reduced patient survival, even after adjusting for age, diabetes, pretransplant dialysis, heart disease, and allograft function. However, normalization of troponin T levels after kidney transplantation was associated with reduced risk.[43]

A similar phenomenon has been observed in LT. Coss and colleagues[44] analyzed 230 LT performed at Mayo Clinic from 1998 to 2001. They assessed multiple potential predictors of CV outcomes, including traditional CVD risk factors, C-reactive protein, serum troponin levels, and echocardiographic parameters. Risk factors for heart disease were common among this population: 60% had a smoking history, 23% were diabetic, 19% had hypertension, 25% had elevated troponin levels, 25% had elevated C-reactive protein, and 16% had preexisting cardiac disease. Over a median follow-up of 8.2 years, there were 59 cardiac events: CAD (63%), myocardial infarction (7%), HF (8.5%), stroke (8.5%), peripheral vascular disease (5%), and CV death (8%). In total 63 recipients died, of whom 7 had a CV cause of death (11%). Multivariate analysis confirmed diabetes, prior smoking, prior CVD, and elevated troponin as independent predictors of posttransplant CV endpoints. Similarly, a prior history of CVD and elevated troponin levels were associated with 1-year posttransplant CV endpoints. Interestingly, the overall 1- and 5-year patient survivals were impacted negatively by a pretransplant troponin of greater than 0.07 ng/mL compared with recipients with normal troponin levels (86.5% and 73% vs 93.5% and 84%; $P = .004$). In a follow-up study including 455 liver transplant recipients, troponin levels of greater than 0.07 ng/mL were once again confirmed to be associated independently with long-term CVD outcomes; other factors identified included age, diabetes, and a history of prior CVD.[45]

Patients with liver cirrhosis have frequent electrocardiographic (ECG) abnormalities, such as prolonged QT interval,[46,47] dyssynchronous electrical and mechanical systole,[48] decreased heart rate variability,[46] and increased QT dispersion.[49–51] The clinical significance of these findings is unclear in patients awaiting a liver transplant, and it is unknown what potential impact they have on cardiac morbidity and mortality after LT.

In a retrospective review of 186 LT recipients from Sweden, Josefsson and colleagues[52] described the main ECG abnormalities and compared them with 92 healthy controls. Cirrhotic patients had an increased prevalence of abnormal QRS axis deviation (21% vs 10%; $P = .02$), prolonged QTc interval (31.5% vs 8%; $P<.001$), Q wave (12% vs 1%; $P = .001$), ST segment depression (5% vs 0%; $P = .02$), a pathologic T wave (10% vs 4%; $P = .07$), and ECG features compatible with CAD (17% vs 5%; $P<.001$). The majority of recipients who developed a posttransplant cardiac event had some abnormality on the pre-LT ECG (69%). Posttransplant cardiac events were associated with prolonged QTc, presence of a Q wave, or the presence of any ECG feature of CAD. Posttransplant mortality was increased in recipients with prolonged QTc interval and the presence of a Q wave, but not with other ECG abnormalities. Others have also described the negative impact of a prolonged QTc interval, including a decreased survival in patients with cirrhosis[53] and its association with peritransplant HF,[54] and more recently with increased post-LT mortality and MACE.[55] In this retrospective study from the Cleveland Clinic, Sonny and colleagues[55] analyzed the pretransplant ECG from 232 adult LT recipients, and almost 60% had a prolonged QTc (>440 ms). The presence of a prolonged QTc interval before LT was found to be associated independently with a composite outcome of death, graft failure and/or MACE (HR, 1.01; 95% CI, 1.00–1.02; $P = .05$).

Cirrhotic cardiomyopathy is a particular form of cardiac dysfunction seen in patients with ESLD. This condition seems to arise as a consequence of the hemodynamic abnormalities that occur in cirrhosis and is characterized by increased cardiac output with a blunted ventricular response to stimuli, systolic and diastolic dysfunction, best appreciated under stress conditions; and ECG abnormalities. Several echocardiographic indicators of diastolic dysfunction have been associated with the development of HF after LT.[54,56,57] Others have described an association between pre-LT diastolic dysfunction and posttransplant mortality, although not all investigators agree.[54,56,58,59] However, in most of these studies, diastolic dysfunction was defined using only 1 or 2 parameters (left atrial volume index > 40, e/e' > 10, e/a < 1, or left ventricular hypertrophy), resulting in errors in the estimation of the true frequency of diastolic dysfunction.

In an effort to determine the prevalence and impact of diastolic dysfunction (as defined by the American Society for Echocardiography) on patients undergoing LT, Sonny and colleagues[55] reviewed the pretransplant echocardiograms of 243 adult LT recipients: 114 had no diastolic dysfunction (46.5%), 113 (46.5%) had grade 1 diastolic dysfunction (impaired relaxation), 16 (6.6%) had grade 2 diastolic dysfunction (pseudonormalization from compensatory increase in filling pressures), and none had grade 3 (restrictive filling pattern). They then compared the findings of diastolic dysfunction with a composite outcome of death, graft failure, and/or MACE (CAD, HF, and/or ischemic stroke) after LT. The presence of diastolic dysfunction was associated with an increased duration of hospital stay after LT (16 ± 13 days vs 12 ± 9 days; $P = .02$); however, it was not associated with the composite outcome at 30 days (7% vs 5.3%; $P = .6$) or at 3 years posttransplantation (25% vs 17%; $P = .1$).

Opposite results were reported by Mittal and colleagues[60] in a large cohort of adult LT recipients from the Henry Ford Hospital in Detroit. In their retrospective analysis of 970 LT recipients, these authors identified diastolic dysfunction in 145 patients (15%): 69 (48%) with grade 1, 44 (30%) with grade 2, and 32 (22%) with grade 3. Recipients with diastolic dysfunction were more commonly diabetic or hypertensive compared with those without diastolic dysfunction. On multivariate analysis, diastolic dysfunction was associated with graft failure (HR, 2.26; 95% CI, 1.46–3.51; $P<.0001$), and there was an incremental effect of the severity of pre-LT diastolic dysfunction on graft failure. After a mean follow-up of 5 years, 270 recipients had died (28% mortality), including 44 deaths among patients with diastolic dysfunction (30% mortality). Patient mortality was increased among recipients with grade 2 (HR, 1.58; 95% CI, 1.04–2.4; $P = .03$) or 3 DD (HR, 1.73; 95% CI, 1.2–2.5; $P = .006$), but not in recipients with grade 1 DD (HR, 0.93; 95% CI, 0.3–2.7; $P = .7$). The main difference in these 2 studies was the prevalence of diastolic dysfunction (15% vs 56%), but more important to the different mortality risk, the severity of diastolic dysfunction was higher in the study by Mittal and associates[60] with 52% of patients diagnosed with diastolic dysfunction had grade 2 or 3, compared with only 7% of patients with grade 2 diastolic dysfunction in the study by Sonny and colleagues[55]

PORTOPULMONARY HYPERTENSION

POPH is a pulmonary vascular complication of portal hypertension that can have an important impact on outcomes before, during, and after LT. POPH may be defined as pulmonary arterial hypertension associated with portal hypertension.[61] Although POPH can be suspected based on transthoracic echocardiography, a diagnosis of POPH requires the presence of portal hypertension and pulmonary hypertension assessed by right heart catheterization. Right heart catheterization criteria include mean pulmonary artery pressure (mean Ppa) of greater than 25 mm Hg at rest, mean pulmonary capillary wedge pressure of greater than 12 mm Hg (to exclude fluid overload), and pulmonary vascular resistance (PVR) of greater than 240 $dyn \cdot s \cdot cm^{-5}$ or greater than 3 Wood units.[62] Although LT can reverse POPH portal hypertension, severe POPH can preclude LT owing to risk of severe right ventricular failure. A mean Ppa of greater than 35 mm Hg and/or a PVR of greater than 250 $dyn \cdot s \cdot cm^{-5}$ are both associated with an LT mortality of approximately 50%. Untreated or refractory POPH has an estimated 1-year survival of around 60%.[62] A mean Ppa of 50 mm Hg or greater and/or a PVR of greater than 250 $dyn \cdot s \cdot cm^{-5}$ are contraindications to LT.

Current liver allocation policies in the United States allow appealing for MELD exception points in patients with an established diagnosis of POPH who have a mean Ppa of less than 35 mm Hg and PVR of less than 400 $dyn \cdot s \cdot cm^{-5}$ and have satisfactory right ventricular function (with or without treatment for POPH).[63] Transesophageal echocardiography should be performed immediately before LT in patients with POPH to confirm satisfactory hemodynamics.

SUMMARY

As a consequence of the success of liver transplant as a therapeutic modality to treat patients with ESLD, we have expanded the criteria for selecting transplant candidates and are now transplanting patients who are older and have more comorbid diseases than ever before. Together with infectious and malignant diseases, CVDs account for the majority of posttransplant deaths.

Patients with liver cirrhosis can develop heart disease through several mechanisms: (1) systemic diseases that affect both the heart and the liver (alcohol use, hemochromatosis), (2) cirrhosis-specific heart disease such as cirrhotic cardiomyopathy, or (3) common CV conditions that affect the general population, such as ischemic heart disease or AF. In an effort to minimize negative outcomes and identify patients at risk for posttransplant CV events, the pretransplant evaluation must include a thorough cardiac evaluation.

No single factor can predict posttransplant CV complications; however, patients with a history of CVD, as well as those with specific abnormalities on echocardiography, electrocardiography, or serum markers of heart disease, seem to be at increased risk of such complications, including cardiac-related death. Pretransplant CV evaluation is essential to detecting these risk factors so their effects can be mitigated through appropriate intervention.

REFERENCES

1. Raval Z, Harinstein ME, Skaro AI, et al. Cardiovascular risk assessment of the liver transplant candidate. J Am Coll Cardiol 2011;58(3):223–31.

2. Albeldawi M, Aggarwal A, Madhwal S, et al. Cumulative risk of cardiovascular events after orthotopic liver transplantation. Liver Transpl 2012;18(3):370–5.
3. VanWagner LB, Lapin B, Skaro AI, et al. Impact of renal impairment on cardiovascular disease mortality after liver transplantation for nonalcoholic steatohepatitis cirrhosis. Liver Int 2015;35(12):2575–83.
4. McElroy LM, Daud A, Davis AE, et al. A meta-analysis of complications following deceased donor liver transplant. Am J Surg 2014;208(4):605–18.
5. Watt KD, Pedersen RA, Kremers WK, et al. Long-term probability of and mortality from de novo malignancy after liver transplantation. Gastroenterology 2009; 137(6):2010–7.
6. Aberg F, Gissler M, Karlsen TH, et al. Differences in long-term survival among liver transplant recipients and the general population: a population-based Nordic study. Hepatology 2015;61(2):668–77.
7. Kowalski HJ, Abelmann WH. The cardiac output at rest in Laennec's cirrhosis. J Clin Invest 1953;32(10):1025–33.
8. Kowalski HJ, Abelmann WH, Mc NW. The cardiac output in patients with cirrhosis of the liver and tense ascites with observations on the effect of paracentesis. J Clin Invest 1954;33(5):768–73.
9. Kotin P, Hall EM. "Cardiac" or congestive cirrhosis of liver. Am J Pathol 1951; 27(4):561–71.
10. Ripoll C, Yotti R, Bermejo J, et al. The heart in liver transplantation. J Hepatol 2011;54(4):810–22.
11. Moller S, Hove JD, Dixen U, et al. New insights into cirrhotic cardiomyopathy. Int J Cardiol 2013;167(4):1101–8.
12. Sola E, Gines P. Renal and circulatory dysfunction in cirrhosis: current management and future perspectives. J Hepatol 2010;53(6):1135–45.
13. Brems JJ, Takiff H, McHutchison J, et al. Systemic versus nonsystemic reperfusion of the transplanted liver. Transplantation 1993;55(3):527–9.
14. Shi XY, Xu ZD, Xu HT, et al. Cardiac arrest after graft reperfusion during liver transplantation. Hepatobiliary Pancreat Dis Int 2006;5(2):185–9.
15. Johnston SD, Morris JK, Cramb R, et al. Cardiovascular morbidity and mortality after orthotopic liver transplantation. Transplantation 2002;73(6):901–6.
16. Eleid MF, Hurst RT, Vargas HE, et al. Short-term cardiac and noncardiac mortality following liver transplantation. J Transplant 2010;2010 [pii:910165].
17. Nicolau-Raducu R, Gitman M, Ganier D, et al. Adverse cardiac events after orthotopic liver transplantation: a cross-sectional study in 389 consecutive patients. Liver Transpl 2015;21(1):13–21.
18. Go AS, Mozaffarian D, Roger VL, et al. Heart disease and stroke statistics–2014 update: a report from the American Heart Association. Circulation 2014;129(3): e28–292.
19. VanWagner LB, Lapin B, Levitsky J, et al. High early cardiovascular mortality after liver transplantation. Liver Transpl 2014;20(11):1306–16.
20. VanWagner LB, Serper M, Kang R, et al. Factors associated with major adverse cardiovascular events after liver transplantation among a national sample. Am J Transplant 2016;16(9):2684–94.
21. Charlton MR, Burns JM, Pedersen RA, et al. Frequency and outcomes of liver transplantation for nonalcoholic steatohepatitis in the United States. Gastroenterology 2011;141(4):1249–53.
22. Vanwagner LB, Bhave M, Te HS, et al. Patients transplanted for nonalcoholic steatohepatitis are at increased risk for postoperative cardiovascular events. Hepatology 2012;56(5):1741–50.

23. Laish I, Braun M, Mor E, et al. Metabolic syndrome in liver transplant recipients: prevalence, risk factors, and association with cardiovascular events. Liver Transpl 2011;17(1):15–22.

24. Raval Z, Harinstein ME, Flaherty JD. Role of cardiovascular intervention as a bridge to liver transplantation. World J Gastroenterol 2014;20(31):10651–7.

25. Martin P, DiMartini A, Feng S, et al. Evaluation for liver transplantation in adults: 2013 practice guideline by the American Association for the Study of Liver Diseases and the American Society of Transplantation. Hepatology 2014;59(3): 1144–65.

26. European Association for the Study of the Liver. Electronic address: easloffice@easloffice.eu. EASL clinical practice guidelines: liver transplantation. J Hepatol 2016;64(2):433–85.

27. Lentine KL, Costa SP, Weir MR, et al. Cardiac disease evaluation and management among kidney and liver transplantation candidates: a scientific statement from the American Heart Association and the American College of Cardiology Foundation. J Am Coll Cardiol 2012;60(5):434–80.

28. Fouad TR, Abdel-Razek WM, Burak KW, et al. Prediction of cardiac complications after liver transplantation. Transplantation 2009;87(5):763–70.

29. Safadi A, Homsi M, Maskoun W, et al. Perioperative risk predictors of cardiac outcomes in patients undergoing liver transplantation surgery. Circulation 2009; 120(13):1189–94.

30. Feinberg WM, Blackshear JL, Laupacis A, et al. Prevalence, age distribution, and gender of patients with atrial fibrillation. Analysis and implications. Arch Intern Med 1995;155(5):469–73.

31. Lloyd-Jones DM, Wang TJ, Leip EP, et al. Lifetime risk for development of atrial fibrillation: the Framingham Heart Study. Circulation 2004;110(9):1042–6.

32. Go AS, Hylek EM, Phillips KA, et al. Prevalence of diagnosed atrial fibrillation in adults: national implications for rhythm management and stroke prevention: the AnTicoagulation and Risk Factors in Atrial Fibrillation (ATRIA) Study. JAMA 2001;285(18):2370–5.

33. Bargehr J, Trejo-Gutierrez JF, Rosser BG, et al. Liver transplantation in patients with atrial fibrillation. Transplant Proc 2013;45(6):2302–6.

34. Baskar S, George PL, Eghtesad B, et al. Cardiovascular risk factors and cardiac disorders in long-term survivors of pediatric liver transplantation. Pediatr Transplant 2015;19(1):48–55.

35. Umphrey LG, Hurst RT, Eleid MF, et al. Preoperative dobutamine stress echocardiographic findings and subsequent short-term adverse cardiac events after orthotopic liver transplantation. Liver Transpl 2008;14(6):886–92.

36. Batra S, Machicao VI, Bynon JS, et al. The impact of left ventricular hypertrophy on survival in candidates for liver transplantation. Liver Transpl 2014;20(6): 705–12.

37. Kia L, Shah SJ, Wang E, et al. Role of pretransplant echocardiographic evaluation in predicting outcomes following liver transplantation. Am J Transplant 2013; 13(9):2395–401.

38. Leithead JA, Kandiah K, Steed H, et al. Tricuspid regurgitation on echocardiography may not be a predictor of patient survival after liver transplantation. Am J Transplant 2014;14(9):2192–3.

39. Bushyhead D, Kirkpatrick JN, Goldberg D. Pretransplant echocardiographic parameters as markers of posttransplant outcomes in liver transplant recipients. Liver Transpl 2016;22(3):316–23.

40. Apple FS, Murakami MM, Pearce LA, et al. Predictive value of cardiac troponin I and T for subsequent death in end-stage renal disease. Circulation 2002; 106(23):2941-5.
41. Deegan PB, Lafferty ME, Blumsohn A, et al. Prognostic value of troponin T in hemodialysis patients is independent of comorbidity. Kidney Int 2001;60(6): 2399-405.
42. Hickson LJ, Cosio FG, El-Zoghby ZM, et al. Survival of patients on the kidney transplant wait list: relationship to cardiac troponin T. Am J Transplant 2008; 8(11):2352-9.
43. Keddis MT, El-Zoghby ZM, El Ters M, et al. Cardiac troponin T before and after kidney transplantation: determinants and implications for posttransplant survival. Am J Transplant 2013;13(2):406-14.
44. Coss E, Watt KD, Pedersen R, et al. Predictors of cardiovascular events after liver transplantation: a role for pretransplant serum troponin levels. Liver Transpl 2011; 17(1):23-31.
45. Fussner LA, Heimbach JK, Fan C, et al. Cardiovascular disease after liver transplantation: when, what, and who is at risk. Liver Transpl 2015;21(7):889-96.
46. Genovesi S, Prata Pizzala DM, Pozzi M, et al. QT interval prolongation and decreased heart rate variability in cirrhotic patients: relevance of hepatic venous pressure gradient and serum calcium. Clin Sci (Lond) 2009;116(12):851-9.
47. Henriksen JH, Gulberg V, Fuglsang S, et al. Q-T interval (QT(C)) in patients with cirrhosis: relation to vasoactive peptides and heart rate. Scand J Clin Lab Invest 2007;67(6):643-53.
48. Henriksen JH, Fuglsang S, Bendtsen F, et al. Dyssynchronous electrical and mechanical systole in patients with cirrhosis. J Hepatol 2002;36(4):513-20.
49. Finucci G, Lunardi F, Sacerdoti D, et al. Q-T interval prolongation in liver cirrhosis. Reversibility after orthotopic liver transplantation. Jpn Heart J 1998;39(3):321-9.
50. Kosar F, Ates F, Sahin I, et al. QT interval analysis in patients with chronic liver disease: a prospective study. Angiology 2007;58(2):218-24.
51. Zambruni A, Trevisani F, Caraceni P, et al. Cardiac electrophysiological abnormalities in patients with cirrhosis. J Hepatol 2006;44(5):994-1002.
52. Josefsson A, Fu M, Bjornsson E, et al. Prevalence of pre-transplant electrocardiographic abnormalities and post-transplant cardiac events in patients with liver cirrhosis. BMC Gastroenterol 2014;14:65.
53. Puthumana L, Chaudhry V, Thuluvath PJ. Prolonged QTc interval and its relationship to autonomic cardiovascular reflexes in patients with cirrhosis. J Hepatol 2001;35(6):733-8.
54. Josefsson A, Fu M, Allayhari P, et al. Impact of peri-transplant heart failure & left-ventricular diastolic dysfunction on outcomes following liver transplantation. Liver Int 2012;32(8):1262-9.
55. Sonny A, Kelly D, Hammel JP, et al. Predictors of poor outcome among older liver transplant recipients. Clin Transplant 2015;29(3):197-203.
56. Dowsley TF, Bayne DB, Langnas AN, et al. Diastolic dysfunction in patients with end-stage liver disease is associated with development of heart failure early after liver transplantation. Transplantation 2012;94(6):646-51.
57. Qureshi W, Mittal C, Ahmad U, et al. Clinical predictors of post-liver transplant new-onset heart failure. Liver Transpl 2013;19(7):701-10.
58. Darstein F, Konig C, Hoppe-Lotichius M, et al. Preoperative left ventricular hypertrophy is associated with reduced patient survival after liver transplantation. Clin Transplant 2014;28(2):236-42.

59. Raevens S, De Pauw M, Geerts A, et al. Prevalence and outcome of diastolic dysfunction in liver transplantation recipients. Acta Cardiol 2014;69(3):273–80.
60. Mittal C, Qureshi W, Singla S, et al. Pre-transplant left ventricular diastolic dysfunction is associated with post transplant acute graft rejection and graft failure. Dig Dis Sci 2014;59(3):674–80.
61. Porres-Aguilar M, Gallegos-Orozco JF, Garcia H, et al. Pulmonary vascular complications in portal hypertension and liver disease: a concise review. Rev Gastroenterol Mex 2013;78(1):35–44.
62. Golbin JM, Krowka MJ. Portopulmonary hypertension. Clin Chest Med 2007; 28(1):203–18, ix.
63. Porres-Aguilar M, Mukherjee D. Portopulmonary hypertension: an update. Respirology 2015;20(2):235–42.

Autoimmune Hepatitis in the Liver Transplant Graft

Eliza W. Beal, MD[a], Sylvester M. Black, MD, PhD[a], Anthony Michaels, MD[b],*

KEYWORDS

- Autoimmune hepatitis • Recurrent autoimmune hepatitis
- De novo autoimmune hepatitis

KEY POINTS

- Recurrent autoimmune hepatitis (AIH) and de novo AIH are two important causes of late graft failure after liver transplantation.
- Recurrent AIH occurs in patients who undergo liver transplantation for AIH.
- De novo AIH occurs in patients who are transplanted for etiologies other than AIH.

RECURRENT AND DE NOVO AUTOIMMUNE HEPATITIS AFTER LIVER TRANSPLANTATION

Autoimmune hepatitis (AIH) is a progressive inflammatory disease of the liver that can lead to acute liver failure and end-stage liver disease requiring liver transplantation (LT) first described by Waldenstrom in 1950.[1,2] This condition, which affects mainly women, is characterized biochemically by increased aspartate aminotransferase (AST) and alanine aminotransferase levels, histologically by interface hepatitis and plasma cell infiltrates, and serologically by non–organ-specific autoantibodies and increased immunoglobulin G (IgG).[3,4] Approximately 2% to 3% of liver transplants performed on children and 4% to 6% of liver transplants performed on adults in Europe and the United States are for AIH.[5]

Recurrent AIH and de novo AIH are 2 important causes of late graft failure after LT. Recurrent AIH occurs in patients who undergo LT for AIH. De novo AIH occurs in patients who are transplanted for etiologies other than AIH.

RECURRENT AUTOIMMUNE HEPATITIS AFTER LIVER TRANSPLANTATION

The first case report describing recurrent AIH, published in 1984, described the case of a 26-year-old woman who underwent LT and developed recurrence of AIH at

Disclosure Statement: The authors have nothing to disclose.
[a] Division of Transplantation, Department of Surgery, The Ohio State University Wexner Medical Center, 395 West 12th Avenue, Suite 100, Columbus, OH 43210, USA; [b] Division of Gastroenterology, Hepatology and Nutrition, The Ohio State University Wexner Medical Center, 395 West 12th Avenue, Suite 200, Columbus, OH 43210, USA
* Corresponding author.
E-mail address: Anthony.Michaels@osumc.edu

Clin Liver Dis 21 (2017) 381–401
http://dx.doi.org/10.1016/j.cld.2016.12.010
1089-3261/17/© 2016 Elsevier Inc. All rights reserved.
liver.theclinics.com

18 months post-LT after corticosteroid reduction. She was treated with azathioprine, discontinuation of cyclosporine, and an increase in corticosteroids and recovered.[6]

The International Autoimmune Hepatitis Group met and developed a set of diagnostic criteria and a scoring system to diagnose AIH.[7] This criteria and scoring system has since been simplified and revised (**Table 1**)[8] and, although this scoring system was designed to diagnose AIH outside of the transplant setting, it is used to diagnose both recurrent and de novo AIH.[9,10] A score of 6 or higher indicates probable AIH, and a score of 7 or higher indicates AIH.[8]

Incidence and Timing of Recurrent Autoimmune Hepatitis

The incidence of recurrent AIH among adult patients undergoing LT reported in the literature is between 7% and 41%[9–23] and a recent systematic review reported a weighted recurrence rate of AIH of 22% (**Table 2**).[24] Timing of recurrence is also variable, but is usually reported to occur more than 12 months after LT.[9–23] The variability in recurrence rates and timing of recurrence reported in the literature may be partially accounted for by variability in study methodology, diagnostic criteria selection, follow-up period, timing of protocol and nonprotocol biopsies, immunosuppression use, and other factors.

The recurrence of AIH may be more common in children. In a small series of 6 children transplanted for AIH between 1985 and 1995, there were 5 recurrences (83.3%) in a mean of 11.4 months, with 3 requiring retransplantation.[25]

Risk Factors for and Pathogenesis of Recurrent Autoimmune Hepatitis

The pathogenesis of, and risk factors for, recurrent AIH are not delineated clearly. Risk factors for recurrent AIH that have been reported in the literature are outlined in **Box 1**.

HLA-DR3 and HLA-DR4 have been identified more commonly in patients with recurrent AIH than in patients without recurrence,[10,11,20,21] although this finding is not consistent in all studies.[9,16,19,23,26,27] An increased risk of recurrent AIH in HLA-DR3 recipients who are transplanted with a graft from an HLA-DR3–negative donor has also been demonstrated.[22,28] Retransplantation for recurrent AIH has also been

Table 1
Diagnostic criteria for AIH

Variable	Cutoff	Points
ANA or SMA	$\geq$1:40	1
ANA or SMA or LKM or SLA	$\geq$1:80	2[a]
IgG	>ULN	1
	>1.1[a] ULN	2
Liver histology (evidence of hepatitis required)	Compatible	1
	Typical	2
Absence of viral hepatitis	Yes	2
$\geq$6; probable AIH		
$\geq$7; definite AIH		

Abbreviations: AIH, autoimmune hepatitis; ANA, antinuclear antibody; Ig, immunoglobulin; LKM, liver kidney microsomal antibody; SLA, Soluble Liver Antigen; SMA, smooth muscle actin; ULN, upper limit of normal.
   [a] Addition of 2 points for all autoantibodies (maximum 2 points).
   Adapted from Hennes EM, Zeniya M, Czaja AJ, et al. Simplified criteria for the diagnosis of autoimmune hepatitis. Hepatology 2008;48(1):171; with permission.

Table 2
Recurrent AIH in adults

Author	Time Period of Study	N Transplanted	Recurred, n (%)	Time to Recurrence
Krishnamoorthy et al,[14] 2016	1999–2014	73	5 (7)	18, 19, 48, 60, 88 mo
Montano-Loza et al,[15] 2009	NR	46	11 (24)	Mean 48 ± 16 mo (range, 9–144; median, 30)
Gonzalez-Koch et al,[10] 2009	1985–1998	41	7 (17)	Mean 4.6 ± 1 y
Vogel et al,[16] 2004	1987–1999	28	9 (32)	Median 12 mo
Duclos-Vallee et al,[11] 2003	1985–1990	17	7 (41)	Mean 2.5 y (range, 0.6–3.0)
Molmenti et al,[9] 2002	1984–1998	55	11 (20)	5/11 (45%) within first year
Yusoff et al,[17] 2002	1985–1999	12	2 (17)	NR
Renz et al,[18] 2002	1988–1997	37	12 (32)	Median 24 mo; mean, 25 ± 22 mo
Reich et al,[26] 2000	1988–1995	32	6/24 (25)	Mean 15 ± 2 mo
Milkiewicz et al,[19] 1999	NR	47	13 (28)	Mean 29 mo (range, 6–63)
Narumi et al,[20] 1999	1988–1997	40	8 (20)	Mean 17.5 ± 12.6 mo
Prados et al,[21] 1998	1984–1996	27	9 (33)	Mean 2.6 ± 1.5 y
Wright et al,[22] 1992	1981–1989	43	11 (26)	NR
Ratziu et al,[23] 1999	1985–1992	25	3/15 (20)	Mean 24 ± 12 mo (range, 12–36)

Abbreviations: AIH, autoimmune hepatitis; NR, not reported.

Box 1
Risk factors for recurrent AIH

HLA-DR3 positive recipient, HLA-DR3 negative donor[22,28]

HLA-DR3 positive[11,20]

HLA-DR3/HLA-DR4 positive recipient[10]

Retransplantation for recurrent AIH[26]

Transplanted for chronic AIH versus fulminant hepatic failure[26]

Concomitant autoimmune disease[15]

Pre-LT high AST[15]

Pre-LT high ALT[15]

Pre-LT high IgG[15]

Explant moderate to severe inflammatory activity[15]

Explant plasma cell infiltrate[15]

Episodes of acute rejection[29]

Abbreviations: AIH, autoimmune hepatitis; ALT, alanine aminotransferase; AST, aspartate aminotransferase; IgG, immunoglobulin G; LT, liver transplantation.

shown to be a risk factor for recurrent AIH[26]; however, this finding has also been refuted.[19,23]

The association of occurrence of acute rejection and later development of recurrent AIH is also controversial with some studies demonstrating an association of episodes of acute rejection and recurrent AIH,[29] whereas others demonstrate a similar incidence and severity of episodes of acute rejection episodes in patients with and without recurrent AIH.[16,20,26]

Montano-Loza and associates[15] completed a retrospective study of 46 patients transplanted for AIH with a focus on determining the risk factors for recurrence of AIH. On univariate analysis they found that pre-LT factors including concomitant autoimmune disease, high AST and alanine aminotransferase levels, high IgG levels, and moderate to severe inflammatory activity and plasma cell infiltrate on explant were associated significantly with recurrence of AIH. On multivariate analysis they found that IgG levels before LT greater than 2 times the upper limit of normal (hazard ratio, 7.5; 95% confidence interval, 1.45–38.45; $P = .02$) and moderate to severe inflammation on explant (hazard ratio, 6.9; 95% confidence interval, 1.76–26.96; $P = .006$) were associated with the recurrence of AIH. Of note, they also found that there was no difference in the risk of recurrence of AIH in patients who had and were treated for episodes of acute rejection. Additionally, they found no difference in pre-LT prednisone use or post-LT immunosuppression regimens. Their study failed to demonstrate a protective effect of prednisone against recurrence of AIH. They also did not find an association between any of the donor factors they tested and recurrence of AIH, and concluded that recurrence risk is limited to recipient factors.[15] Ayata and colleagues[29] confirmed the finding that severe necroinflammatory activity at the time of LT predicts later recurrence. Corticosteroid withdrawal has been reported to play an important role in recurrence of AIH.[19,21,30]

Diagnosis of Recurrent Autoimmune Hepatitis

In recurrent AIH, histologic changes may precede clinical and biochemical evidence of recurrence.[11] Criteria used for diagnosis are the same as those used for patients with AIH who have not undergone LT.[8,31] It is notable that these criteria have not been validated in the post-LT population. These criteria are outlined in **Table 1**.

Although there are no standard, validated criteria for diagnosis of recurrent AIH, the following are often used: elevated serum levels of transaminases, hypergammaglobulinemia or elevated IgG levels, and presence of autoantibodies, consistent histologic features such as lobular and/or periportal interface hepatitis with lymphoplasmacytic infiltrate predominance and steroid responsiveness, in the absence of viral infection or rejection.[32,33]

Recipients with recurrent AIH present with features in common with most other post-LT complications including symptoms such as fever, fatigue, jaundice, abdominal pain, abnormal skin rash, joint pain, and back pain.[4] Biochemical signs of recurrence include elevated alanine aminotransferase and AST.[4] Most patients with recurrent AIH have positive autoantibodies, although several studies have demonstrated that patients who undergo LT for AIH have persistent autoantibodies, but at lower titers than before LT.[26]

Histologic signs of recurrence include interface hepatitis, plasma cell infiltration, acute lobar hepatitis with focal hepatocyte necrosis, acidophil bodies with lymphoplasmacytic cells, and pseudo-rosettes of hepatocytes.[34,35] There may be some differences in histology in recurrent AIH versus AIH in the native liver, including more common presentation with features of acute lobular necrosis in patients with recurrent AIH.[29] Some histologic features of recurrent AIH may overlap with other conditions,

Table 3
Acute rejection, recurrent hepatitis C viral infection, and recurrent autoimmune hepatitis

Acute rejection	Predominantly mixed inflammatory infiltrate, bile duct damage, endothelialitis. Can have small numbers of plasma cells.[88]
Recurrent hepatitis C viral infection	Predominantly lymphocytic portal infiltrate and lobular activity including parenchymal necrosis and apoptotic hepatocytes. Can have small numbers of plasma cells.[89,90]
Recurrent autoimmune hepatitis	Presence of interface hepatitis and significantly increased plasma cells.[11]

but distinctions can be made (**Table 3**).[36] Common histologic features of recurrent AIH are shown in **Fig. 1**.[33]

Monitoring for Recurrence

Duclos-Vallee and coworkers[11] performed a long-term study of 17 women who were transplanted for AIH and performed protocol liver biopsies at 1, 2, 5, and 10 years and as clinically indicated. Four of 7 patients with recurrence demonstrated histologic evidence of recurrence on protocol biopsies including moderate to dense lymphoplasmacytic infiltrate, lobular activity and interface hepatitis. The mean interval between

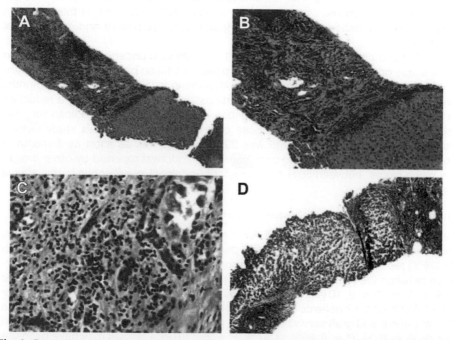

Fig. 1. Recurrent autoimmune hepatitis (*A*) Liver parenchyma with septal fibrosis and a prominent inflammatory infiltrate (stain: hematoxylin and eosin; original magnification, ×100). (*B*) Septal and interface inflammation. Note a bile duct adjacent to the artery and vein (stain: hematoxylin and eosin; original magnification ×200). (*C*) Lymphoplasmacytic infiltrate (stain: hematoxylin and eosin; original magnification, ×600). (*D*) Bridging fibrosis confirmed by trichrome stain (original magnification, ×100). (*Courtesy of* Dr Monica Garcia, Department of Pathology, University of Miami Miller School of Medicine; and *From* Mendes F, Couto CA, Levy C. Recurrent and de novo autoimmune liver diseases. Clin Liver Dis 2011;15(4):860.)

evidence of histologic recurrence and the onset of other signs of recurrence was 9 years (range, 6–14). The authors demonstrated that histologic recurrence precedes biochemical recurrence and advocated for protocol biopsies after LT for AIH.[11] Sakai and colleagues[37] advocate the use of the carboxyflourescein diacetate succinyimidyl ester-mixed lymphocyte reaction (CFSE-MLR) assay to monitor the immune status of AIH patients after LT to optimize immunosuppression and monitor for recurrence. Neither protocol biopsies nor the use of CFSE-MLR assay are currently standard practice.

Management of Recurrent Autoimmune Hepatitis

Treatment of recurrent AIH follows standard treatment for AIH, including increased corticosteroid doses. Cyclosporine-based regimens are often modified to be tacrolimus based. Mycophenolate mofetil can be added in nonresponders.[36] Liver function tests, IgG levels, autoantibody levels, and liver histology should serve as a guide for treatment.[36] Some patients may progress to graft failure and require retransplantation.[26]

Corticosteroid withdrawal for patients who underwent LT for AIH is controversial. Krishnamoorthy and colleagues[14] recently reported on 73 patients transplanted for AIH who were continued on long-term, low-dose corticosteroid therapy with median follow-up of 94 months. The overall 1-, 3-, 5-, and 10-year patient survivals were 92%, 90%, 86%, and 73%. Five patients developed recurrence of AIH (7%). The authors concluded that the use of low-dose corticosteroid treatment in the long term reduced the recurrence of AIH without impacting overall patient and graft survival negatively.[14]

Trouillot and colleagues[38] reported on 21 patients who underwent LT for AIH who were stable on maintenance immunosuppression. Of these patients, 68% were withdrawn from corticosteroids successfully with a mean follow-up period of 22 months (range, 1–34). Patients withdrawn from corticosteroids successfully had a reduction in serum cholesterol levels, decreased use of antihypertensive medications, and reduced use of medications for glucose control.[38] Criticisms of this study include that, although the mean follow-up was 22 months, it was as short as 1 month in some patients.[30] Failure rates of corticosteroid withdrawal reported by other groups are much higher, between 50% and 64%.[19,20] Additional investigation in this area is needed.

Outcomes of Recurrent Autoimmune Hepatitis

Few studies report on outcomes of AIH patients who undergo LT and recur versus those who do not recur. In a study of 46 patients who underwent LT for AIH in which 11 (24%) recurred in a mean of 48 ± 16 months it was noted that there was no difference between the 5- or 10-year survival in patients who did or did not recur (5 years: 82% vs 76%, $P = .9$; 10 years: 77% vs 76%).[15] A study of 41 patients transplanted for type 1 AIH in which 7 patients (17%) recurred noted that there was no difference in the 5-year patient and graft survivals between patients who recurred and those who did not (86% vs 82%, $P = .9$; 86% vs 67%, $P = .5$).[10] These studies may have been underpowered to detect a difference in outcomes between these 2 groups.

DE NOVO AUTOIMMUNE HEPATITIS AFTER LIVER TRANSPLANTATION

Over the past 2 decades, a body of literature has developed regarding LT patients transplanted for non-AIH etiologies who develop increased transaminases, histologic features of plasma cell infiltrate, and typical autoimmune serology after LT. This condition, first described as de novo AIH,[2] has also gone by many other names including post-LT AIH-like hepatitis,[39] graft dysfunction mimicking AIH,[40] posttransplant immune hepatitis,[41] plasma cell hepatitis,[42–44] and de novo immune hepatitis.[45] The presentation is consistent with recurrent AIH; however, this condition occurs in patients who were transplanted for other etiologies.

De novo AIH was first reported in children by Kerkar and colleagues[2] in 1998. In this case series it was noted that 4% of pediatric LT recipients (7/180) presented with de novo AIH. Liver biopsies demonstrated findings consistent with AIH including dense lymphocytic portal tract infiltrate with plasma cells, periportal hepatitis, and bridging collapse. They also had high titers of IgG, the presence of autoantibodies, and met criteria for the diagnosis of AIH. The earliest report in adults was in 1999 when 2 patients transplanted for primary biliary cirrhosis developed an autoimmunelike hepatitis.[46]

Incidence of De Novo Autoimmune Hepatitis

De novo AIH may occur more commonly in children[36] and the incidence of de novo AIH in children has been reported to be variable, between 0.5% and 11%.[2,41,47–55] Time to development of de novo AIH in children is also variable, with the median time to development ranging from 1.2 to 6.9 years.[52,55] Characteristics of children with de novo AIH are detailed in **Table 4**. De novo AIH has an incidence between 0.5% and 3.4% in adults with reported time to development ranging from 0.3 and 7.0 years after LT.[40,56–58]

Histology

As its name implies, de novo AIH shares the biochemical, serologic, and histologic features with AIH and the criteria used to diagnose de novo AIH are very similar to those used to diagnose AIH. These include the International Autoimmune Hepatitis Group scoring systems—revised[31] and simplified.[8] The simplified scoring system is presented in **Table 1**. Other sets of diagnostic criteria have also been set forth, including the one from a review by Edmunds and colleagues,[59] which is detailed in **Box 2**. Criteria for diagnosis have also been outlined by the Banff working group and include at a minimum: interface hepatitis, significant titers of antibodies, hypergammaglobulinemia, and the exclusion of virus-induced or drug-related hepatitis.[34]

Sebagh and colleagues[60] contend that histology assumes a central role in the diagnosis of de novo AIH because, upon biopsy recognition of plasma cell-rich hepatitis with aggressive necroinflammatory activity, full serologic evaluations are not completed. Although studies in both native livers and in de novo AIH suggest plasma cells comprising more than 30% of the infiltrate are diagnostic for AIH and rarely seen in other conditions, precise cutoffs for plasma cell infiltrates have not been defined clearly.[60,61]

Cases of de novo AIH after cadaveric LT with IgG4 positivity have been reported to be associated with more severe histologic activity (**Fig. 2**); however, these cases have been shown to respond to treatment with increased immunosuppression.[44,62] It has been suggested that IgG4-positive de novo AIH and IgG4-negative de novo AIH are in fact separate clinical entities.[44] In contrast, Eguchi and colleagues[63] reported that IgG4 did not play a causal role in de novo AIH after living donor LT in their series, which included 72 living donor LT patients and 4 (5.6%) with de novo AIH.

Although some authors point out the necessity of obtaining a biopsy in a patient with positive autoantibodies before diagnosing de novo AIH, because some patients develop autoantibodies in the absence of histologic changes, other investigators demonstrate that classic histologic features are not always present.[55]

Table 4
De novo AIH in children

Author	Incidence	Sex	Median Age	Median Duration After Surgery	Indications for Transplant	Immunosuppression	Histology	Autoantibodies	Median IgG Titer	Treatment
Pongpaibul et al,[55] 2012	70/685 (10.2%)	19 M, 32 F	4.1 ± 4.2 y	6.9 ± 4.7 y	Primary biliary atresia (53%), fulminant hepatic failure (18%), metabolic liver disease (18%)	Median tacrolimus trough 5.8 ng/mL, median cyclosporine trough 96 ng/mL	Hepatitis (36/51, 71%), variable necroinflammatory activity; lobular hepatitis most common when present, plasma rich infiltrates (16/51, 31%), uncommon central vein endothelitis.	61% ANA (median titer 1:640), 59% ds-DNA antibodies (median titer = 545 IU/mL), 27% SMA (median titer 1:40), 2% LKM (median titer = 1:80).	NR	Continuation of calcineurin inhibitor, addition of mycophenolate mofetil and prednisone (n = 31, 61%), continuation of calcineurin inhibitor and increased in or addition of prednisone (n = 10, 20%), continuation of calcineurin inhibitor and addition of mycophenolate mofetil (n = 9, 18%), other (n = 5, 10%).
Venick et al,[54] 2007	619 (6.6%)	NR	Mean 3.6 ± 0.9 y	Mean 7.0 ± 2 y	Cholestatic liver disease (n = 23), fulminant hepatic failure (n = 13), metabolic liver disease (n = 5)	Pre-1987: cyclosporine, prednisone, 1987: AZA added, 1994: tacrolimus and prednisone, 1995: weaning prednisone	Portal tract infiltrate, periportal hepatitis involving lymphocytes and plasma cells.	24 - ANA, 25 - anti-dsDNA, 10 - SMA, 1 - LKM.	NR	21 mycophenolate mofetil (25 mg/kg/d) and prednisone (1–2 mg/kg/d) tapered over 6 wk, 8 - increased dose of prednisone alone, 7 - Mycophenolate mofetil alone, 3 - mycophenolate mofetil and change from cyclosporine to tacrolimus.

Gibelli et al,[48] 2006	1/205 (0.5%)	1 F	9 y	4 y	Alpha 1-antitrypsin	Cyclosporine and prednisolone	Active chronic hepatitis progressing to cirrhosis, portal lymphocyte aggregates, large number of plasma cells.	Gastric parietal cell antibody, liver–kidney microsomal antibody, anti-hepatic cytosol antibody.	4447 mg/dL	Reduced dose of cyclosporine, increased corticosteroid dose to 1 mg/kg/d tapered to 20 mg every other day, added mycophenolate mofetil 1 g/d and increased to 2 g/d.
Petz et al,[50] 2002	18/155 (11%)	—	1 y	30 mo	Biliary atresia (n = 16), Alagille's syndrome (n = 1), alpha 1-antitrypsin (n = 1)	9 cyclosporine and steroids, 9 tacrolimus and steroids	16 chronic hepatitis with portal mononuclear infiltrate, interface hepatitis, 1 nonspecific changes, biliary ductule proliferation.	53% ANA, 58% SMA, 2 LKM.	1400 (600–2170)	11 steroids (1.5 mg/kg) and AZA (1.5 mg/kg), 5 no therapy owing to rapid normalization of LFTs, 2 no therapy started yet.
Gupta et al,[53] 2001	115 (5%)	2 M, 4 F	2.2 y (0.8–6.0)	8.5 y (3–11)	Biliary atresia (n = 5), propyl thiouracil toxicity (n = 1)	Cyclosporine, AZA, prednisone. AZA discontinued 6 mo post-LT. Prednisone tapered off. All on a single drug at time of graft dysfunction.	Mononuclear infiltrates in portal areas with foci of periportal spillover, portal fibrosis and mild bile ductular proliferation. No infiltration of biliary epithelium, duct damage or loss or endothelialitis. Viral studies all normal.	5 ANA+ (mean, 1226; range, 320–2560), all dsDNA–, 2 SMA, all LKM–.	NR	Prednisone (1–2 mg/kg/d) and AZA (1–2 mg/kg/d). Improvement in liver enzymes. Repeat biopsies in 4 showed progression of fibrosis. Two developed end-stage liver disease, 1 died awaiting retransplantation, 1 underwent successful retransplantation.

(continued on next page)

Table 4
(continued)

Author	Incidence	Sex	Median Age	Median Duration After Surgery	Indications for Transplant	Immunosuppression	Histology	Autoantibodies	Median IgG Titer	Treatment
Spada et al,[52] 2001	5/116 (4.3%)	3 M, 2 F	NR	1.2 y (0.6–18)	Biliary atresia (n = 4), alpha-1 antitrypsin (n = 1)	3 cyclosporine and prednisone, 2 tacrolimus and prednisone	Portal infiltrate, interface hepatitis, lobular necrosis, parenchymal fibrosis.	NR	1800 mg/dL	AZA 1.5–2 mg/kg/d, prednisone 2 mg/kg/d, steroids tapered within 6–8 wk down to 5 mg/kg in responders.
Andries et al,[41] 2001	11/471 (2.4%)	6 M, 5 F	10.5 y (7–13)	115 mo (6.9–182)	Biliary atresia (n = 7), progression familial intrahepatic cholestasis (n = 1), fulminant hepatitis (n = 2)	Pre-1993: cyclosporine, AZA (stopped 1 mo – 1 y), steroids (tapered to 0.25 mg/kg). Post-1993: Tacrolimus as primary	Variable degree of portal and lobular inflammation, piecemeal necrosis, and bridging collapse.	9 ANA (titer 1/80 up to 1/10,000), 1 SMA (1/320), 2 LKM-1 (1/1280).	1365 mg/dL	Did not respond to increasing doses of cyclosporine (n = 10) or tacrolimus (n = 1); 11 received steroids (prednisolone 2 mg/kg/d, then tapered) and AZA (1.5–2.5 mg/kg/d).
Hernandez et al,[49] 1999	5/155 (2.5%)	2 M, 3 F	3.5 y (0.5–14)	5.1 y (1.5–9)	Biliary atresia (n = 4), primary sclerosing cholangitis (n = 1)	Primary immunosuppression with cyclosporine	Patient 1: portal inflammation, plasma cell predominance, patient. Patient 2: lobular infiltrate, plasma cells, interface hepatitis, patient. Patient 3: consistent with AIH, patient. Patient 4: portal infiltrate, plasma cells, portal fibrosis. Patient 5: interface hepatitis, plasma cells, fibrosis.	4 - ANA titers 1:160–1:640, 1 - also SMA 1:80, 1 - elevated total serum protein level.	NR	Standard therapy for AIH; daily steroids and AZA. Cyclosporine doses eliminated in 2 and reduced in 3.

Study	Frequency	Sex	Age	Follow-up	Prior Diagnosis	Treatment	Histology	Autoantibodies	IgG	Outcome
Kerkar et al,[2] 1998	7/180 (4%)	5 M, 2 F	10.3 y (2.0–19.4)	24 mo (6–45)	Biliary atresia (n = 4), Alagille's syndrome (n = 1), drug-induced acute liver failure (n = 1), alpha-1 antitrypsin deficiency (n = 1)	Four on triple with cyclosporine, AZA, prednisolone, and 3 on tacrolimus	Portal and periportal hepatitis with lymphocytes and plasma cells, bridging collapse, perivenular-cell necrosis without changes typical of acute or chronic rejection.	1 ANA, 2 ANA and SMA, 3 atypical LKM, 1 GPC.	22 g/L (17.2–34.4)	All but one responded to prednisolone 2 mg/kg/d and an increase or addition of AZA (1.5 mg/kg/d) within a median of 32 d (range, 7–316).
Miyagawa-Hayashino et al,[51] 2004	13/633 (2.1%)	2 M, 11 F	10 (8 mo–26 y)	3.1 y (0.7–9.5)	NR	NR	Nine definite AIH, 4 probable AIH.	NR	NR	11 patients who underwent follow-up histologic evaluation: 3 retransplantation, 8 similar findings on subsequent biopsies, fluctuations in amount of necroinflammatory activity, increase in fibrosis despite treatment.

Abbreviations: ANA, antinuclear antibody; AZA, azathioprine; GPC, gastric parietal-cell antibody; LKM, liver kidney microsomal antibody; NR, not reported; SMA, smooth muscle antibody.

```
Box 2
Diagnostic criteria for de novo AIH after LT

Liver transplant recipient without history of AIH

Presents with unknown etiology of late graft dysfunction

Elevated aminotransferases

Usually occurs greater than 2 years after transplantation

Graft dysfunction is not due to
   Acute rejection
   Chronic rejection
   Hepatitis B or C virus
   Epstein–Barr virus
   Cytomegalovirus infection
   Vascular problems
   Biliary complications
   Drug toxicity
   Sepsis
   Recurrence of primary disease
   Posttransplant lymphoproliferative disorder

Elevated serum IgG

Positive autoantibody titers
   ANA
   ASMA
   Anti-LKM

Characteristic biopsy findings
   Dense lymphocytic portal tract infiltrate
   Plasma cells
   Interface hepatitis

Abbreviations: AIH, autoimmune hepatitis; ANA, antinuclear antibody; ASMA, anti–smooth
muscle antibody; IgG, immunoglobulin G; LKM, liver kidney microsomal antibody; LT, liver
transplantation.
   Data from United Network for Organ Sharing. Available at: https://www.unos.org/. Accessed
July 20, 2016.
```

Presence of Antibodies in De Novo Autoimmune Hepatitis

Patients transplanted for non-AIH etiologies can develop autoantibodies after LT. The development of autoantibodies has been reported to be associated with the development of chronic hepatitis, chronic rejection, graft dysfunction, graft loss, and death.[64–67] It has also been demonstrated that adults and children can develop autoantibodies in the absence of de novo AIH.[64,66,68,69]

Heneghan and colleagues[40] reported 2 distinct presentations of de novo AIH. Of 7 patients identified, 3 had detectable liver kidney microsomal antibody-1 at high titer in association with a mean AST of 895 IU/L and 4 had positive antinuclear antibody or anti-smooth muscle (ASM) antibodies at low titer and in association with a mean AST level of 209 IU/L. Histology findings included the presence of moderate to severe hepatitis with interface hepatitis, predominantly lymphocyte and plasma cell infiltrate, perivenular cell dropout, bridging necrosis, and collapse. Owing to their failure to recognize the condition originally, they were able to observe the natural history of the disease, which was that histology on serial biopsy progressed from parenchymal bridging collapse to cirrhosis.[40]

Although elevated IgG and autoantibody titers are typically considered to be part of the diagnostic criteria for de novo AIH, there are centers that have reported cases

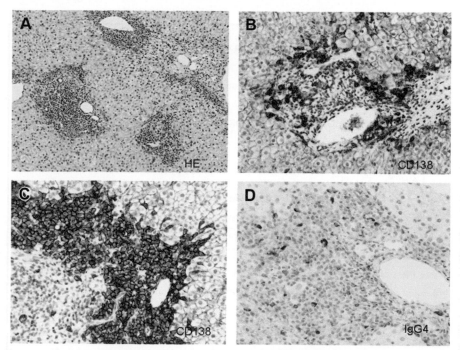

Fig. 2. Pathologic findings of immunoglobulin G4 (IgG4)-associated de novo autoimmune hepatitis after liver transplantation for chronic hepatitis B and C-related cirrhosis and hepatocellular carcinoma. (*A*) Hematoxylin and eosin stain. Portal tracts are enlarged by lymphocytes aggregation with mild centrilobular necrosis. (*B*) Immunologic stain for plasma cells (CD138) shows a cluster of positive plasma cells at the margin of interface hepatitis. At this time there are no IgG4-bearing plasma cells. (*C*) This biopsy with CD138 staining shows more severe plasma cell infiltrates at the margin of interface hepatitis. (*D*) Immunologic stain for IgG4 shows abundant IgG4-bearing plasma cells in a portal tract. (*From* Zhao XY, Rakhda MI, Wang TI, et al. Immunoglobulin G4-associated de novo autoimmune hepatitis after liver transplantation for chronic hepatitis B- and C-related cirrhosis and hepatocellular carcinoma: a case report with literature review. Transplant Proc 2013;45(2):826; with permission.)

of de novo AIH in patients with low IgG levels and absent autoantibodies.[69] Autoantibodies can be present after LT in the absence of de novo AIH and a biopsy must therefore be performed to confirm the diagnosis.[59,66,67,69] Similarly, de novo AIH can be diagnosed in patients without autoantibodies or hypergammaglobulinemia.[69,70]

Risk Factors for the Development of De Novo Autoimmune Hepatitis

Early authors speculated that de novo AIH might be a form of rejection or the consequence of drug- or viral infection-triggered autoimmune injury.[2] Although the pathogenesis of de novo AIH remains unclear, several risk factors have been identified and their roles supported and refuted over the years. These are summarized in **Box 3**.

The development of de novo AIH has been commonly reported in patients who develop hepatitis C virus (HCV) recurrence after LT and who have been treated with pegylated interferon and ribavirin, suggesting that either HCV recurrence or treatment

---

Box 3
Risk factors and protective factors for de novo AIH

Risk Factors

Antiviral therapy for HCV infection with pegylated interferon and ribavarin[43,65,71–77]

Use of antilymphocyte antibodies[72]

Donor and/or recipient HLA-DR3 and/or HLA-DR4 and/or donor/recipient mismatch[2,65,78]

Episodes of acute rejection[51,54,65]

GSTT1 donor/recipient mismatch[56,59]

Type 1 AIH[2,35]

Severe necroinflammatory activity in the explant[4]

Withdrawal of corticosteroids or early withdrawal of corticosteroids[4]

Inadequate immunosuppression secondary to nonadherence[4]

Coexisting autoimmune disorders[4]

Higher titers of autoantibodies at the time of LT[4]

Prolonged course of the underlying AIH associated with prolonged immunosuppression pre-LT[4]

Single immunosuppressive therapy[54]

Protective Factors

Administration of granulocyte colony stimulating factor[72,75]

Abbreviations: AIH, autoimmune hepatitis; HCV, hepatitis C virus; LT, liver transplantation.

---

for HCV recurrence increase risk of developing this condition.[43,71–77] It will be interesting to see if we continue to see similar incidences of de novo AIH after HCV treatment in our current era of interferon-free regimens.

Early studies suggested that de novo AIH is a true autoimmune process after patients with HLA type 1 matches developed the condition.[46] Later studies, however, reported that the condition did not occur more often in patients receiving grafts from living-related donors, where there is increased haplotype matching.[51] It has also been demonstrated that increased matches or mismatches at the HLA-A, -B, and -DR loci are not associated with the development of de novo AIH.[51] Heneghan and colleagues[40] examined the extended HLA haplotypes of donors and recipients and found a mean mismatch score of 5.3 across class I and II alleles, and concluded that increased matching did not lead to an increased risk.

Of the 7 children who developed de novo AIH in the first published study, 5 (71.4%) had donors who were HLA-DR3 or HLA-DR4 positive.[2] Heneghan and colleagues[40] report HLA-DR3 or HLA-DR4 positivity in all donors or recipients. In comparing de novo AIH patients with healthy blood donors, Salcedo and colleagues[57] note that de novo AIH patients showed a higher prevalence of HLA-DR3. Other studies fail to show an association between HLA-DR3 and de novo AIH.[40,78] As noted, some authors report an increased risk of recurrent AIH in HLA-DR3 recipients who are transplanted with a graft from an HLA-DR3–negative donor.[22]

In a single-center study of 788 grafts received by 619 children over a 20-year period, 41 children (6.6%) developed de novo AIH and were compared with a control group. Age, sex, race, initial diagnosis, ischemia time, graft type, Epstein–Barr virus infection, cytomegalovirus infection, HLA haplotype, and immunosuppressive regimens were not different between the groups. Single immunosuppressive therapy, corticosteroid discontinuation, and episodes of allograft rejection were all higher in the de novo AIH group.[54] Miyagawa-Hayashino and associates[51] also report that, among patients who later developed de novo AIH, 69% experienced episodes of acute rejection.

The pathogenesis of de novo AIH is unclear, but may be related to molecular or structural mimicry, uncovering of hidden epitopes, or epitope spreading.[79] Molecular mimicry is an immune response to a non–self-antigen that becomes directed at a similar self-antigen.[80,81]

It has also been suggested that de novo AIH is a form of late cellular rejection. This hypothesis is supported in several ways. First, antibodies are directed against graft antigens (non-self) rather than self-antigens. Second, autoantibodies arise in patients after episodes of acute rejection. Third, acute rejection is a risk factor for development of de novo AIH.[36] Also supporting the de novo AIH as a rejection hypothesis, it has been demonstrated that patients who are glutathione S-transference T1 negative (GSST1-negative) develop antibodies 80% of the time when transplanted with GSST1-positive donors. This is true in all patients who develop AIH.[36]

There is some evidence that de novo AIH is an alloimmune reaction, as opposed to a true autoimmune response. Glutathione S-transferase T1 (GSTT1) is an enzyme involved in the detoxification of electrophilic compounds, including reactive oxygen species, and its role in de novo AIH has been an area of significant interest since when it was first explored.[56,82] The proposed role of GSTT1 is related to a donor–recipient mismatch at this locus.[56] Twenty percent of Caucasians and 11% to 58% of other ethnic groups possess a genetic deletion at the GSTT1 locus[83] and immune sensitization results from a GSTT1-negative recipient receiving a graft from a GSTT1-expressing donor.[45,84] In a study of 35 LT recipients, there was an higher incidence of de novo AIH and of anti-GSTT1 antibodies among those who received tacrolimus (with or without mycophenolate mofetil) than those who received cyclosporine.[85] However, not all patients with a GSTT1 donor–recipient mismatch develop anti-GSTT1 antibodies and not all patients with anti-GSTT1 antibodies have clinically evident de novo AIH. In the population of GSTT1-mismatched patients, male donor sex and non–alcohol-related pre-LT disease were found to be predictive of the development of de novo AIH.[78]

Complement component 4d is generated and deposited during activation of the classical complement pathway. A retrospective analysis of liver biopsies identified C4d-positivity localization in the portal tracts of de novo AIH specimens, whereas in 2 control groups C4d-positivity was present in only 4 of 7 biopsies from patients who experienced rejection and none of the patients who experienced HCV recurrence.[84] The authors, whose significant work in the area of GSTT1 has already provided evidence of donor-specific antibody production, posit that this supports the hypothesis that de novo AIH is a type of rejection.[84] They also demonstrated that IgG1 and IgG4 were the most common IgG subclasses present and noted that IgG4 related diseases are autoimmune diseases, but that the role of anti–GSTT1 IgG4 is currently unknown.[86]

Granulocyte colony stimulating factor given for neutropenia has been reported to be a protective factor against development of de novo AIH.[72,75]

Outcomes

Pongpaibul and colleagues[55] report 70 patients of 685 pediatric LT recipients who developed de novo AIH. The majority of patients who developed de novo AIH showed resolution of laboratory studies after treatment with mean follow-up time after diagnosis of de novo AIH of 6.7 years and 1-, 5-, and 10-year graft survivals in this group were 96%, 89%, and 76%, and patient survivals were 98%, 94%, and 81%, respectively.

Box 4
Treatment recommendations for de novo AIH

Treatment Recommendations for Children

1. Give 1 to 2 mg/kg prednisone or prednisolone (not to exceed 60 mg) and 1 to 2 mg/kg azathioprine daily.

2. Reduce dose of prednisone or prednisolone in weeks 4 to 8 to 5 to 10 mg/d.

3. In absence of response replace azathioprine with up to 40 mg/kg/d of mycophenolate mofetil in up to 2 divided doses.

Treatment Recommendations for Adults

1. Give 30 mg of prednisone or prednisolone and 1 to 2 mg/kg of azathioprine daily.

2. Reduce dose of prednisone or prednisolone to 5 to 10 mg/d.

3. In the absence of response replace azathioprine with 1 g twice daily of mycophenolate mofetil.

Adapted from Liberal R, Longhi MS, Grant CR, et al. Autoimmune hepatitis after liver transplantation. Clin Gastroenterol Hepatol 2012;10(4):346–53.

Treatment

Standard therapy for AIH is corticosteroids and azathioprine in combination. These drugs are effective in approximately 80% of patients. Additional therapies have been tried, including mycophenolate mofetil, D-penicillamine, sirolimus, and anti–T-cell therapies in patients who do not respond to standard therapy.[5] Treatment for de novo AIH is similar to standard treatment for recurrent AIH after LT.

Heneghan and colleagues[40] report in an early study that patients presenting with this condition not currently on corticosteroids were given prednisolone 40 mg/d and then tapered to a maintenance dose of 10 mg/d over 2 months. Patients who had remained on low doses of steroids were increased to 20 mg/d and then tapered to a 10 mg/d maintenance dose. There were no further attempts at corticosteroid withdrawal in this patient population.[40]

Liberal and colleagues,[12] in a comprehensive review, report recommendations for treatment for de novo AIH and these are summarized in **Box 4**. Most cases can be treated effectively, although others may progress to graft failure and require retransplantation.[87]

SUMMARY

Recurrent AIH and de novo AIH are important causes of late graft failure after LT and should be included in the differential diagnosis. Recurrent AIH occurs in patients who undergo LT for AIH. De novo AIH occurs in patients who are transplanted for etiologies other than AIH. Although typically treated with standard treatment for AIH, including corticosteroids and any further adjustments in a patient's immunosuppression, both recurrent and de novo AIH may progress to end-stage liver disease, requiring retransplantation.

REFERENCES

1. Mieli-Vergani G, Vergani D. Autoimmune hepatitis. Nat Rev Gastroenterol Hepatol 2011;8(6):320–9.

2. Kerkar N, Hadzić N, Davies ET, et al. De-novo autoimmune hepatitis after liver transplantation. Lancet 1998;351(9100):409–13.

3. Vergani D, Longhi MS, Bogdanos DP, et al. Autoimmune hepatitis. Semin Immunopathol 2009;31(3):421–35.
4. Kerkar N, Yanni G. 'De novo' and 'recurrent' autoimmune hepatitis after liver transplantation: a comprehensive review. J Autoimmun 2016;66:17–24.
5. Manns MP, Czaja AJ, Gorham JD, et al. Diagnosis and management of autoimmune hepatitis. Hepatology 2010;51(6):2193–213.
6. Neuberger J, Portmann B, Calne R, et al. Recurrence of autoimmune chronic active hepatitis following orthotopic liver grafting. Transplantation 1984;37(4): 363–5.
7. Johnson PJ, McFarlane IG. Meeting report: international autoimmune hepatitis group. Hepatology 1993;18(4):998–1005.
8. Hennes EM, Zeniya M, Czaja AJ, et al. Simplified criteria for the diagnosis of autoimmune hepatitis. Hepatology 2008;48(1):169–76.
9. Molmenti EP, Netto GJ, Murray NG, et al. Incidence and recurrence of autoimmune/alloimmune hepatitis in liver transplant recipients. Liver Transpl 2002; 8(6):519–26.
10. González-Koch A, Czaja AJ, Carpenter HA, et al. Recurrent autoimmune hepatitis after orthotopic liver transplantation. Liver Transpl 2001;7(4):302–10.
11. Duclos-Vallée JC, Sebagh M, Rifai K, et al. A 10 year follow up study of patients transplanted for autoimmune hepatitis: histological recurrence precedes clinical and biochemical recurrence. Gut 2003;52(6):893–7.
12. Liberal R, Longhi MS, Grant CR, et al. Autoimmune hepatitis after liver transplantation. Clin Gastroenterol Hepatol 2012;10(4):346–53.
13. Khalaf H, Mourad W, El-Sheikh Y, et al. Liver transplantation for autoimmune hepatitis: a single-center experience. Transplant Proc 2007;39(4):1166–70.
14. Krishnamoorthy TL, Miezynska-Kurtycz J, Hodson J, et al. Longterm corticosteroid use after liver transplantation for autoimmune hepatitis is safe and associated with a lower incidence of recurrent disease. Liver Transpl 2016;22(1):34–41.
15. Montano-Loza AJ, Mason AL, Ma M, et al. Risk factors for recurrence of autoimmune hepatitis after liver transplantation. Liver Transpl 2009;15(10):1254–61.
16. Vogel A, Heinrich E, Bahr MJ, et al. Long-term outcome of liver transplantation for autoimmune hepatitis. Clin Transplant 2004;18(1):62–9.
17. Yusoff IF, House AK, De Boer WB, et al. Disease recurrence after liver transplantation in Western Australia. J Gastroenterol Hepatol 2002;17(2):203–7.
18. Renz JF, Ascher NL. Liver transplantation for nonviral, nonmalignant diseases: problem of recurrence. World J Surg 2002;26(2):247–56.
19. Milkiewicz P, Hubscher SG, Skiba G, et al. Recurrence of autoimmune hepatitis after liver transplantation. Transplantation 1999;68(2):253–6.
20. Narumi S, Hakamada K, Sasaki M, et al. Liver transplantation for autoimmune hepatitis: rejection and recurrence. Transplant Proc 1999;31(5):1955–6.
21. Prados E, Cuervas-Mons V, de la Mata M, et al. Outcome of autoimmune hepatitis after liver transplantation. Transplantation 1998;66(12):1645–50.
22. Wright HL, Bou-Abboud CF, Hassanein T, et al. Disease recurrence and rejection following liver transplantation for autoimmune chronic active liver disease. Transplantation 1992;53(1):136–9.
23. Ratziu V, Samuel D, Sebagh M, et al. Long-term follow-up after liver transplantation for autoimmune hepatitis: evidence of recurrence of primary disease. J Hepatol 1999;30(1):131–41.
24. Gautam M, Cheruvattath R, Balan V. Recurrence of autoimmune liver disease after liver transplantation: a systematic review. Liver Transpl 2006;12(12):1813–24.

25. Birnbaum AH, Benkov KJ, Pittman NS, et al. Recurrence of autoimmune hepatitis in children after liver transplantation. J Pediatr Gastroenterol Nutr 1997;25(1): 20–5.
26. Reich DJ, Fiel I, Guarrera JV, et al. Liver transplantation for autoimmune hepatitis. Hepatology 2000;32(4 Pt 1):693–700.
27. Götz G, Neuhaus R, Bechstein WO, et al. Recurrence of autoimmune hepatitis after liver transplantation. Transplant Proc 1999;31(1–2):430–1.
28. Balan V, Ruppert K, Demetris AJ, et al. Long-term outcome of human leukocyte antigen mismatching in liver transplantation: results of the National Institute of Diabetes and Digestive and kidney diseases liver transplantation Database. Hepatology 2008;48(3):878–88.
29. Ayata G, Gordon FD, Lewis WD, et al. Liver transplantation for autoimmune hepatitis: a long-term pathologic study. Hepatology 2000;32(2):185–92.
30. Czaja AJ. The immunoreactive propensity of autoimmune hepatitis: is it corticosteroid-dependent after liver transplantation? Liver Transpl Surg 1999; 5(5):460–3.
31. Alvarez F, Berg PA, Bianchi FB, et al. International Autoimmune Hepatitis Group Report: review of criteria for diagnosis of autoimmune hepatitis. J Hepatol 1999;31(5):929–38.
32. Duclos-Vallee JC, Sebagh M. Recurrence of autoimmune disease, primary sclerosing cholangitis, primary biliary cirrhosis, and autoimmune hepatitis after liver transplantation. Liver Transpl 2009;15(Suppl 2):S25–34.
33. Mendes F, Couto CA, Levy C. Recurrent and de novo autoimmune liver diseases. Clin Liver Dis 2011;15(4):859–78.
34. Demetris AJ, Adeyi O, Bellamy CO, et al. Liver biopsy interpretation for causes of late liver allograft dysfunction. Hepatology 2006;44(2):489–501.
35. Hübscher SG. Recurrent autoimmune hepatitis after liver transplantation: diagnostic criteria, risk factors, and outcome. Liver Transpl 2001;7(4):285–91.
36. Schreuder TC, Hübscher SG, Neuberger J. Autoimmune liver diseases and recurrence after orthotopic liver transplantation: what have we learned so far? Transpl Int 2009;22(2):144–52.
37. Sakai H, Urasawa K, Oyama N, et al. Successful covering of a hepatic artery aneurysm with a coronary stent graft. Cardiovasc Intervent Radiol 2004;27(3): 274–7.
38. Trouillot TE, Shrestha R, Kam I, et al. Successful withdrawal of prednisone after adult liver transplantation for autoimmune hepatitis. Liver Transpl Surg 1999; 5(5):375–80.
39. Khettry U, Huang WY, Simpson MA, et al. Patterns of recurrent hepatitis C after liver transplantation in a recent cohort of patients. Hum Pathol 2007;38(3): 443–52.
40. Heneghan MA, Portmann BC, Norris SM, et al. Graft dysfunction mimicking autoimmune hepatitis following liver transplantation in adults. Hepatology 2001;34(3): 464–70.
41. Andries S, Casamayou L, Sempoux C, et al. Posttransplant immune hepatitis in pediatric liver transplant recipients: incidence and maintenance therapy with azathioprine. Transplantation 2001;72(2):267–72.
42. Fiel MI, Schiano TD. Plasma cell hepatitis (de-novo autoimmune hepatitis) developing post liver transplantation. Curr Opin Organ Transplant 2012;17(3):287–92.
43. Ward SC, Schiano TD, Thung SN, et al. Plasma cell hepatitis in hepatitis C virus patients post-liver transplantation: case-control study showing poor outcome and predictive features in the liver explant. Liver Transpl 2009;15(12):1826–33.

44. Castillo-Rama M, Sebagh M, Sasatomi E, et al. "Plasma cell hepatitis" in liver allografts: identification and characterization of an IgG4-rich cohort. Am J Transplant 2013;13(11):2966–77.

45. Aguilera I, Sousa JM, Gavilan F, et al. Glutathione S-transferase T1 genetic mismatch is a risk factor for de novo immune hepatitis in liver transplantation. Transplant Proc 2005;37(9):3968–9.

46. Jones DE, James OF, Portmann B, et al. Development of autoimmune hepatitis following liver transplantation for primary biliary cirrhosis. Hepatology 1999; 30(1):53–7.

47. Evans HM, Kelly DA, McKiernan PJ, et al. Progressive histological damage in liver allografts following pediatric liver transplantation. Hepatology 2006;43(5): 1109–17.

48. Gibelli NE, Tannuri U, Mello ES, et al. Successful treatment of de novo autoimmune hepatitis and cirrhosis after pediatric liver transplantation. Pediatr Transplant 2006;10(3):371–6.

49. Hernandez HM, Kovarik P, Whitington PF, et al. Autoimmune hepatitis as a late complication of liver transplantation. J Pediatr Gastroenterol Nutr 2001;32(2): 131–6.

50. Petz W, Sonzogni A, Bertani A, et al. A cause of late graft dysfunction after pediatric liver transplantation: de novo autoimmune hepatitis. Transplant Proc 2002; 34(5):1958–9.

51. Miyagawa-Hayashino A, Haga H, Egawa H, et al. Outcome and risk factors of de novo autoimmune hepatitis in living-donor liver transplantation. Transplantation 2004;78(1):128–35.

52. Spada M, Bertani A, Sonzogni A, et al. A cause of late graft dysfunction after liver transplantation in children: de-novo autoimmune hepatitis. Transplant Proc 2001; 33(1–2):1747–8.

53. Gupta P, Hart J, Millis JM, et al. De novo hepatitis with autoimmune antibodies and atypical histology: a rare cause of late graft dysfunction after pediatric liver transplantation. Transplantation 2001;71(5):664–8.

54. Venick RS, McDiarmid SV, Farmer DG, et al. Rejection and steroid dependence: unique risk factors in the development of pediatric posttransplant de novo autoimmune hepatitis. Am J Transplant 2007;7(4):955–63.

55. Pongpaibul A, Venick RS, McDiarmid SV, et al. Histopathology of de novo autoimmune hepatitis. Liver Transpl 2012;18(7):811–8.

56. Aguilera I, Wichmann I, Sousa JM, et al. Antibodies against glutathione S-transferase T1 (GSTT1) in patients with de novo immune hepatitis following liver transplantation. Clin Exp Immunol 2001;126(3):535–9.

57. Salcedo M, Vaquero J, Bañares R, et al. Response to steroids in de novo autoimmune hepatitis after liver transplantation. Hepatology 2002;35(2):349–56.

58. Montano-Loza AJ, Vargas-Vorackova F, Ma M, et al. Incidence and risk factors associated with de novo autoimmune hepatitis after liver transplantation. Liver Int 2012;32(9):1426–33.

59. Edmunds C, Ekong UD. Autoimmune liver disease post-liver transplantation: a summary and proposed areas for future Research. Transplantation 2016; 100(3):515–24.

60. Sebagh M, Castillo-Rama M, Azoulay D, et al. Histologic findings predictive of a diagnosis of de novo autoimmune hepatitis after liver transplantation in adults. Transplantation 2013;96(7):670–8.

61. Demetris AJ, Sebagh M. Plasma cell hepatitis in liver allografts: variant of rejection or autoimmune hepatitis? Liver Transpl 2008;14(6):750–5.

62. Zhao XY, Rakhda MI, Wang TI, et al. Immunoglobulin G4-associated de novo autoimmune hepatitis after liver transplantation for chronic hepatitis B- and C-related cirrhosis and hepatocellular carcinoma: a case report with literature review. Transplant Proc 2013;45(2):824–7.

63. Eguchi S, Takatsuki M, Hidaka M, et al. De novo autoimmune hepatitis after living donor liver transplantation is unlikely to be related to immunoglobulin subtype 4-related immune disease. J Gastroenterol Hepatol 2008;23(7 Pt 2):e165–9.

64. Dubel L, Farges O, Johanet C, et al. High incidence of antitissue antibodies in patients experiencing chronic liver allograft rejection. Transplantation 1998; 65(8):1072–5.

65. Liberal R, Mieli-Vergani G, Vergani D. Autoimmune hepatitis: from mechanisms to therapy. Rev Clin Esp 2016;216(7):372–83.

66. Riva S, Sonzogni A, Bravi M, et al. Late graft dysfunction and autoantibodies after liver transplantation in children: preliminary results of an Italian experience. Liver Transpl 2006;12(4):573–7.

67. Avitzur Y, Ngan BY, Lao M, et al. Prospective evaluation of the prevalence and clinical significance of positive autoantibodies after pediatric liver transplantation. J Pediatr Gastroenterol Nutr 2007;45(2):222–7.

68. Foschi A, Zavaglia CA, Fanti D, et al. Autoimmunity after liver transplantation: a frequent event but a rare clinical problem. Clin Transplant 2015;29(2):161–6.

69. Richter A, Grabhorn E, Helmke K, et al. Clinical relevance of autoantibodies after pediatric liver transplantation. Clin Transplant 2007;21(3):427–32.

70. Cho JM, Kim KM, Oh SH, et al. De novo autoimmune hepatitis in Korean children after liver transplantation: a single institution's experience. Transplant Proc 2011; 43(6):2394–6.

71. Cholongitas E, Samonakis D, Patch D, et al. Induction of autoimmune hepatitis by pegylated interferon in a liver transplant patient with recurrent hepatitis C virus. Transplantation 2006;81(3):488–90.

72. Berardi S, Lodato F, Gramenzi A, et al. High incidence of allograft dysfunction in liver transplanted patients treated with pegylated-interferon alpha-2b and ribavirin for hepatitis C recurrence: possible de novo autoimmune hepatitis? Gut 2007;56(2):237–42.

73. Ikegami T, Yoshizumi T, Shirabe K, et al. Frequent plasma cell hepatitis during telaprevir-based triple therapy for hepatitis C after liver transplantation. J Hepatol 2014;60(4):894–6.

74. Aguilera I, Sousa JM, Gómez-Bravo MA, et al. De novo autoimmune hepatitis after interferon treatment in a liver transplant recipient with common variable immunodeficiency. Dig Liver Dis 2014;46(7):663–4.

75. Lodato F, Azzaroli F, Tamè MR, et al. G-CSF in Peg-IFN induced neutropenia in liver transplanted patients with HCV recurrence. World J Gastroenterol 2009; 15(43):5449–54.

76. Kontorinis N, Agarwal K, Elhajj N, et al. Pegylated interferon-induced immune-mediated hepatitis post-liver transplantation. Liver Transpl 2006;12(5):827–30.

77. Selzner N, Guindi M, Renner EL, et al. Immune-mediated complications of the graft in interferon-treated hepatitis C positive liver transplant recipients. J Hepatol 2011;55(1):207–17.

78. Salcedo M, Rodríguez-Mahou M, Rodríguez-Sainz C, et al. Risk factors for developing de novo autoimmune hepatitis associated with anti-glutathione S-transferase T1 antibodies after liver transplantation. Liver Transpl 2009;15(5):530–9.

79. Vanderlugt CL, Miller SD. Epitope spreading in immune-mediated diseases: implications for immunotherapy. Nat Rev Immunol 2002;2(2):85–95.

80. Albert LJ, Inman RD. Molecular mimicry and autoimmunity. N Engl J Med 1999; 341(27):2068–74.
81. Bogdanos DP, Choudhuri K, Vergani D. Molecular mimicry and autoimmune liver disease: virtuous intentions, malign consequences. Liver 2001;21(4):225–32.
82. Aguilera I, Wichmann I, Sousa JM, et al. Antibodies against glutathione S-transferase T1 in patients with immune hepatitis after liver transplantation. Transplant Proc 2003;35(2):712.
83. Sprenger R, Schlagenhaufer R, Kerb R, et al. Characterization of the glutathione S-transferase GSTT1 deletion: discrimination of all genotypes by polymerase chain reaction indicates a trimodular genotype-phenotype correlation. Pharmacogenetics 2000;10(6):557–65.
84. Aguilera I, Sousa JM, Gavilan F, et al. Complement component 4d immunostaining in liver allografts of patients with de novo immune hepatitis. Liver Transpl 2011;17(7):779–88.
85. Aguilera I, Sousa JM, Praena JM, et al. Choice of calcineurin inhibitor may influence the development of de novo immune hepatitis associated with anti-GSTT1 antibodies after liver transplantation. Clin Transplant 2011;25(2):207–12.
86. Aguilera I, Martinez-Bravo MJ, Sousa JM, et al. IgG subclass profile among anti-Glutathione S-transferase T1 antibodies in post-transplant de novo immune hepatitis. Clin Transplant 2016;30(3):210–7.
87. Czaja AJ. Diagnosis, pathogenesis, and treatment of autoimmune hepatitis after liver transplantation. Dig Dis Sci 2012;57(9):2248–66.
88. Banff schema for grading liver allograft rejection: an international consensus document. Hepatology 1997;25(3):658–63.
89. Knodell RG, Ishak KG, Black WC, et al. Formulation and application of a numerical scoring system for assessing histological activity in asymptomatic chronic active hepatitis. Hepatology 1981;1(5):431–5.
90. Ishak K, Baptista A, Bianchi L, et al. Histological grading and staging of chronic hepatitis. J Hepatol 1995;22(6):696–9.

Cholestatic Liver Diseases After Liver Transplant

Nathalie A. Pena Polanco, MD[a], Cynthia Levy, MD[b], Eric F. Martin, MD[b],*

KEYWORDS

- Cholestatic liver disease • Liver transplant • Primary sclerosing cholangitis
- Primary biliary cholangitis • Outcomes • Recurrence

KEY POINTS

- Cholestatic liver disease (CLD) has become an uncommon indication for liver transplant (LT); in general, CLD has the best posttransplant outcomes compared with other indications for LT.
- Disease recurrence is common after LT, but only recurrent primary sclerosing cholangitis (rPSC) seems to negatively affect posttransplant survival.
- Ursodiol (ursodeoxycholic acid [UDCA]) has not been shown to improve posttransplant survival in rPSC or PBC, but UDCA is associated with lower recurrence rates of PBC after LT.
- Acute cellular rejection is more common in autoimmune CLD after LT, but it does not negatively affect patient or graft survival.
- Retransplant is a viable option for patients with disease recurrence who develop graft loss.

INTRODUCTION

Cholestatic liver disease (CLD) comprises a heterogeneous group of disorders characterized by the impairment of bile flow that can progress to cirrhosis. Primary sclerosing cholangitis (PSC) and primary biliary cholangitis (PBC) are the two most common CLD in adults. Other causes of CLD in adults include cholestasis associated with total parenteral nutrition, secondary sclerosing cholangitis, hepatic sarcoidosis, sickle cell hepatopathy, and cystic fibrosis–associated liver disease. Pediatric causes include biliary atresia, Alagille syndrome, and progressive familial intrahepatic cholestasis.

Disclosure: The authors have nothing to disclose.
[a] Division of Internal Medicine, Miller School of Medicine, University of Miami, 1611 Northwest 12th Avenue, Suite Central 600-D, Miami, FL 33136, USA; [b] Division of Hepatology, Miller School of Medicine, University of Miami, 1120 Northwest 14th Street, Suite 1112, Miami, FL 33136, USA
* Corresponding author.
E-mail address: efm10@miami.edu

This article discuss the outcomes after liver transplant (LT) for adult causes of CLD, namely PSC and PBC, with emphasis on the diagnosis of disease recurrence, their associated risk factors, and their impact on patient and graft survival.

PRIMARY SCLEROSING CHOLANGITIS

PSC is a chronic, progressive, immune-mediated CLD characterized by inflammation and fibrosis of intrahepatic and extrahepatic bile ducts, leading to formation of multifocal biliary strictures.[1] PSC may lead to biliary cirrhosis with development of portal hypertension and its complications. Approximately 60% to 80% of patients with PSC have concomitant inflammatory bowel disease (IBD), which is predominately ulcerative colitis (UC).[2] Patients with PSC are at increased risk of developing cholangiocarcinoma (CCA), with a 10-year cumulative incidence estimated at 7% to 9%.[3,4] In addition, the risk of colorectal carcinoma (CRC) in patients with PSC and UC is estimated to be 5-fold higher than in those with UC without PSC.[5]

Indication and Timing of Liver Transplant

LT is the only effective treatment of PSC. Indications for LT for patients with PSC are similar to those with other forms of chronic liver disease and relate primarily to complications of portal hypertension, impaired quality of life (QOL), and chronic liver failure. Unique indications for LT for patients with PSC include intractable pruritus, recurrent bacterial cholangitis, and CCA. Highly selected patients with unresectable perihilar CCA may benefit from LT with protocol-driven application of neoadjuvant therapy established by the Mayo Clinic with 1-year, 3-year, and 5-year patient survivals of 90%, 80%, and 71%, respectively.[6]

Transplant Trends

In general, CLD has become an uncommon indication for LT. Data from the United Network for Organ Sharing (UNOS) show that among 3428 total adult LT in 1995, 16.5% were for PSC and PBC, compared with 10.0% in 2003 and 7.1% in 2015. Although the total number of adult LT from 1995 to 2009 increased by 40.4%, the number of LT for PSC has been fairly stable with an average of 292 LT per year (**Fig. 1**).[7] Thus, the percentage of total LT for PSC performed each year has declined (**Fig. 2**). Although PSC is an uncommon indication for LT in the United States, in Europe, namely the Nordic countries, where there is a lower prevalence of viral hepatitis and alcoholic liver disease, PSC accounted for 15.9% of all LT between 2004 and 2013.[8]

Patients with advanced PSC often manifest their disease with greater increases in bilirubin level than serum creatinine level or International Normalized Ratio and as a result have lower Model for End-stage Liver Disease (MELD) scores than those with other forms of end-stage liver disease, despite being equally sick.[9] As a result, patients with PSC often have disproportionately lower MELD scores that effectively prevent them from receiving a deceased donor LT (DDLT) while extending their waiting time, accumulating increased risks for adverse outcomes, and prolonging their impaired QOL. Consequently, many patients with PSC have undergone live donor LT (LDLT). A recent review of the UNOS database by Goldberg and colleagues[9] revealed that patients with PSC were more likely to obtain an LDLT compared with patients without PSC. Although LDLT account for approximately 5% of all adult LT recipients in the United States each year, nearly 14% of LT recipients with PSC undergo LDLT.

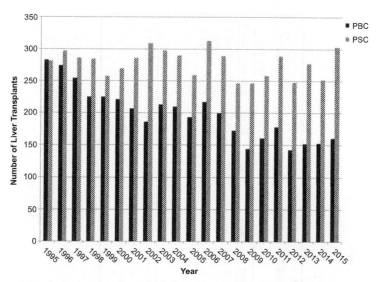

Fig. 1. Number of adult liver transplants performed each year in the United States for PBC and PSC from 1995 to 2015. (*Data from* United Network for Organ Sharing. Available at: https://www.unos.org/. Accessed July 20, 2016.)

Survival After Liver Transplant

In general, CLD have the best posttransplant outcomes compared with other indications for LT.[10,11] LT for PSC is highly successful, with 5-year patient survival rates in the United States exceeding 85% (**Table 1**). Similar results were reported in Europe.[12] An earlier retrospective analysis of the UNOS database by Kashyap and colleagues[13] in 2010 reported similar patient and graft survival for patients with PSC undergoing

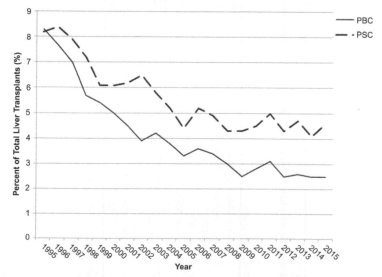

Fig. 2. Percentage of total adult liver transplants performed each year in the United States for PBC and PSC from 1995 to 2015. (*Data from* United Network for Organ Sharing. Available at: https://www.unos.org/. Accessed July 20, 2016.)

Table 1
Patient survival after liver transplant for primary sclerosing cholangitis and primary biliary cholangitis

Indication	Registry	Year	Cohort Size	1 y (%)		3 y (%)		5 y (%)		10 y (%)	
				Patient	Graft	Patient	Graft	Patient	Graft	Patient	Graft
PSC	Mayo Clinic, United States[42]	1985–1996	150	93.7	83.4	92.2 (2-y)	83.4 (2-y)	86.4	79.0	69.8	60.5
	Birmingham, United Kingdom[19]	1986–2006	230	80	75	—	—	68	60	57	50
	UNOS[11]	1994–2009	3854	93.4	86.5	89.7	81.4	87.4	78.0	83.2	71.5
	ELTR[12]	1999–2009	2170	90	83	—	—	82	72	—	—
	UNOS (DDLT)[13]	2002–2006	100	93.0	87.0	87.5	79.7	85.5	79.2	—	—
	UNOS (LDLT)[13]	2002–2006	100	97.2	89.6	95.4	87.1	95.4	87.1	—	—
PBC	UNOS[11]	1994–2009	3052	90.2	85.0	86.7	80.5	84.4	78.1	79.0	71.9
	ELTR[12]	1999–2009	1929	90	85	—	—	83	78	—	—
	UNOS (DDLT)[13]	2002–2006	100	89.6	85.2	87.0	82.5	85.1	80.7	—	—
	UNOS (LDLT)[13]	2002–2006	100	92.8	85.6	90.1	80.9	86.4	77.4	—	—

Abbreviation: ELTR, European Liver Transplant Registry.

LDLT compared with DDLT. However, using multivariate analysis of a more recent review of the UNOS database, Goldberg and colleagues[14] reported that LDLT recipients transplanted at experienced centers with CLD and autoimmune liver disease had significantly lower risks of graft failure compared with all other indications for LT (hazard ratio [HR] 0.75, 95% confidence interval [CI] 0.63–0.84, $P = .004$; and HR 0.56, 95% CI 0.37–0.83, $P = .004$, respectively).

Disease Recurrence

Diagnosis

The diagnosis of recurrent PSC (rPSC) is one of exclusion and, thus, the condition must be distinguished from other causes of biliary strictures of the allograft, namely reperfusion injury, biliary ischemia from hepatic artery thrombosis/stenosis, ABO incompatibility, biliary sepsis, chronic infection, or technical difficulties. The diagnostic criteria for rPSC after LT is outlined in **Table 2**.[15] The exact pathogenesis of rPSC is currently unknown, but is likely multifactorial and influenced by pretransplant and/or posttransplant factors in combination with a genetic predisposition.

Cholangiographic findings

A meta-analysis of 6 studies published in 2010 by Dave and colleagues[16] reported a sensitivity and specificity of magnetic resonance cholangiopancreatography (MRCP) in detecting PSC of 86% and 94%, respectively. However, there are no available studies comparing MRCP with endoscopic retrograde cholangiopancreatography and/or percutaneous transhepatic cholangiography (PTC) in detecting rPSC and, thus, it is not clear whether the sensitivity/specificity is as good as in the primary disease. However, given the rapidly evolving quality of MRCP, noninvasive nature, and reduced cost, MRCP has become the first choice to evaluate intrahepatic and extrahepatic biliary abnormalities after LT. The typical cholangiographic findings in rPSC include multifocal nonanastomotic strictures in both intrahepatic and extrahepatic bile ducts superimposed with segments of normal or dilated ducts.[15] Sheng and colleagues[17] compared the cholangiographic features using PTC of 32 patients with rPSC who developed biliary strictures with the features of 32 patients without PSC who also developed biliary strictures. Intrahepatic strictures were more common in patients with rPSC and the appearance of the strictures was different, with mural irregularity and diverticulumlike outpouchings. Although these cholangiographic changes

Table 2
Diagnostic criteria for recurrent primary sclerosing cholangitis after liver transplant

Inclusion Criteria	Exclusion Criteria

Diagnosis
  Confirmed diagnosis of PSC before LT
Cholangiography
  Nonanastomotic strictures of intrahepatic and/
    or extrahepatic bile ducts with beading and
    irregularities >90 d after LT
Histology
  Fibrous cholangitis and/or fibro-obliterative
    lesions with or without ductopenia, biliary
    fibrosis, or biliary cirrhosis
	Hepatic artery thrombosis/stenosis
	Chronic ductopenic rejection
	Anastomotic strictures
	Nonanastomotic strictures <90 d after LT
	Donor and recipient ABO incompatibility

Adapted from Graziadei IW, Wiesner RH, Batts KP, et al. Recurrence of primary sclerosing cholangitis following liver transplantation. Hepatology 1999;29(4):1050; with permission.

occurred more significantly in patients with rPSC, in most cases, it was impossible to differentiate between rPSC and other conditions based solely on cholangiography.

Histologic findings
Given the high sensitivity and specificity of cholangiography, the use of liver biopsies in diagnosing both PSC and rPSC is considered supplementary to cholangiography. The histologic changes in rPSC are identical to those seen in the native liver with PSC, which often makes it difficult to distinguish rPSC from biliary injury of other causes. The distinction between rPSC and chronic rejection is particularly challenging in that both conditions can result in loss of bile ducts with a subsequent cholestatic pattern of increased levels of liver enzymes. Therefore, it is imperative that the diagnosis of rPSC and chronic rejection be based on a combination of clinical, laboratory, radiographic, and histopathologic findings.

Incidence of recurrent primary sclerosing cholangitis
The incidence of rPSC varies widely based on reports from different centers, which likely reflects differences in diagnostic criteria, study design, length and type of follow-up, and inclusion of protocol biopsies. A systematic review of 22 publications containing data from original studies on the outcomes of LT for PSC identified a recurrence rate of 18.5% (range, 5.7%–59.1%) by 2.6 to 9.1 years.[18] The 7 largest of these studies are listed in **Table 3**.[15,19–24] In the largest series reported to date (n = 230), rPSC occurred in 23.5% of recipients at a median of 4.6 years after LT.[19]

Risk factors for recurrent primary sclerosing cholangitis
Multiple risk factors for rPSC have been identified (**Table 4**).[19,21–30] One of the most studied risk factors for rPSC is concurrent IBD. This risk factor was first described in 2002 in a study by Vera and colleagues,[24] who reported a dramatic reduction in the risk of rPSC if the colon was removed before or at time of LT. Of the 152 patients included in this study, 56 (37%) patients developed rPSC, but only 1 (6%) of 17 patients who underwent colectomy before or at the time of LT developed rPSC. In another study in 2007 by Cholongitas and colleagues[28] evaluating 69 patients with

Table 3
Rates of recurrent primary sclerosing cholangitis after liver transplant

Reference	Time Period	Number of Patients	Recurrence Rate (%)	Median Time to Recurrence (Range)
Graziadei et al,[15] 1999	1985–1996	120	20 (8.3 based on both cholangiographic and histologic features)	36 mo (14–108 mo), histologic criteria; 8.6 mo (3–43 mo), cholangiographic criteria
Alabraba et al,[19] 2009	1986–2006	230	23.5	4.6 y (0.5–12.9 y)
Goss et al,[20] 1997	1984–1996	127	8.6	Not provided
Jeyarajah et al,[21] 1998	1998–1995	118	15.7	21 mo (mean)
Kugelmas et al,[22] 2003	1988–2000	71	21.1	52 mo (mean) (12–110)
Ravikumar et al,[23] 2015	1990–2010	565	14.3	Not provided
Vera et al,[24] 2002	1986–2000	152	37	36 mo (1–120)

Table 4	
Risk factors for recurrent primary sclerosing cholangitis	
HLA-DRB1*08 (in Recipient or Donor)[26]	Use of extended donor criteria grafts[19]
Absence of donor HLA-DR52[21]	Steroid-resistant ACR[26]
Recipient-donor gender mismatch[30]	Use of OKT3[22]
Male recipient[24]	Presence of UC after LT[23]
Younger recipient age[21]	Maintenance of steroid therapy for UC >3 mo[25]
Intact colon before LT[24]	Presence of cholangiocarcinoma before LT[27]
>1 episode of ACR[21]	Concurrent cytomegalovirus infection in recipient[21]
First-degree related donors (LDLT)[29]	

Abbreviations: ACR, acute cellular rejection; HLA, human leukocyte antigen.

PSC who underwent LT, none of the patients with PSC without UC or patients who underwent pre-LT total colectomy developed rPSC. In contrast, rPSC developed in 7 (27%) of those with post-LT UC. These studies suggest that absence of inflammation in the intestine, either by way of the absence of concurrent IBD or colectomy before or during LT, has a protective effect against rPSC.

Multiple studies have also shown acute cellular rejection (ACR) as an independent risk factor for rPSC.[31–33] The exact mechanism explaining the association between ACR and increased risk of rPSC is unknown. The biliary epithelium, by definition, is one of the structures affected in ACR; therefore, it has been suggested that the inflammation of biliary epithelium that occurs in ACR results in an increase in the levels of autoimmune epitopes, which leads to further immune-mediated damage of the bile ducts.[21]

Treatment of recurrent primary sclerosing cholangitis
There is no proven medical therapy for rPSC after LT. Although ursodiol (ursodeoxycholic acid [UDCA]) is used in most transplant centers and improves the liver biochemical profile, its effect on outcomes remains unclear.[31,32] In contrast, the prophylactic use of UDCA may be justified in patients with coexisting UC who may benefit from UDCA by reducing the risk of CRC.[33] In the absence of effective medical therapy, symptomatic management of biliary strictures and their complications, such as cholangitis, remains the only option. As in the nontransplant setting, biliary strictures may be managed by endoscopic or percutaneous methods. Because PSC affects both the intrahepatic and extrahepatic bile ducts, Roux-en-Y choledochojejunostomy after LT was commonly performed.[34] However, this precludes easy endoscopic access to the remnant bile duct because of the length of the Roux limb. Single and double balloon enteroscopy have been reported as safe and efficacious techniques to obtain biliary access in patients with Roux-en-Y choledochojejunostomy after LT.[35,36] In patients with PSC with a disease-free common bile duct, duct-to-duct biliary reconstruction is a safe and effective technique with long-term clinical outcomes comparable with those of Roux-en-Y hepaticojejunostomy.[37–39] In a recent meta-analysis comparing the two techniques, the only clinically significant difference noted was a higher rate of ascending cholangitis in the Roux-en-Y group,[38] which is best explained by bacterial translocation and subsequent colonization inherent in bilioenteric anastomoses.[40]

Rejection
The incidence of rejection after LT overall has declined; however, 20% to 40% of LT recipients still experience ACR that requires additional immunosuppression.[41]

Patients with PSC are commonly thought to have a higher risk of ACR compared with LT recipients with other primary liver diseases. The reported incidence of ACR after LT for patients with PSC is variable between transplant centers and time periods, in large part because of the variable immunosuppressive regimens, inconsistent use of protocol biopsies, and histologic definition of ACR. **Table 5** lists the rates of acute and chronic rejection in patients transplanted for PSC from larger, more recent studies with clearly defined histologic diagnostic criteria.[21,26,42,43]

There are conflicting data on whether the presence of IBD is associated with ACR after LT. Several studies suggest that patients with PSC with concomitant IBD are at increased risk of ACR.[42,44] In a study by Narumi and colleagues,[45] the incidence of moderate or severe rejection in patients with PSC with concomitant IBD was 70% compared with 36% in patients with PSC without IBD and 37% in a matched control group (non-PSC/non-IBD). However, a study by Jeyarajah and colleagues[21] that included 118 LT recipients for PSC showed no association between concomitant IBD and the incidence of ACR.

Importance of Acute Cellular Rejection After Liver Transplant for Primary Sclerosing Cholangitis

Unlike kidney transplant, there is no compelling evidence that early ACR affects long-term graft or patient survival after LT. In contrast, late acute rejection (LAR), which is more common in PBC, PSC, and autoimmune hepatitis (AIH), is associated with worse patient and graft survival.[46]

Retransplant

Earlier studies reported no difference in patient or graft survival among LT recipients with or without rPSC.[20,42] However, more long-term data indicate that rPSC significantly affects graft survival, rate of retransplant, and patient survival.[19,47] Retransplant is a viable option in patients who develop rPSC with subsequent graft loss. In a retrospective review of the UNOS database, the rate of retransplant was significantly higher in patients with PSC compared with patients with PBC (12.4% vs 8.5%) and PSC was identified as an independent predictor for retransplant.[48]

Inflammatory Bowel Disease Activity After Liver Transplant

Recent studies suggest that IBD activity may improve after LT.[49,50] Specifically, in a recent prospective study of patients with PSC with concomitant IBD, LT recipients had significantly lower clinical and histologic IBD activity with lower frequency of

Table 5					
Incidence of rejection after liver transplant for primary sclerosing cholangitis					
Reference	Year	Cohort Size	Rejection Rate (%)	Type of Rejection	Median (Range) Follow-up (mo)
Graziadei et al,[42] 1999	1985–1996	150	69	ACR	55 (10–138)
Brandsaeter et al,[26] 2005	1984–2003	49	71	ACR	77 (17–182)
Jeyarajah et al,[21] 1998	1985–1995	115	39	ACR	Minimal follow-up 12 mo
Graziadei et al,[42] 1999	1985–1996	150	8	Chronic	56 (10–138)
Jeyarajah et al,[21] 1998	1985–1995	115	39	Chronic	Not provided
Milkiewicz et al,[43] 2000	1982–1998	136	7	Chronic	Not provided

backwash ileitis and higher frequency of rectal sparing compared with the nontransplanted group. However, other studies suggest that more than half of patients with PSC with IBD have continued or worsened disease activity despite immunosuppression following LT.[51]

Although there are no data showing an association between post-LT immunosuppression regimen and the risk of rPSC,[22,52] there are data suggesting that immunosuppression affects IBD activity after LT in patients with PSC. Specifically, standard maintenance immunosuppression with tacrolimus (Prograf) and mycophenolate mofetil (CellCept) was associated with worsening IBD activity after LT, whereas combination cyclosporine A and azathioprine was associated with improving IBD activity.[53]

The medical management strategies for IBD after LT are not well defined, but, in general, the underlying principle is no different from IBD in other settings. An important caveat is the concern for increased risk of infection when biologic therapy (eg, infliximab) is added to standard post-LT immunosuppression. Recent case series describe the safety and efficacy of anti–tumor necrosis factor (anti-TNF) therapy in the treatment of IBD after LT.[54–56] In the largest case series, which included 8 patients, nearly 88% of patients started on anti-TNF had a clinical response. However, 50% of patients developed severe infections (*Clostridium difficile* colitis, community-acquired bacterial pneumonia, esophageal candidiasis, and cryptosporidiosis) and 1 patient developed an Epstein-Barr virus–positive polymorphic posttransplant lymphoproliferative disorder after 4 months of anti-TNF therapy.[56] With this in mind, some experts consider azathioprine the preferred immunosuppressive option for patients with moderate to severe IBD in combination with other immunosuppressants, namely tacrolimus. However, for patients who do not respond to azathioprine and/or have severe IBD (eg, fistulizing Crohn disease), anti-TNF therapy should still be considered with close monitoring for potential infectious and malignant complications.

An increased incidence of colon cancer has been reported in patients with PSC transplanted with concomitant IBD, which may be explained by the combined effects of long-standing colitis and post-LT immunosuppression.[57,58] Current American Association For The Study Of Liver Diseases (AASLD) guidelines recommend annual surveillance for colon cancer in patients with PSC after LT.[1]

Bone Mineral Density

Similar to other CLD, patients with PSC have a higher prevalence of metabolic bone disease before and after LT.[59] According to current AASLD guidelines, for the first 5 years after LT, bone mineral density (BMD) should be evaluated every year for osteopenic patients and every 2 to 3 years for patients with normal BMD.[60] The screening and treatment depend on the progression of BMD thereafter.

PRIMARY BILIARY CHOLANGITIS

PBC is an immune-mediated chronic CLD characterized by progressive destruction of intrahepatic bile ducts that may progress to biliary cirrhosis. Although the use of UDCA has been shown to improve biochemical indices, delay histologic progression, and improve transplant-free survival, LT is the only effective treatment of end-stage liver disease caused by PBC.

Indication and Timing of Liver Transplant

The indications for LT for patients with PBC are similar to those with other forms of chronic liver disease. Similar to PSC, intractable pruritus in the setting of PBC may merit consideration for LT. Chronic fatigue is generally not an indication for LT because evidence suggests that it may not improve after LT.[61] Several mathematical models have been developed to estimate survival in patients with PBC. The Mayo PBC Risk Score, which incorporates age, bilirubin level, albumin level, prothrombin time, presence of peripheral edema, and need for diuretic therapy, is a widely used prognostic model and has been shown to be superior to the Child-Pugh Score.[62] However, the Mayo Risk Score is specific for patients with PBC only; thus, the MELD score is often prioritized in all LT candidates. LT should be considered in patients with PBC with a Mayo Risk Score greater than 7.8, bilirubin level greater than 6 mg/dL, and MELD score greater than 12.[63]

Transplant Trends

PBC was the leading indication for LT in the United States during the mid-1980s. In 1995, PBC was the third most common indication for LT in the United States, behind only alcohol and hepatitis C virus (HCV). Despite a 40% increase in the total number of adult LT performed in the United States from 1995 to 2009, the number of LT performed for PBC has steadily decreased during this time by an average of 9.9 cases per year (see **Fig. 1**). Accounting for 2.5% of all adult LT in the United States in 2015, PBC is currently the sixth most common indication for LT in the United States. (see **Fig. 2**).[7] Likewise, deaths related to PBC have also decreased in the last few decades.[64] The decrease in mortality and need for LT closely parallel the increased use of UDCA.[65]

Survival After Liver Transplant

Similar to PSC, post-LT outcomes for PBC are excellent, with 5-year patient survival approaching 85% (see **Table 1**). Similar survival rates were reported in Europe.[66] In a retrospective analysis of the UNOS database from 2002 to 2006, which included 99 patients with PBC who underwent LDLT, patient and graft survival following LDLT were similar to those following DDLT.[13]

Although patient and graft survival are the most often used variables to assess outcomes after LT, improvement of QOL is a compelling variable unique to CLD. Using the National Institute of Diabetes and Digestive and Kidney Diseases Liver Transplant Database Quality of Life Questionnaire, Gross and colleagues[61] assessed 4 aspects of QOL (liver-related symptoms; physical, social, and emotional functioning; health perceptions; and overall QOL) before and after LT for patients with both PBC and PSC. There were no reported differences in QOL parameters between PBC and PSC. QOL following LT was substantially better than before LT, which was observed in all 4 aspects of QOL. In addition, the health-related QOL at 1 year after LT was not associated with pre-LT clinical factors, which suggests that even those who are very ill before LT can make a significant recovery.

Disease Recurrence

Diagnosis
The diagnosis of recurrent PBC (rPBC) is often difficult because the diagnostic criteria before LT are obscured in the post-LT setting by multiple factors. First, only 12% of patients with rPBC report potentially disease-related, but often nonspecific, symptoms.[67] Specifically, fatigue, which is very nonspecific, persists in a large proportion of patients after LT.[68] Second, antimitochondrial antibody (AMA) and immunoglobulin M (IgM) often remain present after LT and, therefore, lose their diagnostic value for rPBC. Likewise, a cholestatic pattern of liver enzymes with increased alkaline phosphatase and gamma glutamyl transpeptidase is also nonspecific after LT and is found in many other conditions (**Table 6**). Because both biochemical and serologic data lack specificity, histology is required in the diagnosis of rPBC. In addition, the characteristic

Table 6
Causes of cholestasis after liver transplant

Early (≤6 mo)	Late (>6 mo)
Extrahepatic	Extrahepatic
Stricture: anastomotic, compressive	Stricture anastomotic
Multiple strictures: ischemic or HAT	Multiple strictures: hepatic artery thrombosis, ischemic, recurrent PSC
Bile leak	Choledocholithiasis
Cholangitis	Intrahepatic
Intrahepatic	Intrahepatic biliary strictures
Ischemia/reperfusion injury	Chronic rejection
ABO incompatibility	Recurrent disease (PSC, PBC, HCV)
HAT/stenosis	ACR
ACR	DILI
Sepsis	De novo AIH
DILI	De novo viral hepatitis
Small for size CBD	
Post-LT infections	

Abbreviations: CBD, common bile duct; DILI, drug-induced liver injury; HAT, hepatic artery thrombosis.

Adapted from Khungar V, Goldberg D. Liver transplantation for cholestatic liver diseases in adults. Clin Liver Dis 2016;20(1):195; with permission.

histologic features of PBC in the nontransplant setting, namely the immune-mediated lymphoplasmacytic injury of small bile ducts and bile duct paucity may be mimicked in the post-LT setting by acute and chronic rejection. Therefore, the diagnosis of rPBC relies on characteristic histologic features and the exclusion of other causes of graft dysfunction (**Table 7**).

Incidence of recurrent primary biliary cholangitis
The overall rates of rPBC range from 0% to 50%, with reported rates of 21% to 37% at 10 years and 43% at 15 years.[69] The median time to rPBC is between 3 and 5.5 years.[69] The reported recurrence rates increase with time but vary in part because of inconsistent use of protocol biopsies and different diagnostic criteria for rPBC.

Risk factors for recurrent primary biliary cholangitis
Several risk factors for rPBC after LT have been identified and are listed in **Table 8**.[70–73] However, their impacts on the development of rPBC are controversial

Table 7
Diagnostic criteria for recurrent primary biliary cholangitis after liver transplant

Inclusion Criteria	Exclusion Criteria
Diagnosis	Acute and chronic rejection
Confirmed diagnosis of PBC in explant histology	Graft-vs-host disease
Serology	Biliary obstruction or cholangitis
Persistence of AMA or AMA-M2	Vascular complications
Histology	Viral hepatitis
Lymphoplasmacytic portal inflammation	DILI
Lymphoid aggregates	
Epithelioid granulomas	
Evidence of bile duct injury	

Table 8
Risk factors for recurrent primary biliary cholangitis

Use of tacrolimus (rather than cyclosporine)[73]	>1 episode of ACR[71]
Prolonged WIT[71]	Recipient age <48 y[70]
Prolonged CIT[71]	Sex mismatch between recipient and donor[70]
Number of HLA mismatches[72]	Pre-LT IgM ≥554 mg/dL[70]

Abbreviations: CIT, cold ischemia time; WIT, warm ischemia time.

based on inconsistent findings. Several, mostly retrospective single-center studies, reported that tacrolimus-based immunosuppression, compared with cyclosporine, was associated with a higher rate and a shorter time of diagnosis of rPBC after LT.[66,74] However, a large meta-analysis by Gautam and colleagues[75] in 2006, which evaluated 16 studies including 1241 patients with PBC who underwent LT, showed no association between the type of immunosuppressive regimen (tacrolimus vs cyclosporine) and rPBC. In addition, Manousou and colleagues[76] suggested that the combination of azathioprine and cyclosporine resulted in the lowest rates of rPBC. However, the impact of human leukocyte antigen mismatches on rPBC following LDLT is unclear.[72,77]

Treatment of Recurrent Primary Biliary Cholangitis

The effective use of UDCA is well established in the treatment of PBC before LT. However, few data are available regarding the use of UDCA in rPBC after LT. In a study of 52 patients with rPBC, Charatcharoenwitthaya and colleagues[78] estimated that, during a 36-month follow-up period, 52% of patients with rPBC who were treated with UDCA experienced normalization in serum alkaline phosphatase and alanine aminotransferase levels compared with only 22% of untreated patients. Although, the use of UDCA did not affect patient or graft survival, longer follow-up is needed to determine the long-term benefit of UDCA in the post-LT setting.

Prevention of Recurrent Primary Biliary Cholangitis

UDCA has also been proposed to have protective properties, and has been studied both in the pretransplant and posttransplant settings. A study by Heathcote and colleagues[79] compared patients with PBC who were treated with UDCA before LT with those who were not. This study reported no difference in post-LT outcomes between the two groups, suggesting that the beneficial effect of UDCA in delaying the need for LT is not associated with a worse outcome after LT becomes necessary.

Results of a recent French multicenter study suggested a beneficial effect of UDCA in preventing rPBC after LT.[80] This study included 90 patients with PBC who underwent LT, 19 of whom were on UDCA since LT, with a mean follow-up of 12 years. rPBC was diagnosed in 48 (53%) patients. In multivariate Cox models, use of UDCA was the only independent factor that affected the risk of rPBC (HR, 0.31; 95% CI, 0.11–0.85). Although this may suggest a role for UDCA as prophylaxis for rPBC after LT, neither rPBC nor use of UDCA affected post-LT patient or graft survival.

Given the increasing survival rates and subsequent life-spans after LT, rPBC may become more clinically relevant in the future. Thus, a growing proportion of patients may live long enough to develop clinically relevant recurrent disease of the liver graft and may benefit from long-term use of UDCA.

Clinical Impact of Recurrent Primary Biliary Cholangitis

Unlike rPSC, most studies conclude that rPBC does not significantly affect long-term patient or graft survival.[47,81] In the 2 largest reported experiences of LT for PBC, a combined 5 out of 639 recipients required retransplant.[78,82] rPBC after second and third LT has been described, but the proportion of graft failure caused by rPBC remains low (7%–14%).[83]

In a recent Japanese study, late graft mortality after LDLT for PBC was predominately the result of a chronic immune-mediated reaction syndrome, including chronic rejection, veno-occlusive disease, and obliterative portal venopathy, and not rPBC.[84]

Rejection

Similar to other forms of autoimmune liver disease, PBC is thought to be associated with an increased risk of rejection after LT.[85] A study by Hayashi and colleagues[86] confirmed that, compared with alcoholic cirrhosis, preexisting autoimmune liver disease is associated with a higher incidence of acute allograft rejection and a trend toward more frequent chronic rejection, but with similar patient and graft survival at 1 and 3 years between both groups. Patients with PBC who underwent LT also have one of the highest risks of LAR, which, unlike ACR, is associated with worsened graft survival.[87] Likewise, chronic rejection is also associated with graft failure. Therefore, some investigators have proposed that the autoimmune component should be recognized in the pathogenesis of chronic rejection, which could in turn have an effect in the development of new strategies for preventing and/or treating chronic rejection following LT.[88]

SUMMARY

Although the number of LT performed for PSC and PBC has declined over the years, post-LT survival for CLD remains among the highest of all indications for liver transplant. As such, a growing proportion of patients are living longer and are at risk for developing clinically relevant recurrent disease and other complications related to chronic immunosuppression. Although UDCA has not been shown to affect post-LT survival in rPSC or rPBC, UDCA is associated with lower recurrence rates of PBC after LT. UDCA was for many years the only US Food and Drug Administration–approved treatment of PBC. Obeticholic acid (Ocaliva), which is a farnesoid X receptor agonist, was approved on May 27, 2016, as only the second drug available for treatment of PBC. Whether this new agent will play a role in the management of recurrent CLD after LT remains to be seen.

REFERENCES

1. Chapman R, Fevery J, Kalloo A, et al. Diagnosis and management of primary sclerosing cholangitis. Hepatology 2010;51(2):660–78.
2. Bambha K, Kim WR, Talwalkar J, et al. Incidence, clinical spectrum, and outcomes of primary sclerosing cholangitis in a United States community. Gastroenterology 2003;125(5):1364–9.
3. Burak K, Angulo P, Pasha TM, et al. Incidence and risk factors for cholangiocarcinoma in primary sclerosing cholangitis. Am J Gastroenterol 2004;99(3):523–6.
4. Claessen MM, Vleggaar FP, Tytgat KM, et al. High lifetime risk of cancer in primary sclerosing cholangitis. J Hepatol 2009;50(1):158–64.
5. Milkiewicz P, Wunsch E, Elias E. Liver transplantation in chronic cholestatic conditions. Front Biosci (Landmark Ed) 2012;17:959–69.

6. Rosen CB, Heimbach JK, Gores GJ. Surgery for cholangiocarcinoma: the role of liver transplantation. HPB (Oxford) 2008;10(3):186–9.

7. United Network for Organ Sharing (UNOS). Available at: https://www.unos.org/. Accessed August 31, 2016.

8. Fosby B, Melum E, Bjoro K, et al. Liver transplantation in the Nordic countries - an intention to treat and post-transplant analysis from the Nordic Liver Transplant Registry 1982-2013. Scand J Gastroenterol 2015;50(6):797–808.

9. Goldberg DS, French B, Thomasson A, et al. Current trends in living donor liver transplantation for primary sclerosing cholangitis. Transplantation 2011;91(10): 1148–52.

10. Futagawa Y, Terasaki PI. An analysis of the OPTN/UNOS liver transplant registry. Clin Transpl 2004;315–29.

11. Singal AK, Guturu P, Hmoud B, et al. Evolving frequency and outcomes of liver transplantation based on etiology of liver disease. Transplantation 2013;95(5): 755–60.

12. Adam R, Karam V, Delvart V, et al. Evolution of indications and results of liver transplantation in Europe. A report from the European Liver Transplant Registry (ELTR). J Hepatol 2012;57(3):675–88.

13. Kashyap R, Safadjou S, Chen R, et al. Living donor and deceased donor liver transplantation for autoimmune and cholestatic liver diseases–an analysis of the UNOS database. J Gastrointest Surg 2010;14(9):1362–9.

14. Goldberg DS, French B, Abt PL, et al. Superior survival using living donors and donor-recipient matching using a novel living donor risk index. Hepatology 2014;60(5):1717–26.

15. Graziadei IW, Wiesner RH, Batts KP, et al. Recurrence of primary sclerosing cholangitis following liver transplantation. Hepatology 1999;29(4):1050–6.

16. Dave M, Elmunzer BJ, Dwamena BA, et al. Primary sclerosing cholangitis: meta-analysis of diagnostic performance of MR cholangiopancreatography. Radiology 2010;256(2):387–96.

17. Sheng R, Campbell WL, Zajko AB, et al. Cholangiographic features of biliary strictures after liver transplantation for primary sclerosing cholangitis: evidence of recurrent disease. AJR Am J Roentgenol 1996;166(5):1109–13.

18. Fosby B, Karlsen TH, Melum E. Recurrence and rejection in liver transplantation for primary sclerosing cholangitis. World J Gastroenterol 2012;18(1):1–15.

19. Alabraba E, Nightingale P, Gunson B, et al. A re-evaluation of the risk factors for the recurrence of primary sclerosing cholangitis in liver allografts. Liver Transpl 2009;15(3):330–40.

20. Goss JA, Shackleton CR, Farmer DG, et al. Orthotopic liver transplantation for primary sclerosing cholangitis. A 12-year single center experience. Ann Surg 1997; 225(5):472–81 [discussion: 481–3].

21. Jeyarajah DR, Netto GJ, Lee SP, et al. Recurrent primary sclerosing cholangitis after orthotopic liver transplantation: is chronic rejection part of the disease process? Transplantation 1998;66(10):1300–6.

22. Kugelmas M, Spiegelman P, Osgood MJ, et al. Different immunosuppressive regimens and recurrence of primary sclerosing cholangitis after liver transplantation. Liver Transpl 2003;9(7):727–32.

23. Ravikumar R, Tsochatzis E, Jose S, et al. Risk factors for recurrent primary sclerosing cholangitis after liver transplantation. J Hepatol 2015;63(5):1139–46.

24. Vera A, Moledina S, Gunson B, et al. Risk factors for recurrence of primary sclerosing cholangitis of liver allograft. Lancet 2002;360(9349):1943–4.

25. Alexander J, Lord JD, Yeh MM, et al. Risk factors for recurrence of primary sclerosing cholangitis after liver transplantation. Liver Transpl 2008;14(2):245–51.
26. Brandsaeter B, Schrumpf E, Bentdal O, et al. Recurrent primary sclerosing cholangitis after liver transplantation: a magnetic resonance cholangiography study with analyses of predictive factors. Liver Transpl 2005;11(11):1361–9.
27. Campsen J, Zimmerman MA, Trotter JF, et al. Clinically recurrent primary sclerosing cholangitis following liver transplantation: a time course. Liver Transpl 2008;14(2):181–5.
28. Cholongitas E, Shusang V, Papatheodoridis GV, et al. Risk factors for recurrence of primary sclerosing cholangitis after liver transplantation. Liver Transpl 2008; 14(2):138–43.
29. Egawa H, Ueda Y, Ichida T, et al. Risk factors for recurrence of primary sclerosing cholangitis after living donor liver transplantation in Japanese registry. Am J Transplant 2011;11(3):518–27.
30. Khettry U, Keaveny A, Goldar-Najafi A, et al. Liver transplantation for primary sclerosing cholangitis: a long-term clinicopathologic study. Hum Pathol 2003; 34(11):1127–36.
31. Carbone M, Neuberger J. Liver transplantation in PBC and PSC: indications and disease recurrence. Clin Res Hepatol Gastroenterol 2011;35(6–7):446–54.
32. Graziadei IW. Recurrence of nonviral liver diseases after liver transplantation. Clin Liver Dis 2014;18(3):675–85.
33. Pardi DS, Loftus EV Jr, Kremers WK, et al. Ursodeoxycholic acid as a chemopreventive agent in patients with ulcerative colitis and primary sclerosing cholangitis. Gastroenterology 2003;124(4):889–93.
34. Welsh FK, Wigmore SJ. Roux-en-Y choledochojejunostomy is the method of choice for biliary reconstruction in liver transplantation for primary sclerosing cholangitis. Transplantation 2004;77(4):602–4.
35. Koornstra JJ. Double balloon enteroscopy for endoscopic retrograde cholangiopancreaticography after Roux-en-Y reconstruction: case series and review of the literature. Neth J Med 2008;66(7):275–9.
36. Saleem A, Baron TH, Gostout CJ, et al. Endoscopic retrograde cholangiopancreatography using a single-balloon enteroscope in patients with altered Roux-en-Y anatomy. Endoscopy 2010;42(8):656–60.
37. Damrah O, Sharma D, Burroughs A, et al. Duct-to-duct biliary reconstruction in orthotopic liver transplantation for primary sclerosing cholangitis: a viable and safe alternative. Transpl Int 2012;25(1):64–8.
38. Pandanaboyana S, Bell R, Bartlett AJ, et al. Meta-analysis of duct-to-duct versus Roux-en-Y biliary reconstruction following liver transplantation for primary sclerosing cholangitis. Transpl Int 2015;28(4):485–91.
39. Sutton ME, Bense RD, Lisman T, et al. Duct-to-duct reconstruction in liver transplantation for primary sclerosing cholangitis is associated with fewer biliary complications in comparison with hepaticojejunostomy. Liver Transpl 2014;20(4): 457–63.
40. Chuang JH, Lee SY, Chen WJ, et al. Changes in bacterial concentration in the liver correlate with that in the hepaticojejunostomy after bile duct reconstruction: implication in the pathogenesis of postoperative cholangitis. World J Surg 2001; 25(12):1512–8.
41. Shaked A, Ghobrial RM, Merion RM, et al. Incidence and severity of acute cellular rejection in recipients undergoing adult living donor or deceased donor liver transplantation. Am J Transplant 2009;9(2):301–8.

42. Graziadei IW, Wiesner RH, Marotta PJ, et al. Long-term results of patients under-going liver transplantation for primary sclerosing cholangitis. Hepatology 1999; 30(5):1121–7.
43. Milkiewicz P, Gunson B, Saksena S, et al. Increased incidence of chronic rejection in adult patients transplanted for autoimmune hepatitis: assessment of risk factors. Transplantation 2000;70(3):477–80.
44. Miki C, Harrison JD, Gunson BK, et al. Inflammatory bowel disease in primary sclerosing cholangitis: an analysis of patients undergoing liver transplantation. Br J Surg 1995;82(8):1114–7.
45. Narumi S, Roberts JP, Emond JC, et al. Liver transplantation for sclerosing cholangitis. Hepatology 1995;22(2):451–7.
46. Uemura T, Ikegami T, Sanchez EQ, et al. Late acute rejection after liver transplantation impacts patient survival. Clin Transpl 2008;22(3):316–23.
47. Rowe IA, Webb K, Gunson BK, et al. The impact of disease recurrence on graft survival following liver transplantation: a single centre experience. Transpl Int 2008;21(5):459–65.
48. Maheshwari A, Yoo HY, Thuluvath PJ. Long-term outcome of liver transplantation in patients with PSC: a comparative analysis with PBC. Am J Gastroenterol 2004; 99(3):538–42.
49. Jorgensen KK, Grzyb K, Lundin KE, et al. Inflammatory bowel disease in patients with primary sclerosing cholangitis: clinical characterization in liver transplanted and nontransplanted patients. Inflamm Bowel Dis 2012;18(3):536–45.
50. Navaneethan U, Choudhary M, Venkatesh PG, et al. The effects of liver transplantation on the clinical course of colitis in ulcerative colitis patients with primary sclerosing cholangitis. Aliment Pharmacol Ther 2012;35(9):1054–63.
51. Verdonk RC, Dijkstra G, Haagsma EB, et al. Inflammatory bowel disease after liver transplantation: risk factors for recurrence and de novo disease. Am J Transplant 2006;6(6):1422–9.
52. Schreuder TC, Hubscher SG, Neuberger J. Autoimmune liver diseases and recurrence after orthotopic liver transplantation: what have we learned so far? Transpl Int 2009;22(2):144–52.
53. Jorgensen KK, Lindstrom L, Cvancarova M, et al. Immunosuppression after liver transplantation for primary sclerosing cholangitis influences activity of inflammatory bowel disease. Clin Gastroenterol Hepatol 2013;11(5):517–23.
54. El-Nachef N, Terdiman J, Mahadevan U. Anti-tumor necrosis factor therapy for inflammatory bowel disease in the setting of immunosuppression for solid organ transplantation. Am J Gastroenterol 2010;105(5):1210–1.
55. Lal S, Steinhart AH. Infliximab for ulcerative colitis following liver transplantation. Eur J Gastroenterol Hepatol 2007;19(3):277–80.
56. Mohabbat AB, Sandborn WJ, Loftus EV Jr, et al. Anti-tumour necrosis factor treatment of inflammatory bowel disease in liver transplant recipients. Aliment Pharmacol Ther 2012;36(6):569–74.
57. Loftus EV Jr, Aguilar HI, Sandborn WJ, et al. Risk of colorectal neoplasia in patients with primary sclerosing cholangitis and ulcerative colitis following orthotopic liver transplantation. Hepatology 1998;27(3):685–90.
58. Vera A, Gunson BK, Ussatoff V, et al. Colorectal cancer in patients with inflammatory bowel disease after liver transplantation for primary sclerosing cholangitis. Transplantation 2003;75(12):1983–8.
59. Trautwein C, Possienke M, Schlitt HJ, et al. Bone density and metabolism in patients with viral hepatitis and cholestatic liver diseases before and after liver transplantation. Am J Gastroenterol 2000;95(9):2343–51.

60. Lucey MR, Terrault N, Ojo L, et al. Long-term management of the successful adult liver transplant: 2012 practice guideline by the American Association for the Study of Liver Diseases and the American Society of Transplantation. Liver Transpl 2013;19(1):3–26.

61. Gross CR, Malinchoc M, Kim WR, et al. Quality of life before and after liver transplantation for cholestatic liver disease. Hepatology 1999;29(2):356–64.

62. Dickson ER, Grambsch PM, Fleming TR, et al. Prognosis in primary biliary cirrhosis: model for decision making. Hepatology 1989;10(1):1–7.

63. European Association for the Study of the Liver. EASL clinical practice guidelines: management of cholestatic liver diseases. J Hepatol 2009;51(2):237–67.

64. Mendes FD, Kim WR, Pedersen R, et al. Mortality attributable to cholestatic liver disease in the United States. Hepatology 2008;47(4):1241–7.

65. Angulo P, Dickson ER, Therneau TM, et al. Comparison of three doses of ursodeoxycholic acid in the treatment of primary biliary cirrhosis: a randomized trial. J Hepatol 1999;30(5):830–5.

66. Liermann Garcia RF, Evangelista Garcia C, McMaster P, et al. Transplantation for primary biliary cirrhosis: retrospective analysis of 400 patients in a single center. Hepatology 2001;33(1):22–7.

67. Silveira MG, Talwalkar JA, Lindor KD, et al. Recurrent primary biliary cirrhosis after liver transplantation. Am J Transplant 2010;10(4):720–6.

68. Carbone M, Bufton S, Monaco A, et al. The effect of liver transplantation on fatigue in patients with primary biliary cirrhosis: a prospective study. J Hepatol 2013;59(3):490–4.

69. Duclos-Vallee JC, Sebagh M. Recurrence of autoimmune disease, primary sclerosing cholangitis, primary biliary cirrhosis, and autoimmune hepatitis after liver transplantation. Liver Transpl 2009;15(Suppl 2):S25–34.

70. Egawa H, Sakisaka S, Teramukai S, et al. Long-term outcomes of living-donor liver transplantation for primary biliary cirrhosis: a Japanese multicenter study. Am J Transplant 2016;16(4):1248–57.

71. Guy JE, Qian P, Lowell JA, et al. Recurrent primary biliary cirrhosis: peritransplant factors and ursodeoxycholic acid treatment post-liver transplant. Liver Transpl 2005;11(10):1252–7.

72. Morioka D, Egawa H, Kasahara M, et al. Impact of human leukocyte antigen mismatching on outcomes of living donor liver transplantation for primary biliary cirrhosis. Liver Transpl 2007;13(1):80–90.

73. Neuberger J, Gunson B, Hubscher S, et al. Immunosuppression affects the rate of recurrent primary biliary cirrhosis after liver transplantation. Liver Transpl 2004; 10(4):488–91.

74. Dmitrewski J, Hubscher SG, Mayer AD, et al. Recurrence of primary biliary cirrhosis in the liver allograft: the effect of immunosuppression. J Hepatol 1996; 24(3):253–7.

75. Gautam M, Cheruvattath R, Balan V. Recurrence of autoimmune liver disease after liver transplantation: a systematic review. Liver Transpl 2006;12(12):1813–24.

76. Manousou P, Arvaniti V, Tsochatzis E, et al. Primary biliary cirrhosis after liver transplantation: influence of immunosuppression and human leukocyte antigen locus disparity. Liver Transpl 2010;16(1):64–73.

77. Hashimoto T, Sugawara Y, Makuuchi M. Impact of human leukocyte antigen mismatching on outcomes of living donor liver transplantation for primary biliary cirrhosis. Liver Transpl 2007;13(6):938–9.

78. Charatcharoenwitthaya P, Pimentel S, Talwalkar JA, et al. Long-term survival and impact of ursodeoxycholic acid treatment for recurrent primary biliary cirrhosis after liver transplantation. Liver Transpl 2007;13(9):1236–45.

79. Heathcote EJ, Stone J, Cauch-Dudek K, et al. Effect of pretransplantation ursodeoxycholic acid therapy on the outcome of liver transplantation in patients with primary biliary cirrhosis. Liver Transpl Surg 1999;5(4):269–74.

80. Bosch A, Dumortier J, Maucort-Boulch D, et al. Preventive administration of UDCA after liver transplantation for primary biliary cirrhosis is associated with a lower risk of disease recurrence. J Hepatol 2015;63(6):1449–58.

81. Jacob DA, Neumann UP, Bahra M, et al. Long-term follow-up after recurrence of primary biliary cirrhosis after liver transplantation in 100 patients. Clin Transpl 2006;20(2):211–20.

82. Jacob DA, Neumann UP, Bahra M, et al. Liver transplantation for primary biliary cirrhosis: influence of primary immunosuppression on survival. Transplant Proc 2005;37(4):1691–2.

83. Jacob DA, Bahra M, Schmidt SC, et al. Mayo risk score for primary biliary cirrhosis: a useful tool for the prediction of course after liver transplantation? Ann Transplant 2008;13(3):35–42.

84. Harimoto N, Ikegami T, Nakagawara H, et al. Chronic immune-mediated reaction syndrome as the cause of late graft mortality in living-donor liver transplantation for primary biliary cirrhosis. Transplant Proc 2014;46(5):1438–43.

85. Berlakovich GA, Imhof M, Karner-Hanusch J, et al. The importance of the effect of underlying disease on rejection outcomes following orthotopic liver transplantation. Transplantation 1996;61(4):554–60.

86. Hayashi M, Keeffe EB, Krams SM, et al. Allograft rejection after liver transplantation for autoimmune liver diseases. Liver Transpl Surg 1998;4(3):208–14.

87. Thurairajah PH, Carbone M, Bridgestock H, et al. Late acute liver allograft rejection; a study of its natural history and graft survival in the current era. Transplantation 2013;95(7):955–9.

88. Carbone M, Neuberger JM. Autoimmune liver disease, autoimmunity and liver transplantation. J Hepatol 2014;60(1):210–23.

The New Era of Hepatitis C Therapy in Liver Transplant Recipients

Ester Coelho Little, MD[a,b], Marina Berenguer, MD[c],*

KEYWORDS

- Hepatitis C virus • Direct antiviral agents • Cirrhosis • Hepatocellular carcinoma
- Liver transplant • Drug-drug interactions • Anti-HCV–positive donors • Waiting list

KEY POINTS

- The use of highly effective and well-tolerated direct antiviral agents against hepatitis C virus (HCV) in the setting of liver transplant has many potential implications.
- With current oral combinations, treatment of patients before and after liver transplant results in sustained viral response rates greater than 95% except in the subset of patients with severely advanced liver disease with portal hypertension.
- The decision to treat before or after liver transplant should take into consideration several variables, particularly the degree of liver and kidney impairment, the presence of hepatocellular carcinoma, the waiting time, the center allocation policy, and the local prevalence of anti-HCV–positive donors.
- Drug-drug interactions, particularly with immunosuppressive agents, need to be considered when treating patients with current oral antivirals both before and after liver transplant.

INTRODUCTION

Until 2011, when the only available treatment of hepatitis C virus (HCV) infection was the combination of pegylated interferon and ribavirin, treatment of HCV in liver recipients was mostly limited to posttransplant, and it was only started if fibrosis was seen on liver biopsy.[1–5] As in the general HCV population, patients who achieved sustained virologic response (SVR) had a better outcome, reflected by reduced and even reversed fibrosis progression and less development of compensated and decompensated cirrhosis, ultimately resulting in improved graft and patient survival.[6–8] Improvement in extrahepatic complications of chronic HCV infection, such as renal function,

Disclosures: Dr M. Berenguer discloses that Ciberehd is partially funded by the Instituto de Salud Carlos III (ISCIII). Dr E.C. Little has nothing to disclose.
[a] Banner Transplant Institute, 1441 North 12th Street, Second floor, Phoenix, AZ 85006, USA; [b] Banner University Medical Center Phoenix, Phoenix, AZ, USA; [c] Servicio de Medicina Digestivo (Torre F-5), La Fe University Hospital, Ciberehd*, University of Valencia, Avda Fernando Abril Martorell n 106, Valencia 46026, Spain
* Corresponding author.
E-mail address: marina.berenguer@uv.es

http://dx.doi.org/10.1016/j.cld.2016.12.012
1089-3261/17/© 2017 Elsevier Inc. All rights reserved.

liver.theclinics.com

was also described.[9] However, SVR rate was limited to 20% to 30% in patients with genotype 1 and 40% to 50% in those with genotype 2 and 3.[1–5] Severity of adverse effects was a major limitation to treatment, with the need for dose reduction seen in 70% of the patients and treatment discontinuation in 30% of them. In addition, interferon was associated with immune-mediated complications, with acute and chronic rejection occurring in 1% to 2% of the patients treated.[1–5,10,11]

With the introduction of the first available NS3/4A protease inhibitors (PI) boceprevir and telaprevir, a meaningful improvement in the SVR rate was seen, but at the expense of significant adverse effects requiring dose reduction, as well as close monitoring of drug levels and drug-drug interaction with the immunosuppressive (IS) medications.[12–14] The use of the first available PIs was short lived because of the emergence of the second wave of the direct-acting antivirals (DAAs).

The discovery of the more potent and better-tolerated DAAs marked a new era in the treatment of HCV infection. With their use, a shift away from HCV as the main reason for liver transplant (LT) is expected to occur in Europe and the United States in the near future.[15] With the advent of the second wave of DAAs came the possibility to rescue posttransplant patients who had progressed to advanced stages of fibrosis and did not tolerate or did not respond to treatment with pegylated interferon/ribavirin or the first wave of PIs. Compassionate use of sofosbuvir and ribavirin in the posttransplant population produced response rates of 59% in this historically difficult-to-treat population.[16] Progressing from compassionate use to small series, and then to larger multicenter clinical trials,[16–33] the DAA reached the status of standard of care for the treatment of HCV in LT patients in a short period of time. At the same time came the realization that patients could also be easily and successfully treated while waiting for LT, thus preventing HCV recurrence post-LT.[34] However, the question of when to treat such patients remains controversial.[35,36]

WHEN TO TREAT HEPATITIS C VIRUS IN PATIENTS WHO NEED LIVER TRANSPLANT

If initiated when there is less severe fibrosis, the response rate to DAAs is superior to that of patients treated at a more advanced stage of the disease, particularly at the stage of decompensated cirrhosis.[30–32] In recent reports, favorable response rates have been achieved, even in those with more advanced cirrhosis, including Child-Turcotte-Pugh (CTP) class B and C, with surprisingly few severe adverse effects[30–32] (Table 1).

The decision to treat patients who are listed for transplant before or after the procedure is still under debate. Clinicians who are in favor of treating these patients before transplant must first consider whether the goal of treatment is to prevent reinfection of the graft[34] or to give the patients a chance to achieve such significant improvement that they will ultimately be removed from the transplant wait list[37–40] (Table 2).

The benefits of HCV eradication in the era of pegylated interferon/ribavirin is well documented. It includes reduction in fibrosis score, hepatic venous pressure, rate of progression of liver failure, rate of liver-related mortality, incidence of hepatocellular carcinoma (HCC), and all cause mortally.[41] Because not much time has elapsed since the advent of the DAAs, evidence that the same benefits will be seen with eradication of HCV with these medications is less robust, but likely to be similar to that of treatment with pegylated interferon/ribavirin.[30,32,38–43] In the early analysis of patients with decompensated cirrhosis who were successfully treated, achieving SVR was associated with improvement in Model for End-stage Liver Disease (MELD) and Child Turcotte Pugh (CTP) scores in a large number of patients.[30–32,43] Overall, 60% in registry trials have shown an improvement in MELD score from baseline to 12 weeks after therapy, but about one-quarter deteriorated despite viral clearance. Furthermore, 2 recent studies

Table 1
Hepatitis C virus treatment after liver transplant: summary of trials

Trial Name	Regimen	N	Genotype (GT)	Duration (wk)	Sustained Viral Response (SVR-12) (Fibrosis Score)	Immunosuppression
CORAL 1	Paritaprevir/ ritonavir/ ombitasvir/ dasabuvir	34	1a and 1b	24	<F2: 97%	Tacrolimus: 85%
SOLAR 1	Sofosbuvir/ ledipasvir/ ribavirin	112	1a, 1b, and 4	12	<F3: 96% CTP A: 96% CTP B: 85% CTP C: 60%	Tacrolimus: 76%
SOLAR 1	Sofosbuvir/ ledipasvir/ ribavirin	111	1a and 1b	24	<F3: 98% CTP A: 96% CTP B: 88% CTP C: 75%	
SOLAR 2	Sofosbuvir/ ledipasvir/ ribavirin	111	1a, 1b, and 4	12	<F3: 93% CTP A: 100% CTP B: 95% CTP C:50%	Tacrolimus: 64%
Solar 2	Sofosbuvir/ ledipasvir/ ribavirin	110	1a and 1b	24	<F4: 100% CTP A: 96% CTP B: 100% CTP C:80%	
ALLY 1	Sofosbuvir/ daclatasvir/ ribavirin	53	1a, 1b, 3 and 6	12	95% GT 1 91% GT 3	Tacrolimus: 83%

Table 2
Advantages and limitations of pre–liver transplant versus post–liver transplant antiviral therapy

	Advantages	Limitations

Pre-LT	High SVR rate
	• Prevent HCV recurrence
	  ○ Simplify post-LT management
	  ○ Improve post-LT outcome
	• Result in MELD and clinical improvement
	  ○ Allow HCC LRT
	  ○ Bridge to LT
	  ○ Delist from WL
	  ○ Spare livers for non-HCV indications
		Lower SVR rate in CHILD C patients
		• Risk of treatment failure caused by RAV with an unknown course post-LT
		DDI (polymedicated)
		Toxicity (almost no data in MELD >20)
		Insufficient MELD improvement; MELD purgatory
		Exclude the option for anti-HCV–positive donors

Post-LT	High SVR rate • Reduce disease progression • Improve graft and patient survival • Improve extrahepatic manifestations of HCV • Improve QOL	Reduced SVR rates in severely decompensated graft cirrhosis DDI (particularly with IS) Difficulty in choosing therapy in the setting of renal impairment

Abbreviations: DDI, drug-drug interactions; HCC, hepatocellular carcinoma; LRT, locoregional therapies; MELD, Model for End-stage Liver Disease; QOL, quality of life; RAV, resistance-associated variants; WL, waiting list.

using data from the English Expanded Access Program, in which decompensated treated patients were compared with a retrospective cohort of similarly decompensated patients who received no treatment for 6 months before the availability of DAAs, showed that treated patients had fewer decompensations, reduced deterioration of MELD score, and overall fewer adverse events.[39,40] In an updated study with longer follow-up (15 months posttherapy), the investigators confirmed their initial findings showing decreasing adverse events rate over time. There were 3% deaths, 5% new liver cancers, 12% LT, and 16% serious decompensations over 15 months among the 317 out of 406 patients who achieved SVR. Compared with the first 6 months from start of treatment and with the group of untreated patients, there was a reduction in incidence of decompensations (7% in months 6–15 and 18% in months 0–6 vs 28% in untreated patients). There was no significant difference in liver cancer incidence (2.5% in months 6–15 and 4% in months 0–6 vs 4% in untreated patients).[40]

Whether or not eradication of HCV treatment with DAAs can result in removing the patient from the LT waiting list is a question with broader implications and limited data at this point.[37–40] Both of the authors of this article have witnessed isolated success stories in their own patient populations. Information derived from a larger number of patients became available with the recent publication of a retrospective, multicenter European study.[38] The authors reported the outcome of 103 consecutive LT candidates with decompensated cirrhosis and no HCC treated with different combinations of DAAs. The cumulative incidences of inactivation and removal from the transplant wait list were seen in 15.5% and 0% of the patients 24 weeks after the start of therapy, in 27.6% and 10.3% of the patients 48 weeks after the start of therapy, and 33% and 19% of the patients 60 weeks after the start of therapy. Using a multivariate competing risk model, 3 variables were identified as predictors of inactivation from the LT waiting list: baseline MELD, delta MELD, and delta albumin. The long-term outcome of the group of patients that was removed from the transplant waiting list and whether similar results will be found by other investigators remain to be seen.

The benefit of any strategy resulting in patients being removed from the waiting list because of significant improvement is irrefutable. In addition to the patients' individual gains, more organs will be available for those who will remain in need of this life-saving procedure.[15] Equally irrefutable is the notion that some of the patients on the transplant waiting list who achieve SVR will continue to progress toward liver failure and/or will develop HCC.[37–40] Depending on the area where they live, these patients will be faced with the fact that there may be a decline in the pool of possible donors, such as those serologically positive for HCV.[44] Although the use of a positive donor could still be an option, retreating patients who have already been treated for HCV is, at least at the current cost, a counterproductive strategy from an economic standpoint.[45]

Another possible scenario in the strategy of treating patients on the waiting list before transplant is the possibility of a decrease in the MELD score not followed by a substantial improvement in the patient's quality of life or even worsening of the complications related to the cirrhosis.[30–32,38–40,43] Depending on the average MELD score at the time of transplant in the area where the patient resides, the decrease in the MELD score following treatment may leave the patient with a MELD score that is less than the average MELD at the time of transplant. This lower score will prolong the time the patient remains on the wait list; the so-called MELD purgatory.[36] This outcome is particularly worrisome for patients who are at an advanced age, in whom the possibility of future decompensation or development of HCC may occur at a time when LT is no longer a viable option.

Waiting to treat the HCV after transplant eliminates both the dilemma of decreasing the pool of donors and the MELD purgatory. More importantly, with the advent of the

DAAs, treatment of posttransplant patients, particularly early on (before progression to more advance stages of fibrosis) has response rates that are similar to those seen in the general HCV population[17–19,23–33] (see **Tables 1** and **2**). These patients are no longer considered part of the population that is difficult to treat and cure. Hence, the choice of treating listed patients solely to prevent the infection of the graft in the era of the new DAAs has less merit.

The dilemma of when to treat HCV in patients listed for transplant could be eliminated if clinicians could identify the patients for whom treatment would allow their removal from the transplant waiting list when it is still likely that the liver functions and the patient's quality of life will be restored to near normal. To be able to accurately identify this group of patients can be considered the Holy Grail of transplant hepatology in the era of DAAs for treatment of HCV. Some factors, such as baseline MELD, delta MELD, baseline albumin level, and age, are helpful,[38–40] but none is 100% accurate in such a complex setting. Until clinicians find the Holy Grail, each treating doctor needs to carefully consider which strategy might be best for which patients. Attention must be given to the patient's age and overall health and nutritional status, the local allocation policy, the average MELD at the time of transplant, and the local prevalence of HCV-positive donors. In addition, it is important to exercise caution when choosing the treatment option in order to avoid the risk of selecting resistance-associated variants (RAVs) of HCV, particularly when treating those who previously failed antiviral therapy.[46]

Based on clinical experience and the currently available data, while waiting for the clearly optimal solution, the authors propose an algorithm based on 3 main factors: baseline MELD score, indication for transplant, and expected response rate to DAAs, intended to guide clinicians facing this challenging dilemma (**Fig. 1**).

A unique subset of patients is those with HCC because these patients are transplanted regardless of their response to antiviral therapy; as long as the cirrhosis is well compensated, waiting to treat them after transplant is likely a wiser choice. In contrast, in those with HCC with more advanced cirrhosis, HCV treatment with possible clinical improvement may be the only opportunity for these patients to receive locoregional therapy as a bridge for LT, with a decreased risk of cancer

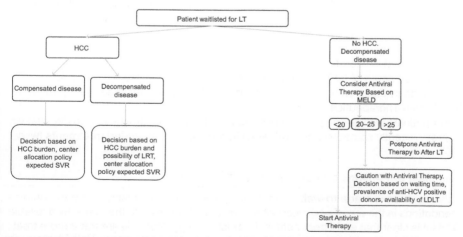

Fig. 1. Management of patients infected with HCV before and after liver transplant. LDLT, live donor liver transplantation; LRT, locoregional therapies.

spread. In this group of patients, HCV treatment before transplant has more clear benefits.

A second unique group is patients with renal failure. In the era of pegylated interferon and ribavirin, patients with HCV and renal insufficiency rarely underwent HCV therapy. Many are now listed for kidney transplant and LT, whereas those with well-preserved liver function are listed for kidney transplant only. For the patients with no cirrhosis or with well-compensated cirrhosis, treatment of HCV before transplant may bring the benefit of improving the liver damage to the point of removing the need for LT. In this case, patients can be moved to the kidney waiting list. The recommended treatment of this group of patients is with elbasvir and grazoprevir.[47] This combination therapy is well tolerated and has an overall response rate that is also in the range of 95% to 100%. For those with more advanced liver disease/decompensated cirrhosis, treatment with the PI grazoprevir is not indicated given the risk of decompensation of the cirrhosis.[48] For these patients, waiting until after the liver/kidney transplant to have HCV treated is the safest and currently only available option, although recent preliminary data suggest that sofosbuvir may be an option in these patients.[49,50]

HOW TO TREAT HEPATITIS C VIRUS IN PATIENTS LISTED FOR LIVER TRANSPLANT
Treatment of Patients with Cirrhosis

The treatment of patients with cirrhosis on the waiting list for transplant is the same as for those not listed. Details of the response rates on this patient population are outside the scope of this review. For patients with genotypes 1 and 4, the combination of sofosbuvir with ledipasvir, daclatasvir, or velpatasvir has high response rates and is well tolerated.[30–32,43] Other options are the combination of elbasvir and grazoprevir; the combination of paritaprevir, ritonavir, ombitasvir, and dasabuvir; and the combination of sofosbuvir and simeprevir in patients with genotype 1b.[50–52]

The severity of the adverse events and risk of further decompensation of cirrhosis in patients treated with the second wave of NS3/4A PI is not as severe as that seen in those treated with pegylated interferon, boceprevir, and telaprevir. Nevertheless, the risk of further decompensation of cirrhosis with 1 death in a clinical trial using the combination of the PI paritaprevir with ombitasvir and dasabuvir resulted in the recommendation in the United States against the use of PIs in patients with advanced cirrhosis (CTP class B and C) and caution when treating patients with cirrhosis CTP class A[52] (www.HCVguidelines.org).

Another concern is that simeprevir is metabolized by the hepatic cytochrome P450 3A system and is excreted by the biliary tract with area under the curve (AUC) values from 0 to 24 hours of 240% and 520% higher in CTP class B and C patients respectively, than in those with normal liver function (Simeprevir package insert; Titusville, NJ. Jansen Therapeutics, 2013).[48,53,54]

For patients with genotypes 2 and 3, the combination of sofosbuvir and daclatasvir, or more recently sofosbuvir and velpatasvir, are the recommended treatments (www. HCV.gov).

Treatment of Hepatitis C Virus After Liver Transplant

If the decision is made to wait to treat the patient after transplant, unlike the recommendations in the era of pegylated interferon and ribavirin, with the currently available DAAs it is clear that early treatment is the best strategy. Not only are there more treatment options available, but the response rate is also more favorable.[17–19,23–33] Nonetheless, there are some issues unique to the treatment of HCV after LT. The first is the risk associated with drug-drug interaction between the DAAs and the IS medications.[48] The cytochrome P450 enzyme system, particularly the 3A4 (CYP3A4) isoenzyme, is responsible for the oxidation of many drugs. Interaction with P-glycoprotein (P-gp) and breast cancer–resistant protein also can potentially affect drug bioavailability. P-gp and CYP450 enzymes are present in the liver and gastrointestinal tract and the DAAs are metabolized through these pathways.[54–56] Changes in drug concentrations affect both the DAAs as well as the IS medications to different degrees. Some of the interactions are significant to the point that their use should be avoided (simeprevir and cyclosporine), whereas others are not clinically significant (cyclosporine and tacrolimus with daclatasvir and sofosbuvir). **Table 3** summarizes these drug-drug interactions.

Another concern is the need to adjust the dose of the IS medications after completion of the HCV treatment, which has been reported in a few studies.[33,57,58] It is speculated that the improvement in liver function explains the increased need for IS medications.[58] Calcineurin inhibitors, mammalian target of rapamycin inhibitors, and antimetabolites are metabolized by the CYP3A4 and the metabolic function of the liver affects the bioavailability of these medications (see Duminda Suraweera and colleagues' article, "Liver Transplantation and Bariatric Surgery: Best Approach," in this issue for more information).

AVAILABLE TREATMENT REGIMENS
Sofosbuvir and Ribavirin

The combinations of sofosbuvir and ribavirin for a period of 24 weeks was first used in patients with genotypes 1 and 4, with fibrosis varying from none/minimal to cirrhosis and an overall response rate of 70% at 12 weeks.[57] The efficacy of this regimen was later proved to be inferior to the combination of sofosbuvir with a second DAA and currently the combination of sofosbuvir and ribavirin is limited to the treatment of patients with HCV genotype 2.

Sofosbuvir and Ledipasvir

The use of sofosbuvir and the NS5A inhibitor ledipasvir in combination with weight-based ribavirin for patients with genotypes 1 and 4 was evaluated in the SOLAR-1 study.[30] A group of posttransplant patients with Metavir fibrosis score from F0 to F3 (n = 111), compensated cirrhosis, CTP class A (n = 51) and decompensated cirrhosis, and CTP class B and C (n = 61) were treated for 12 or 24 weeks. Based on intention to treat analysis SVR was achieved in 96% to 98% of the patients with no cirrhosis or

Table 3				
Need to adjust immunosuppressive medications when using direct antiviral agents				
	Cyclosporine	Tacrolimus	MMF	mTOR
Sofosbuvir	No adjustment	No adjustment	No adjustment	Not available
Simeprevir	Not recommended	No adjustment	No adjustment	Not available
Ledipasvir	No adjustment	No adjustment	No adjustment	Not available
Daclatasvir	No adjustment	No adjustment	No adjustment	Not available
3D[a]	Needs adjustment	Needs adjustment	Needs adjustment	Not available
Grazoprevir/ elbasvir	Not recommended	Needs adjustment	Not available	Not available

Abbreviations: MMF, mycophenolate mofetil; mTOR, mammalian target of rapamycin.
[a] Paritaprevir, ritonavir, ombitasvir, dasabuvir combination.

compensated cirrhosis. Among the patients with decompensated cirrhosis, those with CTP class B had a response rate of 86% to 88%. The group of patients with cirrhosis CTP class C had the lowest response rate: 60% and 75% respectively in patients treated for 12 and 24 weeks. With the exception of the patients with decompensated cirrhosis, the response rate did not vary substantially by the presence or absence of cirrhosis or by treating for 12 or 24 weeks.

In a similarly designed study, SOLAR-2, the posttransplant group comprised patients with no cirrhosis (n = 101), patients with cirrhosis CTP class A (n = 67), CTP class B (n = 45), and CTP class C (n = 8). Among the patients with genotype 1 treated for 12 or 24 weeks the response rate varied from 93% and 100% in all 4 groups.[31]

The number of patients with genotype 1 far exceeded that of those with genotype 4 in both trials. In the 27 patients with genotype 4 included in the SOLAR-2 trial, SVR was achieved in 75% to 100% of them. The rate of adverse events was common in both trials discussed earlier; however, adverse events led to premature discontinuation of therapy in only 4% and 2% of the patients enrolled in the SOLAR-1 and SOLAR-2 trials respectively.

There are limited data on the use of sofosbuvir and ledipasvir combination in genotype 3, and almost no data on the use of this combination in the posttransplant setting,[39] but it is likely that the results will resemble those seen in the general non-transplanted population.[59]

Sofosbuvir and Simeprevir

Multiple sites, including academic and community LT centers, have published their experiences with sofosbuvir and simeprevir with and without ribavirin. All patients had genotype 1 and patients with Metavir score F0 to F4 were included. In 2016, Nguyen and colleagues[25] published a systematic review and meta-analysis that included 325 patients treated in the United States with a combination of sofosbuvir and simeprevir with and without ribavirin for 12 weeks. Most patients included in the study were male, white, and had genotype 1, and the mean age was 60 years. The pooled SVR rate was 88% (95% confidence interval, 83.4%–91.5%). Although some patients treated with the sofosbuvir and simeprevir combination also received ribavirin, neither the addition of ribavirin nor the duration of treatment affected the response rate. The only difference in response rate was seen when comparing patients with less (Metavir score F0-2) and those with more (Metavir score F3-4) advanced stages of fibrosis: 95% and 82% respectively. Treatment was well tolerated and the most common adverse effects were headache, fatigue, infection, and anemia.

Sofosbuvir and Daclatasvir

With the combination of sofosbuvir, daclatasvir, and ribavirin in a cohort of 53 posttransplant patients the response rate was 94% in genotype 1 and 91% in genotype 3.[32] When used in combination with simeprevir, with and without ribavirin, the response rate decreased to 67% to 72%. With either sofosbuvir or simeprevir, daclatasvir is well tolerated except for anemia when used in combination with ribavirin. When calcineurin inhibitor was the IS used in patients treated with daclatasvir, there was an increase in the AUC of daclatasvir; however, there was no clinical relevance associated with this. As seen in the use of other DAAs in the posttransplant setting, the severity of the disease before initiation of treatment was the major determinant of response rate when patients were treated with daclatasvir.[28,32,60]

In HCV infections with genotype 2 without advanced disease the combination of sofosbuvir and daclatasvir with ribavirin for 12 weeks is recommended, and the duration of treatment is prolonged to 24 weeks in patients who cannot tolerate ribavirin.

For patients with genotype 3, the currently recommended therapy is the combination of sofosbuvir and daclatasvir with ribavirin for 12 weeks. For ribavirin-ineligible patients, the treatment is prolonged to 24 weeks.[32,61]

Paritaprevir, Ritonavir, Ombitasvir, and Ribavirin

The combination of paritaprevir, ritonavir, ombitasvir, and ribavirin was used in 34 posttransplant patients with genotype 1 infection.[33] All patients had Metavir fibrosis score F0 to F2. The medications were administrated on a fixed dose for 24 weeks. The response rate was 97% and the most common adverse effects were fatigue, headache, and cough. Only 1 of the patients discontinued treatment because of adverse effects. Because of drug-drug interaction between ritonavir and calcineurin inhibitors, dose adjustment was needed during the treatment. As mentioned earlier, this combination treatment is not indicated for patients with decompensated cirrhosis given the risk of worsening the cirrhosis and concerns for hepatotoxicity.

Other Combinations

The excellent results with use of sofosbuvir and velpatasvir in the nontransplant population coupled with its pangenotypic properties make this a promising regimen for patients with HCV recurrence posttransplant.[43] Its pharmacokinetic profile is similar to that of ledipasvir and therefore significant drug-drug interactions are not expected. However, there are no available data on the use of sofosbuvir and velpatasvir in the posttransplant setting.

The use of a fixed-dose combination of elbasvir and grazoprevir in patients with HCV genotypes 1 and 4, and in particular its safety on patients with renal insufficiency, brought significant gain to the population of patients infected with HCV. However, there is limited experience with its use in patients with more advanced disease and none in the posttransplant population.[47] Given that a PI is part of this combination, it is not recommended for patients with advanced decompensated liver disease, and drug-drug interactions with the IS agents are expected.[48]

The combination of 3 different DAAs (1 NS3/4A, 1 NS5a, and 1 NS5b) is also a promising alternative but is not yet approved by the United States or Europe,[46] particularly for patients failing DAA therapy.

FIBROSING CHOLESTATIC HEPATITIS

Fibrosing cholestatic hepatitis (FCH), characterized by rapid progression of portal fibrosis and cholestasis following transplant, is estimated to occur in 2% to 10% of patients. It is suggested that FCH results from the effects of direct viral toxicity in the context of immunosuppression.[62] The prognosis of FCH is poor (50%–90% mortality in 2 years) and, given the nature of the disease, retransplant of the affected patients is controversial.

The early attempts to treat FCH with pegylated interferon–based therapies resulted in serious adverse events, including sepsis and death.[13]

The advent of the second-generation DAAs changed the course of this severe complication of HCV in posttransplant patients. In the initial reports, patients were treated with sofosbuvir and ribavirin; more recent reports used a combination of 2 DAAs (ie, sofosbuvir with ledipasvir and sofosbuvir with daclatasvir). As seen in the general HCV-infected population, the best indicator of response is the severity of the fibrosis; hence early treatment is the key factor. Data derived from small series showed SVR-12 (Sustained Viral Response) in up to 100% of the patients when treatment was started early, with very significant clinical improvement.[29–32]

RESISTANCE-ASSOCIATED VARIANTS

When properly chosen and properly taken, the current, more potent, DAAs rarely fail to achieve eradication of the HCV virus. Nonadherence, especially during the early phase of treatment, is associated with the emergency of RAVs.[63] Although there are some circumstances in which failure to achieve SVR is not associated with the virus itself, the emergence of RAVs is the main reason for failure to eradicate the virus. It is estimated that 53% to 91% of patients with virologic relapse harbor HCV isolates that are resistant to 1, 2, or 3 DAAs.[46,63]

There are no current data on the emergency of RAVs in the posttransplant population, but data from studies in the general HCV population can be used to guide choices and avoid pitfalls when treating posttransplant patients.[64]

Not all viruses with RAVs are fit. RAVs associated with the use of PIs disappear after treatment withdrawal; in contrast, RAVs associated with NS5A tend to remain present long after treatment discontinuation. Although the clinical relevance of the HCV RAVs is not completely understood, care must be exercised when retreating patients who failed to respond to one of the DAAs.[45,63]

SUMMARY

The advent of the DAAs has revolutionized transplant hepatology with an expected shift away from HCV as the main reason for LT in Europe and the United States in the near future.

With the exception of patients with genotype 2, who can be successfully treated with sofosbuvir and ribavirin, the combination of 2 DAAs with or without ribavirin is the mainstay in the treatment of patients with HCV posttransplant.

Sofosbuvir in combination with ledipasvir, daclatasvir, or simeprevir with or without ribavirin has excellent response rates in the posttransplant population. Caution needs to be exercised when treating patients with cirrhosis with PI, and this class of drugs is contraindicated in those with decompensated cirrhosis (CTP B or C).

Drug-drug interaction needs attention when treating HCV posttransplant, particularly with regard to the need to adjust the dose of the IS medications.

The decision of when to treat patients listed for LT is unresolved. There are potential benefits associated with treatment before transplant, with the possibility of achieving not only SVR but also clinical improvement that will allow the removal of some patients from the LT waiting list. How to identify those who will benefit from this strategy remains a puzzle.

Treatment of HCV with DAAs after the LT is better and safer than ever before. It should be initiated early in the course of the disease before progression to more advanced stages of fibrosis.

The decision of when to treat these patients should be made carefully and taking into consideration the characteristics of each individual patient as well as those of the transplant center.

REFERENCES

1. Samuel D, Forns X, Berenguer M, et al. Report of the monothematic EASL conference on liver transplantation for viral hepatitis (Paris, France, January 12-14, 2006). J Hepatol 2006;45:127–43.

2. Wang CS, Ko HH, Yoshida EM, et al. Interferon-based combination therapy for hepatitis C virus after liver transplantation: a review and quantitative analysis. Am J Transplant 2006;6:1586–99.

3. Berenguer M. Systematic review of the treatment of established recurrent hepatitis C with pegylated interferon in combination with ribavirin. J Hepatol 2008; 49(2):274–87.

4. Xirouchakis E, Triantos C, Manousou P, et al. Pegylated interferon and ribavirin in liver transplant candidates and recipients with HCV cirrhosis: systematic review and meta-analysis of prospective studies. J Viral Hepat 2008;15:699–709.

5. Berenguer M, Aguilera V, Rubín A, et al. Comparison of two non-contemporaneous HCV-liver transplant cohorts: strategies to improve the efficacy of antiviral therapy. J Hepatol 2012;56(6):1310–6.

6. Bizollon T, Pradat P, Mabrut JY, et al. Benefit of sustained virological response to combination therapy on graft survival of liver transplanted patients with recurrent chronic hepatitis C. Am J Transplant 2005;5(8):1909–13.

7. Picciotto FP, Tritto G, Lanza AG, et al. Sustained virological response to antiviral therapy reduces mortality in HCV reinfection after liver transplantation. J Hepatol 2007;46:459–65.

8. Berenguer M, Palau A, Aguilera V, et al. Clinical benefits of antiviral therapy in patients with recurrent hepatitis C following liver transplantation. Am J Transplant 2008;8(3):679–87.

9. Blé M, Aguilera V, Rubín A, et al. Improved renal function in liver transplant recipients treated for hepatitis C virus with a sustained virological response and mild chronic kidney disease. Liver Transpl 2014;20(1):25–34.

10. Selzner N, Guindi M, Renner EL, et al. Immune-mediated complications of the graft in interferon-treated hepatitis C positive liver transplant recipients. J Hepatol 2011;55(1):207–17.

11. Levitsky J, Fiel MI, Norvell JP, et al. Risk for immune-mediated graft dysfunction in liver transplant recipients with recurrent HCV infection treated with pegylated interferon. Gastroenterology 2012;142(5):1132–9.

12. Forns X, Didier S, Mutimer D, et al. Efficacy of telaprevir-based therapy in stable liver transplant patients with chronic genotype 1 hepatitis C. Ann Hepatol 2016; 15(4):512–23.

13. Coilly A, Roche B, Dumortier J, et al. Safety and efficacy of protease inhibitors to treat hepatitis C after liver transplantation: a multicenter experience. J Hepatol 2014;60(1):78–86.

14. Verna EC, Saxena V, Burton JR Jr, et al. Telaprevir- and boceprevir-based triple therapy for hepatitis C in liver transplant recipients with advanced recurrent disease: a multicenter study. Transplantation 2015;99(8):1644–51.

15. Jena AB, Stevens W, Gonzalez YS, et al. The wider public health value of HCV treatment accrued by liver transplant recipients. Am J Manag Care 2016;22(6 Spec No):SP212–9.

16. Forns X, Charlton M, Denning J, et al. Sofosbuvir compassionate use program for patients with severe recurrent hepatitis C following liver transplantation. Hepatology 2015;61(5):1485–94.

17. Pungpapong S, Aqel B, Leise M, et al. Multicenter experience using simeprevir and sofosbuvir with or without ribavirin to treat hepatitis C genotype 1 after liver transplant. Hepatology 2015;61(6):1880–6.

18. Saab S, Greenberg A, Li E, et al. Sofosbuvir and simeprevir is effective for recurrent hepatitis C in liver transplant recipients. Liver Int 2015;35(11):2442–7.

19. Gutierrez JA, Carrion AF, Avalos D, et al. Sofosbuvir and simeprevir for treatment of hepatitis C virus infection in liver transplant recipients. Liver Transpl 2015; 21(6):823–30.

20. Brown RS Jr, O'Leary JG, Reddy KR, et al, Hepatitis C Therapeutic Registry Research Network Study Group. Interferon-free therapy for genotype 1 hepatitis C in liver transplant recipients: real-world experience from the hepatitis C therapeutic registry and research network. Liver Transpl 2016;22(1):24–33.

21. Crittenden NE, Buchanan LA, Pinkston CM, et al. Simeprevir and sofosbuvir with or without ribavirin to treat recurrent genotype 1 hepatitis C virus infection after orthotopic liver transplantation. Liver Transpl 2016;22(5):635–43.

22. Jackson WE, Hanouneh M, Apfel T, et al. Sofosbuvir and simeprevir without ribavirin effectively treat hepatitis C virus genotype 1 infection after liver transplantation in a two-center experience. Clin Transplant 2016;30(6):709–13.

23. Faisal N, Bilodeau M, Aljudaibi B, et al. Sofosbuvir-based antiviral therapy is highly effective in recurrent hepatitis c in liver transplant recipients: Canadian multicenter "real-life" experience. Transplantation 2016;100(5):1059–65.

24. Ciesek S, Proske V, Otto B, et al. Efficacy and safety of sofosbuvir/ledipasvir for the treatment of patients with hepatitis C virus re-infection after liver transplantation. Transpl Infect Dis 2016;18(3):326–32.

25. Nguyen NH, Yee BE, Chang C, et al. Tolerability and effectiveness of sofosbuvir and simeprevir in the post-transplant setting: systematic review and meta-analysis. BMJ Open Gastroenterol 2016;3(1):e000066.

26. Coilly A, Fougerou-Leurent C, de Ledinghen V, et al, ANRS C023 CUPILT Study Group. Multicentre experience using daclatasvir and sofosbuvir to treat hepatitis C recurrence after liver transplantation - the CO23 ANRS CUPILT study. J Hepatol 2016;65(4):711–8.

27. Dumortier J, Leroy V, Duvoux C, et al. Sofosbuvir-based treatment of hepatitis C with severe fibrosis (METAVIR F3/F4) after liver transplantation: results from the CO23 ANRS CUPILT study. Liver Transpl 2016;22(10):1367–78.

28. Fontana RJ, Brown RS, Moreno-Zamora A, et al. Daclatasvir combined with sofosbuvir or simeprevir in liver transplant recipients with severe recurrent hepatitis C infection. Liver Transpl 2016;22(4):446–58.

29. Leroy V, Dumortier J, Coilly A, et al, Agence Nationale de Recherches sur le SIDA et les Hépatites Virales CO23 Compassionate Use of Protease Inhibitors in Viral C in Liver Transplantation Study Group. Efficacy of sofosbuvir and daclatasvir in patients with fibrosing cholestatic hepatitis C after liver transplantation. Clin Gastroenterol Hepatol 2015;13(11):1993–2001.

30. Charlton M, Everson GT, Flamm SL, et al. Ledipasvir and sofosbuvir plus ribavirin for treatment of HCV infection in patients with advanced liver disease. Gastroenterology 2015;149:649–59.

31. Manns M, Samuel D, Gane EJ, et al, SOLAR-2 Investigators. Ledipasvir and sofosbuvir plus ribavirin in patients with genotype 1 or 4 hepatitis C virus infection and advanced liver disease: a multicentre, open-label, randomised, phase 2 trial. Lancet Infect Dis 2016;16(6):685–97.

32. Poordad F, Schiff ER, Vierling JM, et al. Daclatasvir with sofosbuvir and ribavirin for hepatitis C virus infection with advanced cirrhosis or post-liver transplantation recurrence. Hepatology 2016;63(5):1493–505.

33. Kwo PY, Mantry PS, Coakley E, et al. An interferon-free antiviral regimen for HCV after liver transplantation. N Engl J Med 2014;371(25):2375–82.

34. Curry MP, Forns X, Chung RT, et al. Sofosbuvir and ribavirin prevent recurrence of HCV infection after liver transplantation: an open-label study. Gastroenterology 2015;148(1):100–7.

35. Bunchorntavakul C, Reddy KR. Treat chronic hepatitis C virus infection in decompensated cirrhosis - pre- or post-liver transplantation? The ironic conundrum in the era of effective and well-tolerated therapy. J Viral Hepat 2016;23(6):408–18.

36. Barsa JE, Branch AD, Schiano TD. A pleasant dilemma to have: to treat the HCV patient on the waiting list or to treat post-liver transplantation? Clin Transplant 2015;29(10):859–65.

37. Ruiz I, Feray C, Pawlotsky JM, et al. Patient with decompensated hepatitis C virus-related cirrhosis delisted for liver transplantation after successful sofosbuvir-based treatment. Liver Transpl 2015;21:408–9.

38. Belli LS, Berenguer M, Cortesi PA, et al, for the European Liver and Intestine Association (ELITA). Delisting of liver transplant candidates with chronic hepatitis C after viral eradication: a European study. J Hepatol 2016. http://dx.doi.org/10.1016/j.jhep.2016.05.010.

39. Foster GR, Irving WL, Cheung MC, et al, HCV Research, UK. Impact of direct acting antiviral therapy in patients with chronic hepatitis C and decompensated cirrhosis. J Hepatol 2016;64(6):1224–31.

40. Cheung M, Walker AJ, Hudson BE, et al. Outcomes after successful direct-acting antiviral therapy for patients with chronic hepatitis C and decompensated cirrhosis. J Hepatol 2016;65(4):741–7.

41. Van Der Meer J, Berenguer M. Reversion of disease manifestations after HCV eradication. J Hepatol 2016;65(1 Suppl):S95–108.

42. Martini S, Sacco M, Strona S, et al. Impact of viral eradication with sofosbuvir-based therapy on the outcome of post-transplant hepatitis C with severe fibrosis. Liver Int 2016;37(1):62–70.

43. Curry MP, O'Leary JG, Bzowej N, et al, ASTRAL-4 Investigators. Sofosbuvir and velpatasvir for HCV in patients with decompensated cirrhosis. N Engl J Med 2015;373(27):2618–28.

44. Ellingson K, Seem D, Nowicki M, et al, For the Organ Procurement Organization Nucleic Acid Testing Yield Project Team. Estimated risk of human immunodeficiency virus and hepatitis C virus infection among potential organ donors from 17 organ procurement organizations in the United States. Am J Transplant 2011;11:1201–8.

45. Coilly A, Samuel D. Pros and cons: usage of organs from donors infected with hepatitis C virus – revision in the direct-acting antiviral era. J Hepatol 2016;64:226–31.

46. Pawlotsky JM. Hepatitis C virus resistance to direct-acting antiviral drugs in interferon-free regimens. Gastroenterology 2016;151:70–86.

47. Roth D, Nelson DR, Bruchfeld A, et al. Grazoprevir plus elbasvir in treatment-naive and treatment-experienced patients with hepatitis C virus genotype 1 infection and stage 4-5 chronic kidney disease (the C-SURFER study): a combination phase 3 study. Lancet 2015;386(10003):1537–45.

48. Smolders EJ, de Kanter CT, van Hoek B, et al. Pharmacokinetics, efficacy, and safety of hepatitis C virus drugs in patients with liver and/or renal impairment. Drug Saf 2016;39(7):589–611.

49. Desnoyer A, Pospai D, Lê MP, et al. Pharmacokinetics, safety and efficacy of a full dose sofosbuvir-based regimen given daily in hemodialysis patients with chronic hepatitis C. J Hepatol 2016;65(1):40–7.

50. Saxena V, Nyberg L, Pauly M, et al. Safety and efficacy of simeprevir/sofosbuvir in hepatitis C-infected patients with compensated and decompensated cirrhosis. Hepatology 2015;62:715–25.

51. Aqel BA, Pungpapong S, Leise M, et al. Multicenter experience using simeprevir and sofosbuvir with or without ribavirin to treat hepatitis C genotype 1 in patients with cirrhosis. Hepatology 2015;62(4):1004–12.

52. Modi AA, Nazario H, Trotter JF, et al. Safety and efficacy of simeprevir plus sofosbuvir with or without ribavirin in patients with decompensated genotype 1 hepatitis C cirrhosis. Liver Transpl 2016;22(3):281–6.

53. Stine JG, Intagliata N, Shah NL, et al. Hepatic decompensation likely attributable to simeprevir in patients with advanced cirrhosis. Dig Dis Sci 2015;60:1031–5.

54. Dresser GK, Spence JD, Bailey DG. Pharmacokinetic-pharmacodynamic consequences and clinical relevance of cytochrome P450 3A4 inhibition. Clin Pharmacokinet 2000;38:41–57.

55. Marquez B, Van Bambeke F. ABC multidrug transporters: target for modulation of drug pharmacokinetics and drug-drug interactions. Curr Drug Targets 2011;12: 600–20.

56. Dick TB, Lindberg LS, Ramirez DD, et al. A clinician's guide to drug-drug interactions with direct-acting antiviral agents for the treatment of hepatitis C viral infection. Hepatology 2016;63:634–43.

57. Charlton M, Gane E, Manns MP, et al. Sofosbuvir and ribavirin for treatment of compensated recurrent hepatitis C virus infection after liver transplantation. Gastroenterology 2015;148(1):108–17.

58. Saab S, Rheem J, Jimenez M, et al. Curing hepatitis C in liver transplant recipients is associated with changes in immunosuppressant use. J Clin Transl Hepatol 2016;4(1):32–8.

59. Gane EJ, Hyland RH, An D, et al. Efficacy of ledipasvir and sofosbuvir, with or without ribavirin, for 12 weeks in patients with HCV genotype 3 or 6 infection. Gastroenterology 2015;146:1454–61.

60. Herzer K, Papadopoulos-Köhn A, Walker A, et al. Daclatasvir, simeprevir and ribavirin as a promising interferon-free triple regimen for HCV recurrence after liver transplant. Digestion 2015;91:326–33.

61. Leroy V, Angus P, Bronowicki JP, et al. Daclatasvir, sofosbuvir, and ribavirin for hepatitis C virus genotype 3 and advanced liver disease: a randomized phase III study (ALLY-3+). Hepatology 2016;63(5):1430–41.

62. Narang TK, Ahrens W, Russo MW, et al. Post-liver transplant cholestatic hepatitis C: a systematic review of clinical and pathological findings and application of consensus criteria. Liver Transpl 2010;16:1228–35.

63. Roche B, Coilly A, Roque-Afonso AM, et al. Interferon-free hepatitis C treatment before and after liver transplantation: the role of HCV drug resistance. Viruses 2015;7:5155–68.

64. Berenguer M. Last gasps of the HCV dragon: direct antiviral failures and HCV positive donors. Liver Transpl 2016;22(S1):47–51.

Liver Retransplantation
How Much Is Too Much?

 CrossMark

Jennifer Berumen, MD*, Alan Hemming, MD

KEYWORDS

- Hepatic retransplantation • Primary transplant • Model for End-Stage Liver Disease
- Hepatitis C • Retransplant models

KEY POINTS

- Outcomes for hepatic retransplantation have improved over time, but continue to be significantly worse than with primary transplant.
- Retransplant is surgically challenging with a high need for arterial and biliary reconstruction.
- Several factors, including high Model for End-Stage Liver Disease score and older donor age continue to be risk factors for poor outcomes with retransplant.
- Hepatitis C has been a controversy in retransplant, but with new medications for hepatitis C this may change.

INTRODUCTION

Since the early days of liver transplantation, retransplantation has been recognized as a technical and surgical challenge. The first reports of retransplantation were by Starzl and colleagues[1] at the University of Pittsburgh in 1982 in his article entitled Evolution of Liver Transplantation. The first retransplant he reported was completed in 1968 in his series of more than 350 transplants from 1968 to 1981, in which 27 patients required retransplant. Only 6 of those survived over 6 months, and most deaths were from sepsis. Shaw and colleagues[2] at the University of Colorado later reported another series of 170 transplants from 1963 to 1980, of which 21 required retransplant. Rejection was the most common reason for retransplant at that time before the revolutionary introduction of cyclosporine, and the major reasons for death and graft failure remained multisystem organ failure and sepsis.[2] Both noted that retransplant operations were technically challenging with poor outcomes; however, retransplant remained the only option for patient survival in some situations. With the goal to "avoid futile transplantation," many centers have studied retransplantation, and several

The authors have nothing to disclose.
Department of Abdominal Transplantation and Hepatobiliary Surgery, University of California, San Diego, La Jolla, CA 92037, USA
* Corresponding author.
E-mail address: jberumen@ucsd.edu

Clin Liver Dis 21 (2017) 435–447
http://dx.doi.org/10.1016/j.cld.2016.12.013
1089-3261/17/Published by Elsevier Inc.

models have been proposed to determine risk and under what circumstances hepatic retransplant should be considered.[3]

In the studies and models involving retransplant, only one thing remains constant: patient and graft survival with retransplantation is worse than with primary liver transplant. Prolonged hospital stays, increased intensive care unit stays, resource use, and increased cost also come with this increased mortality.[4–6] Survival for pediatric retransplant is superior to that of adult, however, still inferior to that of initial transplant.[2,7] The outcomes of retransplant have improved over time but still remain worse than those of primary transplant.[5,8–11] In their initial report, Shaw and colleagues[2] reported a 60% 1-year survival rate in children and a 45% 1-year survival rate in adults. In 1997, the 1-year survival rate for retransplant was reported in one study to be 50% versus 80% for that of initial transplant,[4] and one model estimates a 1.93 increase in risk of death with retransplant.[12] In a United Network for Organ Sharing (UNOS) study from 1996 to 2005, the initial transplant 1-, 3-, and 5-year survival rates were reported at 83%, 75%, and 69% versus 67%, 60%, and 53% for retransplant, respectively.[13] Another UNOS database study in 2009 of 3977 retransplants reported a 37.8% graft failure rate at 1 year with retransplant.[14] Early mortality is typically caused by sepsis and multisystem organ failure but has also been attributed to poorly functioning grafts and even aggressive hepatitis B or C recurrence before the use of hepatitis B immune globulin and the introduction of antiviral agents.[2,15] The timing of retransplant may also affect outcomes, with periods including early, intermediate, and late retransplants or urgent, acute, and elective as described by Shaw and colleagues.[2] The retransplant rate has decreased over time,[9] and more current studies of the UNOS database found retransplant rates of about 12%[12] with 7.9% of listed liver transplant candidates waiting for retransplant in 2005. Only 1% of those candidates were older than 65,[13] as candidates listed for retransplant tend to be younger with higher Model for End Stage Liver Disease (MELD) scores (21 vs 15).[16,17]

Indications for retransplant are varied and have also changed with time.[9] About 70% of the graft losses within the first year seem to be early secondary to primary nonfunction (PNF) and vascular thrombosis. After 1 year, more than 50% are caused by chronic rejection and recurrent hepatitis or primary disease recurrence.[6,13] In several studies, there are now fewer retransplants for acute and chronic rejection and less for ischemic complications and disease recurrence, but PNF rates have remained about the same.[5,9] Rates for hepatic arterial thrombosis (HAT), as reported by Kashyap and colleagues,[9] decreased over 17 years from 8.1% to 3.7%, but Pfitzmann and colleagues[5] reported that retransplant rates for HAT increased in their population, possibly because of the use of more marginal liver donors and performing transplants in sicker patients. There is also a shift away from attempting to manage early HAT expectantly with management of biliary complications toward early retransplantation.

There is no clear consensus about whether it is the reason for graft failure or the initial cause of liver disease that affects retransplant mortality. Many studies show significant effects and some have shown no difference in outcomes.[7] Hepatitis C virus (HCV) recurrence shows significance for worse outcomes in several studies and is a common reason for retransplant. Unlike HCV, alcoholic liver disease and nonalcoholic steatohepatitis rarely necessitate retransplant.[6]

TECHNICAL CONSIDERATIONS

Retransplantation presents a much more technically challenging operation than primary transplant.[18] Arterial collateralization of the liver and scar formation make dissection difficult, especially in late retransplantation.[2,19] Several studies indicate an increased mortality rate in retransplant with the increased need for blood transfusions,[5] and Pfitzmann and colleagues[5] estimated a 3% increase in mortality rate with each unit of blood needed. Venovenous bypass may be used to help alleviate the need for blood transfusions, especially in late retransplantation.[18] Techniques for the recipient hepatectomy must be considered, including mass clamping of the hilum with subsequent high transection of the porta hepatis[20] or careful high hilar dissection to preserve structures.[19,21] Venous cuffs can be retained from the prior liver graft and used for reanastomosis.[2,19] The graft artery cannot be used at the same point because of vascular infiltration and the risk of failure or thrombosis,[2] and a more proximal vascular anastomosis or aortic jump graft is required.[1] Reports indicate a 28.2% to 60.5% need for aortic conduits in reconstruction and a 26.8% to 29.2% need for biliary reconstruction, including hepaticojejunostomy.[5,7,21] The University of Miami reported that in cases of multiple retransplantations (more than 2 grafts), they use the technique of mass clamping of the porta hepatis. With this procedure, all patients require biliary reconstructions with hepaticojejunostomy because the recipient bile duct is oversewn once it is identified in the clamping. All also required aortic jump grafts.[20] Adequate vascular grafts are needed from the donor to facilitate this, and the use of gastroepiploic grafts has also been described for arterial reconstruction.[2,21]

FACTORS AFFECTING OUTCOMES

Several factors have been identified as significant predictors of mortality and graft loss with retransplant. Only some of these factors remain important across multiple studies. These factors include the use of older donors (age >60), renal failure, and high recipient MELD score (greater than 25 or 30). Several studies were completed before widespread use of the MELD score but show that factors related to the MELD, including creatinine level, international normalized ratio (INR), and bilirubin level contribute to outcomes. In other reviews, factors predictive of poor survival include multiple prior transplants, transplants within 7 to 30 days after the primary transplant, increased MELD score, cold ischemic time greater than 12 hours, increased donor age, split livers, or deceased after cardiac death (DCD) donor livers.[6]

When looking at large database reviews, a UNOS study by Yoo and colleagues[22] from 1988 to 2001 with 761 retransplants for PNF and 3428 for other causes indicated a decreased survival associated with increased creatinine. Poor outcomes with increased creatinine levels have been indicated in many other studies as well.[4,15,22–25] Another UNOS study by Ghabril and colleagues[8] from 1994 to 2005 found that mortality increased with patient age, MELD score greater than 25, transplant within 1 year of the original, and warm ischemic time of more than 75 minutes. Donor age greater than 60 was also associated with mortality only in HCV-positive recipients[8] and in another study in all recipients.[26] Others showed increased mortality with older age, recipients older than 50, preoperative ventilator support, inpatient status, elevated bilirubin levels, and the use of intraoperative blood products.[4,5,15,24,25] Before the use of MELD score, Child Pugh score was found to indicate worse outcomes. A Childs class of C was shown by Yao and colleagues[15] to have worse survival with encephalopathy as a significant indicator. With hepatic encephalopathy the 1- and 5-year survival rates were 38% and 30%, respectively, compared with 91% and 84% without.[15]

The effect of MELD score on outcomes has been a well-studied indicator in retransplant. MELD score shows good concordance with pretransplant mortality on the list for retransplant candidates but a poor concordance with postoperative mortality when excluding exception MELD points and comparing with primary transplants.[16] However, in one study of relisted patients, the pretransplant mortality rate was higher than that for primarily listed patients but because they were listed at a higher MELD score.[16] Another study by Maduka and colleagues[27] found that retransplant recipients who were listed with MELD exception points were much more likely to undergo retransplant than patients listed at their actual MELD score (85.2% vs 69.4%). Relisted candidates who did not receive exception points were more likely to be removed from the list because of death (19.4% vs 5.6%). Alternatively, patients who were initial recipients of DCD grafts that required relisting had a lower mortality rate than those who were relisted after receiving a brain-dead donor. This finding is likely owing to the higher use of MELD exceptions for DCD recipients, even with excluding patients listed for HAT within 14 days who received automatic exceptions.[27] Another study of the UNOS database by Allen and colleagues[28] also excluding relisting after the first 14 days found that DCD recipients had a better survival rate on the waitlist, and they were listed with lower biological MELD scores than brain-dead donor recipients. The graft survival rates with retransplant after a DCD primary transplant was similar to their first graft survival rates.[28]

The actual MELD score, however, clearly correlates to postoperative survival after retransplant, with a higher biological MELD score resulting in lower survival rates. Excluding exception points, MELD score greater than 25 was found to have consistently worse survival. Watt and colleagues[29] found a 42% 1-year and 21% 5-year survival with a MELD score greater than 30, and McCashland and colleagues[30] reported that a MELD score greater than 30 has a 50% perioperative survival rate. An alternate study that did not exclude MELD exception points actually showed a higher survival rate at higher MELD scores. This finding is difficult to interpret without looking at the biological MELD scores that may be attributable to the high retransplant rate with exception points.[17]

Better outcomes are found with retransplant for PNF, high total bilirubin level, a high factor II level,[23] donor younger than 25, and MELD score less than 23[31] or MELD score less than 10.[3] Center volume does not seem to affect overall survival rate, but Reese and colleagues[14] reported an improved 1-year survival rate at high volume centers (more than 88 transplants a year) only if the transplant was done at less than 160 days.

The timing of retransplant may also affect survival rate. The best survival is found with early retransplant (<7 days) and late retransplant. Multiple studies indicated an increased mortality rate if retransplant occurs between 8 and 30 days after the initial transplant, although not all studies used this interval to define the timing of transplant.[7,10,32–34] In 2005, a study at the University of California Los Angeles (UCLA) indicated a relatively low mortality rate with a relative risk of death of 1 at retransplant less than 7 days after initial, 0.858 at more than 30 days, and the worst (1.37) from 8 to 30 days.[10] This study was a follow-up to their earlier study of 356 retransplants up to 1996, in which 89% of their retransplant deaths were within 1 year, still with the worst survival at 8 to 30 days.[7] Another study indicated 67% perioperative mortality rate when operating between 8 and 30 days.[33] One study found only worse outcomes with retransplant at 30 days or less[35]; however, another report out of France found the highest mortality rate with retransplant for chronic rejection between 31 and 360 days.[36]

The indication for retransplant does not clearly affect outcomes, although there are many different conclusions from studies involving the transplant primary and retransplant indication. A European 6-center study found that non-PNF outcomes did not affect survival.[37] However, the UNOS study reported by Yoo and colleagues[22] from

1988 to 2001 found decreased survival with HCV and PNF. In other studies, PNF has not been a factor.[23] Recurrent disease is found to be a risk factor over retransplants for ischemic-type biliary lesions or rejection.[5] HCV as a risk factor is slightly controversial and was found in some studies to be significant but not in others. Watt and colleagues[29] found it only to be significant when compared with retransplant for hepatitis B virus (HBV) or autoimmune hepatitis but not other causes.

RETRANSPLANT FOR HEPATITIS C OR HUMAN IMMUNODEFICIENCY VIRUS

One of controversies in liver transplantation involves the issue of outcomes with HCV. HCV almost always reinfects the graft within 48 hours, and there is a 5% to 30% chance of cirrhosis within 5 years of transplant.[38] The results with retransplantation for HCV have been variable depending on the study. No difference in outcomes when retransplanting for recurrent HCV were seen in several studies, including a multicenter European study that showed no effect on outcomes regardless of HCV recipient status[37] and no difference in 1- and 3-year survival rates when compared with other primary diseases at retransplant at greater than 90 days out.[30] Another study found decreased survival rates with HCV retransplant when done before 90 days and worse outcomes if done at or after 90 days.[8] Others reported improved outcomes over the years of experience with transplanting for recurrent hepatitis C, with decreased outcomes only secondary to retransplant for HBV and autoimmune disease but not other causes of liver disease.[29] Better outcomes were seen with HCV retransplant in patients with better preoperative physical status.[39]

Despite this finding, multiple contradictory studies reported worse outcomes for patient survival when retransplanting for HCV.[29,40,41] The risk of death in these studies, in addition to being worse with HCV status, was increased with increasing creatinine, donor age older than 60, clinical HCV recurrence, graft failure caused by cirrhosis, or early aggressive HCV recurrence.[40,42] These studies reported 66% of patients dying with a median of 2.2 months after retransplant for HCV. An UNOS database study from 1997 to 2002 by Pelletier and colleagues[43] reported a 30% higher mortality rate with HCV retransplant compared with other causes, in which the highest risk was between 3 and 24 months after initial transplant with recipient ages from 18 to 39. However, more consistently, donor age older than 60 seems to be a persistent risk factor for death with HCV retransplantation in multiple studies.[40,42,44]

Newer work with HCV is focused on obtaining a sustained viral response (SVR) to HCV treatment, which is shown to improve overall transplant outcomes. Results are best if SVR is obtained, with a 95.2% 5-year survival rate reported with SVR, an 87.5% 5-year survival in relapsers, and a significantly lower 49.9% 5-year survival in nonresponders.[41] The best option second to eradicating HCV before transplant[38] may be to treat the virus as early as possible to prevent the need for retransplant, along with modifying factors that may accelerate HCV recurrence. Factors found to accelerate HCV recurrence include older donor age, posttransplant diabetes, and high-dose steroid use.[45] Therefore, better perioperative management may improve HCV transplant outcomes on its own and prevent the need for retransplant. In addition, the use of the recently released direct-acting antivirals combined with protease inhibitors to treat HCV may provide broader SVR with treatment and decrease the potential need for retransplantation for HCV. Posttransplant treatment with these new medications is found to stabilize fibrosis and improve graft survival, especially with SVR,[46] with the American Association for the Study of Liver Disease recommending treatment strategies after transplant with these medications.[38]

Recently, discussions regarding human immunodeficiency virus (HIV) transplantation have become more common, and a multicenter study by Agüero and colleagues[47] reported experience with performing retransplant on patients with HIV.[47] A total of 600 patients with HIV underwent transplant in this group, and 6% (37 patients) underwent retransplant. The main indications for retransplant included technical complications such as HAT and PNF. Patients with HIV who were candidates for transplant had well-controlled HIV and were divided into 3 groups: HCV with an active viral load, HCV without detectable viral load at the time of transplant, and HBV infection. The patients with HCV without detectable viral load or HBV infection did about the same as other groups undergoing retransplant. Outcomes were clearly worse when co-infected with HIV and active HCV, with the increased risk of death coming from recurrent HCV and death typically within 1 year of transplant. Only a small percentage of the retransplanted patients in this cohort underwent retransplant for recurrent HCV, which likely reflects the hesitance of surgeons to perform retransplant with recurrent HCV because of the expected poor outcome with active co-infection of HCV/HIV. None of these patients died of complications from HIV.[47]

MODELS TO PREDICT OUTCOMES

Several different models have been developed to help centers determine the risks when dealing with retransplantation and improve outcomes.[6] Most models were developed before the widespread use of MELD scores. Rosen and colleagues[48] in 1999 proposed a model after analyzing the UNOS database from 1990 to 1996 for 1356 retransplants. They further validated the model in 2003 by evaluating 281 patients over 6 centers in Europe. His group found that recipient age, bilirubin level, creatinine level, and interval after the primary liver transplant were predictive of survival after retransplant. Although HCV status and donor age were significant with univariate analysis of outcome, they did not have a significant effect when put into the multivariate model. There was also no change in outcomes seen compared with non–PNF failure.[37] This finding was later further validated by a second European study showing that lower Rosen scores had better outcomes and recommended retransplant only if the Rosen score was less than 20.5. Again, no difference in outcomes by HCV status was found.[18]

UCLA proposed a model in 1999 after evaluating 150 retransplant cases. They reported 5 independent variables that predicted survival: age group (pediatric vs adult), preoperative mechanical ventilation, cold ischemic time greater than 12 hours, preoperative creatinine, and preoperative bilirubin.[49] Another model developed by Linhares and colleagues[50] published in 2006 evaluated 30 variables from 139 patients and reported a model from 4 independent variables: recipient age, creatinine, urgency of retransplant, and early failure of the initial transplant. They reported that with higher scores, there were significantly worse outcomes. Scores greater than 32 had a 1-, 3-, and 5-year survival rates of 21%, 19%, and 16% compared with 85%, 82%, and 77% if the score was less than 24.[50] Another group at the University of California San Francisco also has proposed a retransplant donor risk index after evaluating 1327 retransplants in the UNOS database from 2002 on. They also found no difference when the recipients had HCV and added the cause of graft failure to the risk index of the donor. They found the highest survival rate in non–extended criteria donors and non-HCV groups overall but no difference in outcomes in the other groups evaluated.[51]

Several other models were later proposed after these, including one specifically to address the risk of retransplant in HCV and one in pediatric patients.[52,53] These models along with specifics are summarized in **Table 1**.[6]

Table 1
Prediction models for hepatic retransplant

Author	Retransplant Prediction Model	Risk Categories	1-y Survival (%)
Markmann et al,[49] 1999	Give 1 point for: total bilirubin level ≥13 mg/dL, Cre ≥1.6 mg/dL, preoperative ventilator requirement, cold ischemia ≥12 h, transplant into adult recipient	Very low risk (score = 1) Low risk (score = 2) Medium risk (score = 3) High risk (score = 4) Very high risk (score = 5)	83 67–72 43–53 20–27 6
Rosen et al,[48] 1999	RS = 0.024× (recipient age) + 0.112×√(bilirubin in mg/dL) + 0.230×(log$_e$ Cre in mg/dL) – 0.974×(cause of graft failure) + UNOS coefficient Cause of graft failure: 1 if PNF, 0 for non-PNF UNOS coefficient: Status 1 = −0.261, Status 2 = −0.463, Status 3 = −1.07	Low risk: R <0.75 Medium risk: R = 0.75–1.46 High risk: R ≥1.47	70–76 49–59 28–40
Azoulay et al,[23] 2002	R = 0.04×(recipient age) + 0.89×(log$_e$ Cre in μmol/L) – 1.28×(1 if PNF is indication, 0 if non-PNF) + 1.38×(1 if emergent, 0 if nonemergent) + 1.27×(1 if urgent, 0 if nonurgent) – 0.23×√(total bilirubin in μmol/L) – 1.38×(log$_e$ factor II level) + 0.05×(√[total bilirubin] × log$_e$ [factor II level])	Low risk: R = −0.6 Medium risk: R = 0.42 High risk: R = 1.7	88 70 26
Rosen et al,[37] 2003	R = 10 × (0.0236×[recipient age] + 0.125×√[bilirubin in mg/dL] + 0.438× [log$_e$ Cre in mg/dL] – 0.234 [interval to retransplant, 0 for 15–60 d, 1 for >60 d])	Low risk: R <16 Medium risk: R = 16–20 High risk: R >20	75 58 42
Linhares et al,[50] 2006	Give 14 points for urgent/emergent retransplant Give 4 points for every 10-y increment in recipient age Give 4 points for every 100 μmol/L increment in Cre Subtract 10 points if retransplant required within 7 d	Low risk: <24 points Medium risk: 24–32 points High risk: >32 points	85 69 21
Maggi et al,[55] 2008	Log (odds of death in 1 y) = −4.81 + 2.23×(recipient sex, 1 for male, 0 for female) + 1.86×(donor age, 0 for <40 y, 1 for 40–59 y, 2 for≥60 y) + 1.60×(MELD score, 0 for <26, 1 for ≥26)		—
Davis et al,[53] 2009	Pediatric retransplant RS: Assign 1 point for neonatal cholestasis/paucity of bile ducts, being on life support at time of retransplant, receiving a split-liver graft Subtract 1 point for: age 5–18 y at time of retransplant, acute rejection as indication for retransplant	Low risk: <0 points Medium risk: 0 points High risk: 1–3 points	82 62 49

(continued on next page)

Author	Retransplant Prediction Model	Risk Categories	1-y Survival (%)

Table 1
(continued)

Author	Retransplant Prediction Model	Risk Categories	1-y Survival (%)
Hong et al,[54] 2011	Assign 2 RS points for intraoperative pRBC >30 units, more than 1 prior liver transplant, mechanical ventilation before retransplant, or interval from prior transplant to retransplant of 15–30 d Assign 1 RS point for interval from prior transplant to retransplant of 31–180 d, donor age >45 y, MELD score >27, serum albumin level <2.5 g/dL at time of retransplant, recipient age >55 y	PIC I: RS = 0 Category II: RS = 1–2 Category III: RS = 3–4 Category IV: RS = 5–12	84 75 63 33
Andres et al,[52] 2012	Specifically for HCV-positive retransplant candidates: RS = 0.23×(donor age) + 4.86×log (Cre) − 2.45×log (interval between transplants in days) + 2.69×INR + 0.1×(recipient age) − 3.27×(serum albumin) + 40	Low risk: RS <30 Medium risk: RS 30–40 High risk: RS >40	72.2–87.3 62.5–71.7 50

Abbreviations: Cre, creatinine; PIC, predictive index category; pRBC, packed red blood cells; RS, risk score.

Adapted from Kitchens WH, Yeh H, Markmann JF. Hepatic retransplant: what have we learned? Clin Liver Dis 2014;18(3):741–2; with permission.

MULTIPLE RETRANSPLANTS

The need for retransplantation can also lead to further retransplantation, with some series reporting more than 5 grafts for individual patients. Most studies, but not all, indicate worse outcomes with repeated retransplants.[1,2,7,10,18–20,36,56] In the UCLA series from 1984 to 1996, no patient who underwent 3 transplants survived to 1 year,[7] and a more inclusive UCLA series from 1981 to 2001 confirmed progressively worse outcomes with multiple transplants.[10] Another study indicated that in 2437 transplants over 25 years there were 1-, 3-, 5-, and 10-year survival rates for 193 retransplants of 66%, 61%, 57%, and 47%, respectively, compared with second retransplant survival rates in 23 patients of 45%, 40%, 40%, and 25%, respectively. Of 6 patients who underwent a third retransplant, there was a 24% 1-year survival rate with none surviving 3 years at the time of publication.[31] Of 39 retransplant patients reported by Akpinar and colleagues,[20] 32 had 3 grafts, 5 had 4 grafts, and 2 had 5 with subsequent perioperative mortality rates of 25%, 14%, and 50%, respectively, with a 1-year patient survival rate of 76%.[20] A French multicenter study found that of 399 retransplant patients, 45 required a third graft for HAT and chronic rejection with a 17% perioperative mortality rate. Eight of those needed 4 grafts for chronic rejection with a 50% perioperative mortality rate, and 1 patient needed 5 for Budd Chiari syndrome. That patient survived to only 20 months after the fifth transplant.[19] The study by Memeo and colleagues[19] indicated that 90-day postoperative mortality for repeat retransplant could be predicted by the need for vasopressor support, preoperative sepsis, PNF, increasing MELD score, urgency of retransplant, creatinine level, and INR.[19] A separate review of 5596 liver transplants from the Eurotransplant registry found a retransplant rate of 7% overall with the biggest gap in survival outcomes between the first and second liver transplant but not much worse with the third or fourth transplant.[56]

Others have reported patients with varying percentages of retransplants who underwent subsequent multiple retransplants but have not indicated the outcomes. Rates vary from one report of 21.1% of 54 retransplants requiring a third graft[36] to another with 774 retransplant patients with 148 undergoing a third (19%), 20 a fourth (2.5%), and 5 having more than 4 grafts (0.6%).[9] Another study in Europe with 108 retransplants found 9 patients needing 3 grafts, and 1 patient needing a fourth,[18] and the UNOS study by Yoo and colleagues[22] from 1988 to 2001 showed 4189 retransplants, 10.6% of which required a third transplant.[22] Reasons for multiple retransplant have been similar to those for the second transplant with indications including PNF, HAT, chronic rejection, and cryptogenic liver failure.

SUMMARY

With liver retransplantation, "when is too much too much?" remains an open question. With the goal to avoid futile transplantation, many ethical issues come into play with retransplant.[57] Although trends over time have shown improved outcomes in graft and patient survival rates,[5,8–11] retransplant results still remain significantly worse than those for primary transplant.[8] At least 1 of every 12 livers is used for retransplantation, which potentially takes a liver away from a primary transplant candidate who will have a better outcome.[12] Avoiding late retransplantation with MELD scores greater than 25, patients on ventilators, renal insufficiency, or advanced age and avoiding retransplant between 8 to 30 days seem to be prudent.[32] With current median MELD scores at time of transplant in some regions exceeding 30, however, retransplantation may be prohibitive in patients not receiving MELD exception points. The highest risk recipients seem to be older recipients with higher MELD scores (higher creatinine and bilirubin levels before MELD). Very few liver retransplant candidates who also received a simultaneous liver and kidney transplant have been reported. Only 5 combined liver retransplant and kidney transplant recipients were reported in a report by Yao and colleagues,[15] but their individual outcomes were not reported.

HCV virus was found to potentially change outcomes but has not reached significance to make any of the models predicting risk. In addition, there are now new direct-acting antiviral and protease inhibitor combination treatments for HCV, which may reduce the need for retransplants, modulate retransplant outcomes, and potentially even decrease the primary need for transplant for HCV. Given this finding, it does not seem necessary to include HCV as a contraindication to retransplant, as the prognosis of HCV may improve over time.

Donors should be carefully considered for retransplant recipients. Worse outcomes have been seen with older donors and extended criteria donors, and it is recommended not to use donors older than 70 years for retransplant if possible.[58] DCD donors also have worse outcomes, including a 40% increase in graft failure and 15% increase in death, so DCD livers should be avoided in retransplant candidates unless emergent retransplant is needed.[28] The increased risk of marginal donors may be difficult to avoid, however, as marginal donors are the only way in many areas to perform transplant or retransplant at MELD scores less than 30 without exception points. The liver allocation system was changed in June 2013 to introduce liver sharing regionally for patients with MELD scores of 35 or above, known as "Share 35". With this, in many regions, the best quality livers are being allocated to the sickest patients with MELD scores greater than 35, with more marginal livers going to patients with MELD scores less than 35. This creates a difficult dilemma for retransplantation without exception points, as retransplantation at MELD scores of greater than 30 is prohibitive in terms of morbidity and mortality, and yet only marginal livers are being offered for MELD scores less than 35 and may force retransplant with marginal donors. Our selection and management of extended criteria donors has also improved over time, and this may allow transplantation with extended criteria donors in select cases.[26]

In the final analysis, liver transplant teams need to carefully assess the individual patient that requires retransplantation and the organ that becomes available for that retransplant in a multidisciplinary fashion. High-risk recipients include patients with high MELD scores, renal failure, and poor preoperative status (on the ventilator). High-risk donors include extended criteria donors, donors older than 60 years, and DCD donors. Although there are guides to prognosis, liver transplant teams must balance the need of the individual patient with the overall utility of using a given liver in a high-risk situation.

REFERENCES

1. Starzl TE, Iwatsuki S, Van Thiel DH, et al. Evolution of liver transplantation. Hepatology 1982;2(5):614–36.
2. Shaw BW, Gordon RD, Iwatsuki S, et al. Hepatic retransplantation. Transplant Proc 1985;17(1):264–71.
3. Ghobrial RM. Retransplantation for recurrent hepatitis C in the model for end-stage liver disease era: how should we or shouldn't we? Liver Transpl 2003;9: 1025–7.
4. Wong T, Devlin J, Rolando N, et al. Clinical characteristics affecting the outcome of liver retransplantation. Transplantation 1997;64:878–82.
5. Pfitzmann R, Benscheidt B, Langrehr JM, et al. Trends and experiences in liver retransplantation over 15 years. Liver Transpl 2007;13(2):248–57.
6. Kitchens WH, Yeh H, Markmann JF. Hepatic retransplant: what have we learned? Clin Liver Dis 2014;18(3):731–51.
7. Markmann JF, Markowitz JS, Yersiz H, et al. Longterm survival after retransplantation of the liver. Ann Surg 1997;226:408–20.
8. Ghabril M, Dickson R, Wiesner R. Improving outcomes of liver retransplantation: an analysis of trends and the impact of Hepatitis C infection. Am J Transplant 2008;8:404–11.
9. Kashyap R, Jain A, Reyes J, et al. Causes of retransplantation after primary liver transplantation in 4000 consecutive patients: 2–19 years follow-up. Transplant Proc 2001;33:1486–7.
10. Busuttil RW, Farmer DG, Yersiz H, et al. Analysis of longterm outcomes of 3200 liver transplantations over two decades: a single-centre experience. Ann Surg 2005;241:905–16.
11. Bellindo CB, Martinez JM, Artacho GS, et al. Have we changed the liver retransplantation survival? Transplant Proc 2012;4:1526–9.
12. Ghobrial RM, Gornbein J, Steadman R, et al. Pretransplant model to predict posttransplant survival in liver transplant patients. Ann Surg 2002;236:315–22 [discussion: 322–3].
13. Magee JC, Barr ML, Basadonna GP, et al. Repeat organ transplantation in the United States, 1996–2005. Am J Transplant 2007;7:1424–33.
14. Reese PP, Yeh H, Thomasson AM, et al. Transplant center volume and outcomes after liver retransplantation. Am J Transplant 2009;9(2):309–17.

15. Yao FY, Saab S, Bass NM, et al. Prediction of survival after liver retransplantation for late graft failure based on preoperative prognostic scores. Hepatology 2004; 39:230–8.
16. Edwards E, Harper A. Does MELD work for relisted candidates? Liver Transpl 2004;10(Suppl):10–6.
17. Kim HJ, Larson JJ, Lim YS, et al. Impact of MELD on waitlist outcome of retransplant candidates. Am J Transplant 2010;10:2652–7.
18. Marti J, Charco R, Ferrer J, et al. Optimization of liver grafts in liver retransplantation: a European single-center experience. Surgery 2008;144(5):762–9.
19. Memeo R, Laurenzi A, Pittau G, et al. Repeat liver retransplantation: rationale and outcomes. Clin Transplant 2016;30(3):312–9.
20. Akpinar E, Selvaggi G, Levi D, et al. Liver retransplantation of more than two grafts for recurrent failure. Transplantation 2009;88(7):884–90.
21. Kim H, Lee KW, Yi NJ, et al. Outcome and technical aspects of liver retransplantation: analysis of 25-year experience in a single major center. Transplant Proc 2015;47(3):727–9.
22. Yoo HY, Maheshwari A, Thuluvath PJ. Retransplantation of liver: primary graft nonfunction and hepatitis C virus are associated with worse outcome. Liver Transpl 2003;9:897–904.
23. Azoulay D, Linhares MM, Huguet E, et al. Decision for retransplantation of the liver: an experience- and cost-based analysis. Ann Surg 2002;236:713–21 [discussion: 721].
24. Facciuto M, Heidt D, Guarrera J, et al. Retransplantation for late liver graft failure: predictors of mortality. Liver Transpl 2000;6:174–9.
25. Jimenez M, Turrion VS, Alvira LG, et al. Indications and results of retransplantation after a series of 406 consecutive liver transplantations. Transplant Proc 2002;34:262–3.
26. Marti J, Fuster J, Navasa M, et al. Effects of graft quality on non-urgent liver retransplantation survival: should we avoid high-risk donors? World J Surg 2012; 36(12):2914–22.
27. Maduka RC, Abt PL, Goldberg DS. Use of model for end-stage liver disease exceptions for donation after cardiac death graft recipients relisted for liver transplantation. Liver Transpl 2015;21:554–60.
28. Allen AM, Kim WR, Xiong H, et al. Survival of recipients of livers from donation after circulatory death who are relisted and undergo retransplant for graft failure. Am J Transplant 2014;14:1120–8.
29. Watt KD, Lyden ER, McCashland TM. Poor survival after liver retransplantation: is hepatitis C to blame? Liver Transpl 2003;9:1019–24.
30. McCashland T, Watt K, Lyden E, et al. Retransplantation for hepatitis C: results of a U.S. multicenter retransplant study. Liver Transpl 2007;13:1246–53.
31. Marudanayagam R, Shanmugam V, Sandhu B, et al. Liver retransplantation in adults: a single-centre, 25-year experience. HPB (Oxford) 2010;12(3):217–24.
32. Zimmerman MA, Ghobrial RM. When shouldn't we retransplant? Liver Transpl 2005;11(Suppl 2):14–20.
33. Chen GH, Fu BS, Cai CJ, et al. A single-centre experience of retransplantation for liver transplant recipients with a failing graft. Transplant Proc 2008;40:1485–7.
34. Shen ZY, Zhu ZJ, Deng YL, et al. Liver retransplantation: report of 80 cases and review of literature. Hepatobiliary Pancreat Dis Int 2006;5(2):180–4.
35. Abdelfattah MR, Al-Sebayel M, Broering D. An analysis of outcomes of liver retransplant in adults: 12-year's single-center experience. Exp Clin Transplant 2015;13(Suppl 1):95–9.

36. Pérez-Saborido B, Menéu-Díaz JC, de los Galanes SJ, et al. Short- and long-term overall results of liver retransplantation: "Doce de Octubre" Hospital Experience. Transplant Proc 2014;41(6):2441–3.
37. Rosen HR, Prieto M, Taltavull TC, et al. Validation and refinement of survival models for liver retransplantation. Hepatology 2003;38:460–9.
38. Righi E, Londero A, Carnelutti A, et al. Impact of new treatment options for hepatitis C virus infection in liver transplantation. World J Gastroenterol 2015;21: 10760–75.
39. Neff GW, O'Brien CB, Nery J, et al. Factors that identify survival after liver retransplantation for allograft failure caused by recurrent hepatitis C infection. Liver Transpl 2004;10:1497–503.
40. Martí J, De la Serna S, Crespo G, et al. Graft and viral outcomes in retransplantation for hepatitis C virus recurrence and HCV primary liver transplantation: a case-control study. Clin Transplant 2014;28:821–8.
41. Tanaka T, Selzner N, Therapondos G, et al. Virological response for recurrent hepatitis C improves long-term survival in liver transplant recipients. Transpl Int 2013; 26:42–9.
42. Carmiel-Haggai M, Fiel MI, Gaddipati HC, et al. Recurrent hepatitis C after retransplantation: factors affecting graft and patient outcome. Liver Transpl 2005; 11:1567–73.
43. Pelletier SJ, Schaubel DE, Punch JD, et al. Hepatitis C is a risk factor for death after liver retransplantation. Liver Transpl 2005;11:434–40.
44. Roayaie S, Schiano TD, Thung SN, et al. Results of retransplantation for recurrent hepatitis C. Hepatology 2003;38:1428–36.
45. Carrión JA, Navasa M, Forns X. Retransplantation in patients with hepatitis C recurrence after liver transplantation. J Hepatol 2010;53:962–70.
46. Verna EC, Abdelmessih R, Salomao MA, et al. Cholestatic hepatitis C following liver transplantation: an outcome-based histological definition, clinical predictors, and prognosis. Liver Transpl 2013;19:78–88.
47. Agüero F, Rimola A, Stock P, et al. Liver retransplantation in patients with HIV-1 infection: an international multicenter cohort study. Am J Transplant 2016;16: 679–87.
48. Rosen HR, Madden JP, Martin P. A model to predict survival following liver retransplantation. Hepatology 1999;29:365–70.
49. Markmann JF, Gornbein J, Markowitz JS, et al. A simple model to estimate survival after retransplantation of the liver. Transplantation 1999;67:422–30.
50. Linhares MM, Azoulay D, Matos D, et al. Liver retransplantation: a model for determining long-term survival. Transplantation 2006;81:1016–21.
51. Northup PG, Pruett TL, Kashmer DM, et al. Donor factors predicting recipient survival after liver retransplantation: the retransplant donor risk index. Am J Transplant 2007;7(8):1984–8.
52. Andres A, Gerstel E, Combescure C, et al. A score predicting survival after liver retransplantation for hepatitis C virus cirrhosis. Transplantation 2012;93(7): 717–22.
53. Davis A, Rosenthal P, Glidden D. Pediatric liver retransplantation: outcomes and a prognostic scoring tool. Liver Transpl 2009;15(2):199–207.
54. Hong JC, Kaldas FM, Kositamongkol P, et al. Predictive index for long-term survival after retransplantation of the liver in adult recipients. Ann Surg 2011;254(3): 444–9.
55. Maggi U, Consonni D, Bertoli P, et al. A risk score and a flowchart for liver retransplantation. Transplant Proc 2008;40(6):1956–60.

56. Pollard S, Lerut J, Paul A, et al. Evolution of indications and results of liver transplantation in Europe. A report from the European Liver Transplant Registry (ELTR). J Hepatol 2012;57(3):675–88.
57. Biggins SW. Futility and rationing in liver retransplantation: when and how can we say no? J Hepatol 2012;56(6):1404–11.
58. Segev DL, Maley WR, Simpkins CE, et al. Minimizing risk associated with elderly liver donors by matching to preferred recipients. Hepatology 2007;46:1907–18.

Moving?

Make sure your subscription moves with you!

To notify us of your new address, find your **Clinics Account Number** (located on your mailing label above your name), and contact customer service at:

Email: journalscustomerservice-usa@elsevier.com

800-654-2452 (subscribers in the U.S. & Canada)
314-447-8871 (subscribers outside of the U.S. & Canada)

Fax number: 314-447-8029

Elsevier Health Sciences Division
Subscription Customer Service
3251 Riverport Lane
Maryland Heights, MO 63043

*To ensure uninterrupted delivery of your subscription, please notify us at least 4 weeks in advance of move.

Printed and bound by CPI Group (UK) Ltd, Croydon, CR0 4YY

03/10/2024

01040398-0009